CLINICS IN CHEST MEDICINE

Venous Thromboembolism

VICTOR F. TAPSON, MD, GUEST EDITOR

VOLUME 24 • NUMBER 1 • MARCH 2003

W.B. SAUNDERS COMPANY
A Division of Elsevier Inc.
PHILADELPHIA   LONDON   TORONTO   MONTREAL   SYDNEY   TOKYO

W.B. SAUNDERS COMPANY
A Division of Elsevier Inc.

The Curtis Center • Independence Square West • Philadelphia, Pennsylvania 19106

http://www.wbsaunders.com

CLINICS IN CHEST MEDICINE
March 2003
Editor: Sarah E. Barth

Volume 24, Number 1
ISSN 0272-5231

Reprints: For copies of 100 or more, of articles in this publication, please contact the Commercial Reprints Department, Elsevier Inc., 360 Park Avenue South, New York, New York 10010-1710. Tel. (212) 633-3813 Fax: (212) 633-3820 e-mail: reprints@elsevier.com.

The ideas and opinions expressed in *Clinics in Chest Medicine* do not necessarily reflect those of the Publisher. The Publisher does not assume any responsibility for any injury and/or damage to persons or property arising out of or related to any use of the material contained in this periodical. The reader is advised to check the appropriate medical literature and the product information currently provided by the manufacturer of each drug to be administered to verify the dosage, the method and duration of administration, or contraindications. It is the responsibility of the treating physician or other health care professional, relying on independent experience and knowledge of the patient, to determine drug dosages and the best treatment for the patient. Mention of any product in this issue should not be construed as endorsement by the contributors, editors, or the Publisher of the product or manufacturers' claims.

Clinics in Chest Medicine (ISSN 0272-5231) is published quarterly by W.B. Saunders Company. Corporate and editorial offices: The Curtis Center, Independence Square West, Philadelphia, PA 19106-3399. Accounting and circulation offices: 6277 Sea Harbor Drive, Orlando, FL 32887-4800. Periodicals postage paid at Orlando, FL 32887, and additional mailing offices. Subscription price is $176.00 per year (domestic individuals), $241.00 per year (domestic institutions), $195.00 per year (Canadian individuals), $288.00 per year (Canadian institutions), $222.00 per year (international individuals), and $288.00 per year (international institutions). International air speed delivery is included in all *Clinics* subscription prices. All prices are subject to change without notice. POSTMASTER: Send address changes to *Clinics in Chest Medicine* (ISSN 0272-5231), W.B. Saunders Company, Periodicals Fulfillment, Orlando, FL 32887-4800. **Customer Service: 1-800-654-2452 (US). From outside of the US, call 1-407-345-4000.**

Clinics in Chest Medicine is covered in *Index Medicus, Current Contents/Clinical Medicine, EMBASE/Excerpta Medica, Science Citation Index,* and *ISI/BIOMED.*

Printed in the United States of America.

GUEST EDITOR

VICTOR F. TAPSON, MD, Associate Professor of Medicine, Director, Pulmonary Hypertension Center, Division of Pulmonary and Critical Care Medicine, Duke University Medical Center, Durham, North Carolina

CONTRIBUTORS

SELIM M. ARCASOY, MD, FCCP, Associate Professor of Clinical Medicine, Pulmonary, Allergy, and Critical Care Division, Columbia University College of Physicians and Surgeons; and Medical Director, Lung Transplantation Program, New York Presbyterian Hospital of Columbia and Cornell University, New York, New York

BRIAN F. GAGE, MD, MSC, Assistant Professor of Medicine, Division of General Medical Sciences, Washington University School of Medicine, and Barnes-Jewish Hospital, St. Louis, Missouri

IAN A. GREER, MD, FRCP (Glas)(Ed)(Lond), FRCOG MFFP, Regius Professor of Obstetrics and Gynaecology; Chairman, Division of Developmental Medicine, University of Glasgow, Glasgow Royal Infirmary, Glasgow, Scotland, United Kingdom

JOHN A. HEIT, MD, Professor of Medicine, Division of Cardiovascular Diseases, Section of Vascular Diseases; Director, Mayo Clinic Special Coagulation Laboratories, Division of Hematology, Section of Hematology Research; and Director, Mayo Clinic Thrombophilia Center, Department of Internal Medicine, Mayo Clinic and Foundation, Rochester, Minnesota

CLIVE KEARON, MB, MRCPI, FRCP(C), PhD, McMaster Clinic, Henderson General Hospital, Hamilton, Ontario, Canada

FRANKLIN A. MICHOTA, MD, Assistant Professor of Medicine, Section Head of Hospital Medicine, Department of General Internal Medicine, The Cleveland Clinic Foundation, Cleveland, Ohio

TIMOTHY A. MORRIS, MD, Associate Professor of Medicine, Division of Pulmonary and Critical Care Medicine, University of California, San Diego Medical Center, San Diego, California

NESTOR L. MÜLLER, MD, PhD, Professor and Head of Department, Department of Radiology, University of British Columbia, Vancouver General Hospital, Vancouver, British Columbia, Canada

THOMAS L. ORTEL, MD, PhD, Associate Professor of Medicine, Division of Hematology; Assistant Professor of Pathology; and Medical Director, Clinical Coagulation and Platelet Antibody Laboratories, Duke University Medical Center, Durham, North Carolina

STEPHANIE L. PERRY, MD, Fellow, Divisions of Hematology and Medical Oncology, Duke University Medical Center, Durham, North Carolina

TOM POWELL, FFR (RCSI), Clinical Fellow in Thoracic Radiology, Department of Radiology, University of British Columbia, Vancouver General Hospital, Vancouver, British Columbia, Canada

ANA T. ROCHA, MD, Pulmonary and Critical Care Fellow, Division of Pulmonary and Critical Care Medicine, Duke University Medical Center, Durham, North Carolina

MARC RODGER, MD, FRCP(C), MSc, Department of Medicine, Ottawa Hospital and the University of Ottawa, Ottawa, Ontario, Canada

VICTOR F. TAPSON, MD, Associate Professor of Medicine, Director, Pulmonary Hypertension Center, Division of Pulmonary and Critical Care Medicine, Duke University Medical Center, Durham, North Carolina

ANIL VACHANI, MD, Fellow, Pulmonary, Allergy and Critical Care Division, University of Pennsylvania School of Medicine, Philadelphia, Pennsylvania

PHILIP S. WELLS, MD FRCP(C), MSc, Department of Medicine, Ottawa Hospital and the University of Ottawa, Ottawa, Ontario, Canada

ROGER D. YUSEN, MD, MPH, Assistant Professor of Medicine, Divisions of Pulmonary and Critical Care Medicine and General Medical Sciences, Washington University School of Medicine, and Barnes-Jewish Hospital, St. Louis, Missouri

CONTRIBUTORS

CONTENTS

The epidemiology and clinical features of thrombophilia are discussed, as well as the underlying pathogenesis (when known). The authors present their approach to the clinical and laboratory evaluation of patients with venous thromboembolism and their family members and discuss how this information can be used to guide therapeutic decision making.

FORTHCOMING ISSUES

RECENT ISSUES

CLINICS
IN CHEST
MEDICINE

Clin Chest Med 24 (2003) xi–xiii

Preface
Venous thromboembolism

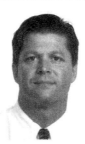

Victor F. Tapson
Guest Editor

This issue on venous thromboembolism offers an overview that is based on the research and experience of seasoned clinicians and researchers who are intensely interested in this important disease entity. Although the work presented herein is predominantly North American, it offers experienced perspectives from both sides of the Atlantic and is provided by a multidisciplinary group of contributors. Many concepts have evolved since the last time an issue of the *Clinics in Chest Medicine* was devoted to venous thromboembolism (in 1995). A concept that is pivotal to both the suspicion and prevention of venous thromboembolism is the recognition of risk factors. Although von Virchow very insightfully hypothesized his triad well over 100 years ago, we continue to learn more. Dr. John Heit has investigated the importance of various risk factors for thrombosis, and he presents a detailed review of this topic based on his own research and other data. The importance of genetic–environmental interactions in this multifactorial disease process is emphasized, since improved understanding in this realm offers a better opportunity to identify individuals at risk. Not only is it important to recognize well-described risk factors (eg, surgery), but institutionalization—whether defined as the hospital, nursing home, or other chronic care facility confinement—is also an independent risk factor for venous thromboembolism. In fact, autopsy studies indicate that more than 75% of

fatal pulmonary embolism cases occur in nonsurgical inpatients.

Previously, diagnostic considerations included whether or not spiral computed tomography scanning was sensitive enough to be used in the setting of suspected pulmonary embolism. At present, this technique is used more commonly than the ventilation–perfusion scan at many hospitals in the United States, Canada, Europe, and other areas around the world. The sensitivity is still debated, although it clearly improves as the size of the emboli increase. The technology is clearly improving as well. Drs. Powell and Müller have accomplished the task of objectively reviewing the role of computed tomography and, while noting its potential limitations, conclude that this technique should replace the ventilation–perfusion scan for suspected pulmonary embolism. The advantages of multiple-detector row scanners and the use of the narrowest possible detector aperture within the constraints imposed by the duration of the contrast material bolus and the breath-holding capability of the patient are emphasized in this excellent review. Dr. Philip Wells has pioneered the concept of pretest probability, and his article very nicely compliments the diagnostic concepts outlined above. The strategy of using a scoring system to rate the clinical probability of deep venous thrombosis and pulmonary embolism has been shown to reduce the need for imaging studies when rigorously applied.

Over the past decade, nothing has affected the prevention and treatment of thrombotic disorders more than the advent and use of low molecular heparin preparations. These anticoagulants have clear advantages over standard, unfractionated heparin, including improved bioavailability, subcutaneous delivery for all indications, and no requirement for monitoring in the vast majority of therapeutic settings. Dr. Timothy Morris, a pulmonologist, has offered a detailed discussion of the pharmacology of these drugs and how they differ from their predecessor, unfractionated heparin, which has served as the dominant parenteral anticoagulant for more than 50 years. Dr. Roger Yusen, also a pulmonologist, presents the background data that have led to increased use of low molecular weight heparin for outpatient therapy of established acute deep venous thrombosis, a practice that has radically changed the approach to its treatment. The cost savings associated with outpatient therapy is stressed as well. Another much-debated therapeutic concept involves the appropriate duration of therapy. Dr. Clive Kearon, a clinical trialist from the McMaster Clinic and Hamilton Research Centre, presents the available data and an insightful viewpoint based on his own extensive experience investigating this subject.

Massive pulmonary embolism requires a rapid but detailed clinical assessment with careful attention to indications and contraindications to thrombolytic therapy. This therapeutic modality tends to generate more interest and controversy than perhaps any area involving thromboembolic disease. Drs. Selim Arcasoy and Anil Vachani present a detailed review of this topic, including the most recent data published.

Because of the frequent presence of associated disease processes, the risk of therapy, and the risk of venous thromboembolism itself, the approach to venous thromboembolism must be cautious and balanced. Perhaps no other area involving this disease is as challenging as when the affected or at-risk patient is pregnant. Dr. Ian Greer, a professor of obstetrics, has studied this area in depth and provides a perspective emphasizing the importance of thrombotic disease in pregnancy and how this "acquired" risk factor and major cause of maternal death can be prevented and managed.

The importance of prophylaxis in the medically ill population is stressed by Dr. Franklin Michota, a hospitalist, who offers a systematic approach to preventing venous thromboembolism in this patient population. Several recent and ongoing clinical trials have focused on medical patients, and the data that are accumulating indicate that most hospitalized medical patients require prophylaxis. A complex setting in which the typical rules of diagnosis, treatment, and prevention of thromboembolism management cannot always be applied is intensive care. Dr. Ana Rocha's discussion of this setting emphasizes the importance of recognizing the risk factors in this heterogeneous patient population and outlines important diagnostic and management issues. The critical balance between thrombosis and bleeding is of particular concern in these patients.

The increasing recognition of thrombophilic disorders has both aided in patient management and made it more complex. Drs. Stephanie Perry and Thomas Ortel offer a perspective on the recognition and approach to these disorders. Unfortunately, difficulties exist in determining which patients require prolonged primary or secondary prophylaxis and how long it should be offered, because in many settings inadequate sample sizes make it impossible to perform studies that are large enough to obtain answers. These issues, as well as the often difficult question of who should be tested for inherited or acquired thrombophilias, are discussed in detail.

Consensus guidelines have been published regarding the prevention and treatment of venous thromboembolism. None have had as much impact as the American College of Chest Physicians Consensus Conference on Antithrombotic Therapy, an evidence-based statement that has been evolving since 1986. The evolution of this statement and its impact are discussed in the final article of this issue, which was kindly reviewed by Dr. Jack Hirsh.

Many questions remain to be answered with regard to the diagnosis, treatment, and prevention of venous thromboembolism, a disease that contributes to the death of 100,000 to 200,000 patients per year, a number that probably exceeds the mortality from breast cancer, highway fatalities, and HIV-related disease combined. Although it is common, the diagnosis is commonly missed and the medical literature continues to document the underuse of prophylaxis. Continued research is crucial and will help guide such issues as: (1) exactly who needs no further evaluation if the spiral computed tomography scan is negative; (2) who should receive thrombolytic therapy for pulmonary embolism; (3) the impact of various thrombophilias on the duration of prophylaxis; (4) the duration of prophylaxis for general medical patients; (5) when outpatient prophylaxis should be considered; and (6) the intensity of long-term treatment with oral anticoagulants. Such information will serve as the basis for future evidence-based recommendations.

Finally, heightened awareness must be encouraged. Although not every patient admitted to the hospital requires venous thromboembolism prophylaxis, the vast majority do. Certainly every patient admitted should be considered for prophylaxis.

Victor F. Tapson
Duke University Medical Center
Division of Pulmonary and Critical Care Medicine
Room 351, Bell Building, Box 27710
Durham, NC 27710, USA
E-mail address: tapso001@mc.duke.edu

Clin Chest Med 24 (2003) 1–12

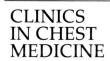

Risk factors for venous thromboembolism

John A. Heit, MD[a,b,c,*]

[a]*Division of Cardiovascular Diseases, Section of Vascular Diseases, Mayo Clinic and Foundation, 200 First Street SW,*
Rochester, MN 55905,USA
[b]*Division of Hematology, Section of Hematology Research, Stabile 610, Mayo Clinic and Foundation,*
200 First Street SW, Rochester, MN 55905, USA
[c]*Department of Internal Medicine, Mayo Clinic and Foundation, 200 First Street SW, Rochester, MN 55905, USA*

Venous thromboembolism is a common disease, with an average annual incidence of more than 1 case per 1000 person-years [1]. It also is a lethal disease, mostly owing to pulmonary embolism. Almost one quarter of all pulmonary embolisms present as essentially sudden death [2]. For these patients, available time is insufficient to recognize, diagnose, and begin therapy in an attempt to alter the course of the disease. Pulmonary embolism is an independent predictor of reduced survival for as long as 3 months after the event [2]. Patients who have deep vein thrombosis often sustain serious and costly long-term complications. Serious venous stasis syndrome develops in almost 30% of patients within 10 years [3,4] at an estimated cost of more than $4000 per episode in 1997 United States dollars [5]. To improve survival, prevent complications, and reduce health care costs, the occurrence of venous thromboembolism must be reduced. Nevertheless, despite a great deal of effort, the incidence of venous thromboembolism has remained relatively constant since about 1980 (Fig. 1) [1,6]. The failure to reduce the incidence of venous thromboembolism may reflect an increase in the population at risk (eg, an increase in the average

population age), exposure of the population to more or new risk factors (eg, an increase in surgical procedures) [7], inadequate identification of all high-risk populations, underuse of appropriate prophylaxis [8,9], or prophylaxis failure. To provide appropriate prophylaxis, persons at risk for venous thromboembolism must be identified. This article discusses clinical (environmental) exposures that are independent risk factors for venous thromboembolism, including estimates of the magnitude of risk and the burden of disease in the community (eg, population attributable risk) that can be accounted for by each exposure. In addition, other diseases that have been associated with venous thromboembolism are discussed.

Risk factors for venous thromboembolism

Age

The incidence of venous thromboembolism increases dramatically with advancing age (Fig. 2) [1,10–13], ranging from about 1 case per 1 million person-years for children aged less than 15 years to nearly 1 case per 100 person-years for adults aged more than 85 years. In one study, older age was an independent risk factor for deep vein thrombosis [14]. With the exception of catheter-induced thrombosis [15], venous thromboembolism is extremely uncommon among children. In a large population-based study that identified all community residents with incident venous thromboembolism over a 25-year period (n = 2218), only four patients were less than

The work was funded, in part, by grants from the National Institutes of Health (HL 60279, HL66216) and the Centers for Disease Control and Prevention (TS306), by the US Public Health Service, by the Doris Duke Charitable Foundation Innovation in Clinical Research, and by the Mayo Foundation.

* Hematology Research, Stabile 610, Mayo Clinic, 200 First Street SW, Rochester, MN 55905.

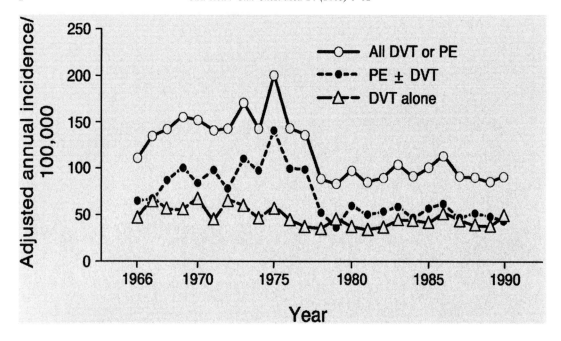

Fig. 1. Age- and sex-adjusted annual incidence of all venous thromboembolism, DVT alone, and PE with or without DVT among Olmsted County, Minnesota, residents by calendar year, 1966 to 1990. DVT, deep vein thrombosis; PE, pulmonary embolism. (*From* Silverstein MD, Heit JA, Mohr DN, Petterson TM, O'Fallon WM, Melton LJ. Trends in the incidence of deep vein thrombosis and pulmonary embolism: a 25-year population-based, cohort study. Arch Intern Med 1998;158:585–93; with permission.)

15 years of age at the time of deep vein thrombosis or pulmonary embolism [1]. The effect of age on venous thromboembolism risk is extremely important and should always be considered when estimating the risk in the individual patient. Moreover, the relative proportion of venous thromboembolisms presenting as pulmonary embolisms also increases with age (Fig. 2). This finding predicts that, as the average United States population age increases, the number of pulmonary embolisms (with associated poor survival) will also increase.

Gender

The risk imparted by gender remains uncertain. In a large population-based study, the incidence of venous thromboembolism was higher among males (male-to-female ratio, 1.2:1), especially for older ages (Fig. 3) [1]. Other studies have reported no difference in autopsy-discovered pulmonary embolism by gender [16], an increase in the risk for pulmonary embolism and deep vein thrombosis among men [14,17], or an increase in the risk for pulmonary embolism among obese women [18]. The weight of the evidence suggests a higher incidence among

females during the childbearing years, whereas the incidence in older age groups is higher among males [1].

Other independent risk factors for venous thromboembolism include surgery, trauma, hospital or nursing home inpatient status, a malignant neoplasm with or without concurrent chemotherapy, central vein catheterization or transvenous pacemaker, prior superficial vein thrombosis, varicose veins, and neurologic disease with extremity paresis (Table 1) [19].

Surgery

The highest risk for venous thromboembolism is imparted by hospitalization for surgery, with a 6 to 22 fold increased risk [19–21]. The risk among surgery patients can be stratified further based on patient age, the type of surgery, and the presence of malignant neoplasm [22,23]. The incidence of postoperative venous thromboembolism is increased for surgery patients who are 65 years of age or older. High-risk surgical procedures include neurosurgery, major orthopedic surgery of the leg, thoracic, abdominal, or pelvic surgery for malignancy, renal transplantation, and cardiovascular surgery. Other

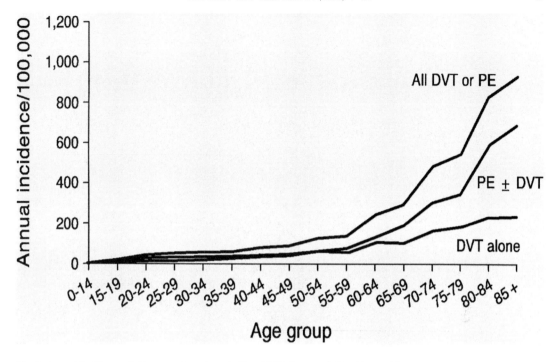

Fig. 2. Annual incidence of all venous thromboembolism, DVT alone, and PE with or without DVT among Olmsted County, Minnesota, residents, 1966 to 1990, by age. DVT, deep vein thrombosis; PE, pulmonary embolism. (*From* Silverstein MD, Heit JA, Mohr DN, Petterson TM, O'Fallon WM, Melton LJ. Trends in the incidence of deep vein thrombosis and pulmonary embolism: a 25-year population-based, cohort study. Arch Intern Med 1998;158:585–93; with permission.)

high-risk procedures include transfemoral angiography or angioplasty with stenting, and placement of an upper-extremity arteriovenous shunt for hemodialysis (a risk factor for innominate, subclavian, and axillary vein thrombosis). A recent study identified obesity (body mass index $\geq 25 \text{ kg/m}^2$) as an independent risk factor for venous thromboembolism after total hip arthroplasty [24]. Although previous investigators have suggested that the risk from surgery is less with neuraxial (spinal or epidural) anesthesia when compared with general anesthesia [25], in a multivariate analysis, the type of anesthesia was not an independent risk factor for venous thromboembolism after controlling for surgery [19].

Trauma

Recent trauma imparts the next most potent risk for venous thromboembolism, with nearly a 13-fold increase in risk [19,21]. Prospective studies document a high incidence of asymptomatic deep vein thrombosis among trauma patients, especially among patients sustaining head trauma, spinal injury, and fractures of the pelvis, femur, and tibia [26].

Hospitalization for acute medical illness or nursing home confinement

Institutionalization, defined as hospital, nursing home, or other chronic care facility confinement, is an independent risk factor for venous thromboembolism, imparting about an eightfold increased risk [19,21]. Autopsy studies show that more than 75% of fatal pulmonary embolisms occur in nonsurgical inpatients [27,28]. These data support providing appropriate prophylaxis for this high-risk population [20,29]. The increased risk associated with hospital confinement most likely reflects immobilization [17,20,30–32] and the acuity and severity of illness.

Malignant neoplasm

The risk among patients with malignancy is increased fourfold [19,21]. Malignancy is an independent risk factor for outpatient-acquired deep vein thrombosis [14,23]. Potential causes of thrombosis among cancer patients include direct vein compression or invasion, abnormal production of procoagulants (eg, tumor cell expression of tissue factor or

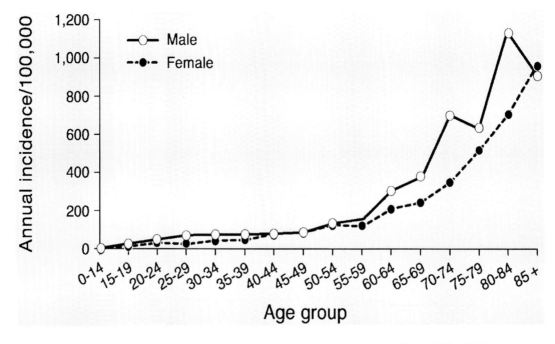

Fig. 3. Annual incidence of venous thromboembolism among Olmsted County, Minnesota, residents, 1966 to 1990, by age-group and gender. (*From* Silverstein MD, Heit JA, Mohr DN, Petterson TM, O'Fallon WM, Melton LJ. Trends in the incidence of deep vein thrombosis and pulmonary embolism: a 25-year population-based, cohort study. Arch Intern Med 1998;158:585–93; with permission.)

other circulating procoagulants), and increased circulating levels of normal procoagulant factors (eg, fibrinogen, factor VIII) [33,34]. Cancer patients receiving immunosuppressive or cytotoxic chemotherapy are at even higher risk for venous thromboembolism [19,35–37]. Chemotherapy with L-asparaginase is a well-recognized risk factor for venous thromboembolism [38], possibly owing to

reduced plasma antithrombin activity [39]. Recently, an increased risk of venous thromboembolism has been reported for patients with multiple myeloma receiving chemotherapy and thalidomide [40]. A routine examination for occult malignancy is warranted for patients presenting with idiopathic venous thromboembolism, especially among patients in whom venous thromboembolism recurs [41–45].

Table 1
Independent risk factors for deep vein thrombosis or pulmonary embolism

Baseline characteristic	Odds ratio	95% Confidence interval
Institutionalization with or without recent surgery		
No institutionalization or recent surgery	1.00	—
Institutionalization without recent surgery	7.98	4.49–14.18
Institutionalization with recent surgery	21.72	9.44–49.93
Trauma	12.69	4.06–39.66
No malignancy	1.00	
Malignancy without chemotherapy	4.05	1.93–8.52
Malignancy with chemotherapy	6.53	2.11–20.23
Prior central venous catheter or transvenous pacemaker	5.55	1.57–19.58
Prior superficial vein thrombosis	4.32	1.76–10.61
Neurologic disease with extremity paresis	3.04	1.25–7.38
Serious liver disease	0.10	0.01–0.71

Data from Heit SA, Silverstein MD, Mohr DN, et al. Risk factors for deep vein thrombosis and pulmonary embolism: a population-based case–control study. Arch Intern Med 2000;160:809–15.

Neurologic disease

Patients with neurologic disease and extremity paresis or plegia have a threefold increased risk for venous thromboembolism that is independent of hospital confinement [19]. The prevalence of pulmonary embolism is increased among autopsied patients dying with paraplegia or quadriplegia [16], and the risk of deep vein thrombosis among neurologic patients with paralyzed legs [46,47] and among nonambulatory stroke patients is increased [48].

Central venous catheters and transvenous pacemakers

The risk for upper-extremity deep vein thrombosis among patients with a current or recent central venous catheter or a transvenous pacemaker is increased about sixfold [19]. The increasing use of central venous catheters for hemodynamic monitoring and parenteral alimentation; for cancer, antibiotic, or antifungal therapy; and for hemodialysis has precipitated an epidemic of catheter-related, upper-extremity venous thrombosis. Central venous access via femoral vein catheters is associated with a higher incidence of venous thrombosis when compared with subclavian vein catheterization [49].

Superficial vein thrombosis

Prior superficial vein thrombosis is an independent risk factor for subsequent deep vein thrombosis or pulmonary embolism remote for the episode of superficial thrombophlebitis [19]. Superficial vein thrombosis is most likely a phenotypic expression of an underlying thrombophilia. In support of this hypothesis, prior superficial vein thrombosis also is an independent risk factor for deep vein thrombosis and pulmonary embolism during pregnancy or postpartum [50].

Varicose veins

The risk for deep vein thrombosis imparted by varicose veins is uncertain and seems to vary by patient age [19]. One study found that 45-year-old patients with varicose veins had a fourfold increased risk of venous thromboembolism compared with a twofold risk for 60-year-old patients and no increased risk for 75-year-old patients with varicose veins. In contrast, varicose veins were not an independent predictor of major pulmonary embolism discovered at autopsy in the Framingham study [18]. Similarly, varicose veins were not an independent risk factor for deep vein thrombosis among outpatients with no recent trauma, surgery, or immobilization [14].

Liver disease

Serious liver disease is associated with a 90% decrease in the risk for venous thromboembolism [19]. This finding is biologically plausible. Patients with serious liver disease often have prolonged clotting times, reduced clearance of fibrin degradation products, and thrombocytopenia. These impairments of normal hemostasis may protect patients from venous thromboembolism.

Additional risk factors

Among women, additional risk factors for venous thromboembolism include oral contraceptive use [20,23,51,52], pregnancy and the postpartum period [20,23,53], hormone replacement therapy [54–58], and tamoxifen therapy [59] or therapy with other selective estrogen receptor modulators (eg, raloxifene).

Oral contraceptives

Most oral contraceptives contain an estrogen (eg, ethinylestradiol or mestranol) and a progestogen (eg, norethindrone, levonorgestrel, desogestrel, gestodene, or norgestimate). First-generation oral contraceptives contained at least 50 μg or more of estrogen, and the progestogen was norethindrone. First-generation oral contraceptives increased the risk for venous thromboembolism about four to eight fold [60,61]. Because of a dose–response between the content of estrogen (mestranol) and the risk for venous thromboembolism [62,63], second-generation oral contraceptives were developed in which the estrogen content was reduced to 35 μg or less and combined with a different progestogen (levonorgestrel). When compared with first-generation oral contraceptives, the risk for venous thromboembolism with the use of second-generation oral contraceptives is reduced [64] but still substantial, with approximately a fourfold increased risk [65]. More recently, third-generation oral contraceptives have been introduced that contain newer progestogens (desogestrel, gestodene, or norgestimate), which have fewer androgenic metabolic effects and do not adversely affect lipid levels. These newer progestogens more strongly suppress ovarian activity, allowing a further reduction in estrogen content to 20 μg; however, several studies have shown that oral contraceptives containing desogestrel and gestodene confer a twofold higher risk for venous thrombosis than do formulations containing levonorgestrel [56,66–69].

Pregnancy and the puerperium

About 1 in 2000 women experience thrombosis during pregnancy. This risk is about tenfold the risk for nonpregnant women of the same age [53,70,71]. The risk is also increased during the puerperium, with most studies finding a higher risk than during pregnancy.

Hormone replacement therapy

Among postmenopausal women who have not undergone a hysterectomy, the most common form of hormone replacement therapy is oral conjugated equine estrogen (0.625 mg) plus medroxyprogesterone (2.5 mg) once daily. In addition to oral administration, estrogen may be replaced via transdermal patches. Hormone replacement therapy is associated with a two to four fold increased risk of venous thrombosis [21,55–57]. Given the apparent lack of benefit of hormone replacement therapy in preventing coronary events [72–74] and the availability of other nonhormonal therapies for osteoporosis and postmenopausal symptoms, the use of hormone replacement therapy will most likely diminish.

Statin therapy

A subgroup analysis of the Heart Estrogen/progestin Replacement Study (HERS) found a 50% risk reduction for venous thromboembolism among postmenopausal women receiving 3-hydroxy-3-methylglutaryl coenzyme A reductase inhibitors (statins) [21]. A retrospective cohort study found a 22% relative risk reduction for deep vein thrombosis among selected individuals aged 65 years or older and receiving statin therapy [75]. If these findings are confirmed, these studies may provide novel insights into the pathogenesis of venous thromboembolism based on the ability of statins to decrease thrombus formation and improve fibrinolysis [76], reduce inflammation [77], and enhance the anticoagulant protein C system via modification of neutral plasma lipids [78].

Body mass index

Body mass index and current or past tobacco smoking are not independent risk factor for venous thromboembolism [19,21]. Although previous studies have reported an increased risk owing to obesity [14,16,30,79] and smoking [79], these studies failed to control for hospital confinement or other risk factors. Chronic obstructive pulmonary disease and renal failure also are not independent risk factors for venous thromboembolism [14,17,19]. The risk for venous thromboembolism associated with congestive heart failure, independent of hospitalization, is uncertain. After controlling for hospitalization, congestive heart failure or other cardiac disease was not an independent risk factor for venous thromboembolism [19,21]. In contrast, autopsy studies have demonstrated an increased prevalence of pulmonary embolism among patients dying with cardiac disease, especially cardiac disease causing congestive heart failure [16,30]. In addition, other case–control studies have found heart failure to be an independent risk factor for deep vein thrombosis among outpatients with no recent trauma, surgery, or immobilization [14,23].

Other conditions associated with venous thromboembolism include heparin-induced thrombocytopenia and thrombosis, myeloproliferative disorders (especially polycythemia rubra vera and essential thrombocythemia), intravascular coagulation and fibrinolysis (disseminated intravascular coagulation), nephrotic syndrome, paroxysmal nocturnal hemoglobinuria, thromboangiitis obliterans (Buerger's disease), thrombotic thrombocytopenic purpura, Behçet's syndrome, systemic lupus erythematosus, and inflammatory bowel disease.

Although the relative risk for venous thromboembolism imparted by the exposures discussed previously is increased, the absolute risk (eg, incidence rate) is much lower. Surgery patients have the highest relative risk for venous thromboembolism, yet the current incidence among some of the highest risk surgery groups (eg, total knee or hip replacement) may be as low as 1.5% to 3.4% [80,81]. These data beg the question, "What is different about the patient with a risk factor in whom venous thromboembolism develops when compared with the patient with the same risk factor in whom it does not?" Recent evidence regarding the role of inherited or acquired thrombophilia (defined as a predisposition to thrombosis) has provided new answers to this question. Familial reductions in plasma antithrombin, protein C, or protein S activity are strongly associated with venous thromboembolism; however, altogether, the prevalence of these recognized familial thrombophilias among patients with venous thromboembolism is approximately 5% [82].

The discovery of activated protein C resistance and the factor V Leiden mutation has provided exciting new insights into the etiology of venous thromboembolism [83,84]. The carrier frequency of factor V Leiden or the prevalence of activated protein C resistance among incident venous thromboembolism cases is 12% to 20% [85,86]. In case–control studies, heterozygous factor V Leiden carriers have an eightfold increased risk for venous thromboembolism, whereas homozygotes have an 80 to 100 fold increased risk for venous thromboembolism [87]. The risk for venous thromboembolism is compounded by genetic interaction between factor V Leiden and other inherited disorders, such as antithrombin III, protein C, or protein S deficiency [88–90]. Genetic and environmental exposures also interact to increase the risk for venous thromboembolism. The risk for venous thromboembolism increases 30-fold among women who are carriers of heterozygous factor V Leiden and who receive oral contraceptive therapy [91]. Similarly, the risk for symptomatic venous thromboembolism is increased fivefold among factor V Leiden carriers undergoing total hip replacement [92]. Together, these data suggest that venous thromboembolism is a complex (multifactorial) disease.

Population attributable risk

To address the potential impact of universal prophylaxis or modification of currently recognized risk factors (if either were possible) on the incidence of venous thromboembolism in the community, data from a population-based, case–control study [19] were used to estimate the population attributable risk (defined as the percentage of all cases of a disease in a population that can be attributed to a risk factor) for

venous thromboembolism associated with specific risk factors. Proper interpretation of population attributable risk requires the establishment of causality between the risk factor and the disease; however, causality is a complex concept. It is not easy to establish that a factor causes a disease. This fact notwithstanding, it is logical that further research should be planned around factors that are associated with large attributable risk.

The attributable risk estimates associated with the independent risk factors for venous thromboembolism are shown in Table 2 [94]. Hospitalization and nursing home residence (current or recent) together account for almost 60% of all venous thromboembolism disease in the community. The incidence of venous thromboembolism is more than 150-fold higher among hospitalized patients when compared with community residents [93]. Hospitalization for medical illness and hospitalization for surgery account for almost equal proportions of venous thromboembolism (22% and 24%, respectively), emphasizing the need to provide prophylaxis to both of these risk groups. Nursing home residence independently accounts for more than one-tenth of all venous thromboembolism disease in the community. Additional studies are needed to identify risk factors for venous thromboembolism among nursing home residents (independent of cancer, congestive heart failure, or neurologic disease with extremity paresis) such that prophylaxis can be targeted to those patients at highest risk.

Malignant neoplasm accounts for almost one-fifth of all venous thromboembolism disease in the com-

Table 2
Population attributable risk[a] associated with independent risk factors for venous thromboembolism

Risk factor	Attributable risk	95% Confidence interval
Hospitalization or nursing home	58.8	53.4–64.2
Hospitalization with surgery	23.8	20.3–27.3
Hospitalization without surgery	21.5	17.3–25.6
Nursing home	13.3	9.9–16.8
Active malignant neoplasm	18.0	13.4–22.6
Malignant neoplasm with chemotherapy	6.4	3.9–9.0
Malignant neoplasm without chemotherapy	11.6	7.6–15.5
Trauma	12.0	9.0–14.92
Congestive heart failure	9.5	3.3–15.8
Prior central venous catheter or pacemaker	9.1	5.7–12.6
Neurologic disease with extremity paresis	6.9	3.5–10.2
Prior superficial vein thrombosis	5.4	3.0–7.7
Varicose veins/vein stripping	0	0–10.2

[a] Adjusted for age, sex, year of event, and terms in final model.
Data from Heit JA, O'Fallon WM, Petterson TM, et al. Relative impact of risk factors for deep vein thrombosis and pulmonary embolism: a population-based study. Arch Intern Med 2002;162:1245–8.

munity. Among cancer patients, malignant neoplasm not requiring cytotoxic or immunosuppressive chemotherapy accounted for almost twice the incidence of venous thromboembolism when compared with the incidence associated with cancers requiring chemotherapy. Additional studies are needed to identify risk factors for venous thromboembolism among cancer patients. Trauma, congestive heart failure, and placement of a central venous catheter or transvenous pacemaker lead accounted for similar proportions of venous thromboembolism in the community. The burden of disease accounted for by central venous catheters (9%) is particularly noteworthy as a relatively recent risk factor and emphasizes the need for additional studies addressing prophylaxis in this patient group.

The percentages of incident venous thromboembolism cases attributed to combinations of individual risk factors (adjusting for the final model) are illustrated in Fig. 4. All eight risk factors together accounted for 74% (95% confidence interval, 70%–79%) of all venous thromboembolism cases observed. If all of these eight risk factors could be eliminated, approximately 25% of the venous thromboembolism cases in the community would still be unexplained.

Summary

Venous thromboembolism is a common and potentially lethal disease. Patients who have pulmonary embolism are at especially high risk for death. Death owing to pulmonary embolism is independent of other comorbid conditions (eg, cancer, chronic heart disease, or lung disease). Sudden death is often the first clinical manifestation. Only a reduction in the incidence of venous thromboembolism can reduce

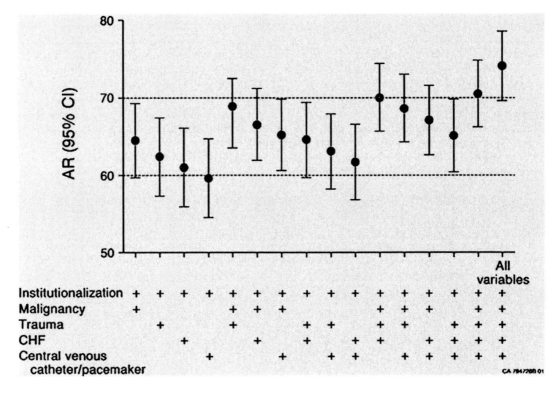

Fig. 4. Age-, sex-, event year-, main effects-, and interactions-adjusted population attributable risk associated with the six most important independent risk factors (institutionalization [hospitalization with or without surgery, or nursing home confinement], active malignant neoplasm [with or without chemotherapy], trauma, congestive heart failure [CHF], or prior central venous catheter or pacemaker), or all eight independent risk factors for first lifetime definite venous thromboembolism, among Olmsted County, Minnesota, residents diagnosed 1976 to 1990. (*Data from* Heit JA, O'Fallon WM, Petterson TM, et al. Relative impact of risk factors for deep vein thrombosis and pulmonary embolism: a population-based study. Arch Intern Med 2002;162: 1245–8.)

sudden death owing to pulmonary embolism and venous stasis syndrome owing to deep vein thrombosis. The incidence of venous thromboembolism has been relatively constant since about 1980. Improvement in the incidence of venous thromboembolism will require better recognition of persons at risk, improved estimates of the magnitude of risk, the avoidance of risk exposure when possible, more widespread use of safe and effective prophylaxis when risk is unavoidable, and targeting of prophylaxis to those persons who will benefit most. Recognition of venous thromboembolism as a multifactorial disease with genetic and genetic–environmental interaction has provided significant insights into its epidemiology and offers the possibility of improved identification of persons at risk for incident and recurrent venous thromboembolism.

References

[1] Silverstein MD, Heit JA, Mohr DN, Petterson TM, O'Fallon WM, Melton LJ. Trends in the incidence of deep vein thrombosis and pulmonary embolism: a 25-year population-based, cohort study. Arch Intern Med 1998;158:585–93.

[2] Heit JA, Silverstein MD, Mohr DN, Petterson TM, O'Fallon WM, Melton LJ. Predictors of survival after deep vein thrombosis and pulmonary embolism: a population-based, cohort study. Arch Intern Med 1999; 159:445–53.

[3] Prandoni P, Lensing AWA, Cogo A, et al. The long-term clinical course of acute deep vein thrombosis. Ann Intern Med 1996;125:1–7.

[4] Ridker PM, Miletich JP, Stampfer MJ, Goldhaber SZ, Lindpaintner K, Hennekens CH. Factor V Leiden and risks of recurrent idiopathic venous thromboembolism. Circulation 1995;92:2800–2.

[5] Bergqvist D, Jendteg S, Johansen L, Persson U, Ödegaard K. Cost of long-term complications of deep venous thrombosis of the lower extremities: an analysis of a defined patient population in Sweden. Ann Intern Med 1997;126:454–7.

[6] Heit JA, Melton LJI, Lohse CM, et al. Incidence of venous thromboembolism in hospitalized patients versus community residents. Mayo Clin Proc 2001;76: 1102–10.

[7] Madhok R, Lewallen DG, Wallrichs SL, Isltrup DM, Kurland RL, Melton LJI. Trends in the utilization of primary total hip arthroplasty, 1969 through 1990: a population-based study in Olmsted County, Minnesota. Mayo Clin Proc 1993;68:11–8.

[8] Anderson FA, Wheeler HB, Goldberg RJ, Hosmer DW, Forcier A, Patwardhan NA. Physician practices in the prevention of venous thromboembolism. Ann Intern Med 1991;115:591–5.

[9] Bratzler DW, Raskob G, Murray CK, Bumpus LJ, Piatt DS. Underuse of venous thromboembolism prophylaxis for general surgery patients in the community. Arch Intern Med 1998;158:1909–12.

[10] Coon WW, Willis PW, Keller JB. Venous thromboembolism and other venous disease in the Tecumseh community health study. Circulation 1973;48:839–46.

[11] Kierkegaard A. Incidence of acute deep vein thrombosis in two districts: a phlebographic study. Acta Chir Scand 1980;146:267–9.

[12] Anderson FA, Wheeler HB, Goldberg RJ, et al. A population-based perspective of the hospital incidence and case-fatality rates of deep vein thrombosis and pulmonary embolism: the Worcester DVT Study. Arch Intern Med 1991;151:933–8.

[13] Nordström M, Lindblad B, Bergqvist D, Kjellström T. A prospective study of the incidence of deep-vein thrombosis within a defined urban population. J Intern Med 1992;232:155–60.

[14] Cogo A, Bernardi E, Prandoni P, et al. Acquired risk factors for deep vein thrombosis in symptomatic outpatients. Arch Intern Med 1994;154:164–8.

[15] Massicote MP, Dix D, Monagle P, Adams M, Andrew M. Central venous catheter related thrombosis in children: analysis of the Canadian Registry of Venous Thromboembolic Complications. J Pediatr 1998;133: 770–6.

[16] Coon WW. Risk factors in pulmonary embolism. Surgery Gynecology and Obstetrics 1976;143:385–90.

[17] Quinn DA, Thompson BT, Terrin ML, et al. A prospective investigation of pulmonary embolism in women and men. JAMA 1992;268:1689–96.

[18] Goldhaber SZ, Savage DD, Garrison RJ, et al. Risk factors for pulmonary embolism: the Framingham study. Am J Med 1983;74:1023–8.

[19] Heit JA, Silverstein MD, Mohr DN, Petterson TM, O'Fallon WM, Melton LJ. Risk factors for deep vein thrombosis and pulmonary embolism: a population-based case-control study. Arch Intern Med 2000;160: 809–15.

[20] Rosendaal FR. Risk factors for venous thrombotic disease. Thromb Haemost 1999;82:610–9.

[21] Grady D, Wenger NK, Herrington D, et al. Postmenopausal hormone therapy increases the risk for venous thromboembolic disease. Ann Intern Med 2000;132: 689–96.

[22] Geerts WH, Heit JA, Clagett GP, et al. Prevention of venous thromboembolism: Sixth American College of Chest Physicians Consensus Conference on Antithrombotic Therapy. Chest 2001;119:132S–75S.

[23] Samama M-M. An epidemiologic study of risk factors for deep vein thrombosis in medical outpatients. Arch Intern Med 2000;160:3415–20.

[24] White RH, Gettner S, Newman JM, Romano PS. Predictors of rehospitalization for symptomatic venous thromboembolism after total hip arthroplasty. N Engl J Med 2000;343:1758–64.

[25] Sharrock NE, Haas SB, Hargett MJ, Urguhart B, Insall JN, Scuderi G. Effects of epidural anesthesia on the

incidence of deep vein thrombosis after total knee replacement. J Bone Joint Surg Am 1991;73A:502–6.

[26] Geerts WH, Code KI, Jay RM, Chen E, Szalai JP. A prospective study of venous thromboembolism after major trauma. N Engl J Med 1994;331:1601–6.

[27] Havig Ö. Pulmonary thromboembolism: clinicopathological correlations and multiple regression analysis of possible risk factors. Acta Chir Scand 1977;478:48–80.

[28] Sandler DA, Martin JF. Autopsy proven pulmonary embolism in hospital patients: are we detecting enough deep vein thrombosis? J R Soc Med 1989;82:203–5.

[29] Lederle FA. Heparin prophylaxis for medical patients? Ann Intern Med 1998;128:768–70.

[30] Coon WW, Coller FA. Some epidemiologic considerations of thromboembolism. Surgery Gynecology and Obstetrics 1959;109:487–501.

[31] Gibbs NM. Venous thrombosis of the lower limbs with particular reference to bed rest. Br J Surg 1957;191: 209–36.

[32] Gross JS, Neufield RR, Libow LW, Gerber I, Rodstein M. Autopsy study of the elderly institutionalized patient: review of 234 autopsies. Arch Intern Med 1988; 148:173–6.

[33] Zurborn KH, Duscha H, Gram J, Bruhn HD. Investigations of the coagulation system and fibrinolysis in patients with disseminated adenocarcinomas and non-Hodgkin lymphomas. Oncology. 1990;45:608–12.

[34] Bick RL. Coagulation abnormalities in malignancy: a review. Semin Thromb Hemost 1992;18:353–69.

[35] Goodnough LT, Saito H, Manni A, Jones PK, Pearson OH. Increased incidence of thromboembolism in stage IV breast cancer patients treated with a five-drug chemotherapy program. Cancer 1984;54:1264–8.

[36] Levine MN, Gent M, Hirsch J, et al. The thrombogenic effect of anti-cancer drug therapy in women with stage II breast cancer. N Engl J Med 1988;318:404–7.

[37] Weijl NI, Rutten MF, Zwinderman AH. Thromboembolic events during chemotherapy for germ cell cancer: a cohort study and review of the literature. J Clin Oncol 2000;18:2169–78.

[38] Kucek O, Kwaan HC, Gunnak W, Vasquez RM. Thromboembolic complications associated with L-asparaginase therapy. Cancer 1985;55:702.

[39] Liebman HA, Wada JK, Patch MJ, McGehee W. Depression of functional and antigenic plasma antithrombin III due to therapy with L-asparaginase. Cancer 1982;50:451.

[40] Zangari M, Anaissie E, Barlogie B, et al. Increased risk of deep vein thrombosis in patients with multiple myeloma receiving thalidomide and chemotherapy. Blood 2001;98:1614–5.

[41] Prandoni P, Lensing AW, Büller HR. Deep vein thrombosis and the incidence of subsequent symptomatic cancer. N Engl J Med 1992;327:1128–33.

[42] Nordström M, Lindblad B, Anderson H, Bergqvist D, Kjellström T. Deep venous thrombosis and occult malignancy: an epidemiological study. BMJ 1994;308: 891–4.

[43] Sorensen HT, Mellemkjaer L, Steffensen FH, Olsen JH, Nielsen GL. The risk of a diagnosis of cancer after primary deep venous thrombosis or pulmonary embolism. N Engl J Med 1998;338:1169–73.

[44] Hettiarachchi RJ, Lok J, Prins MH, Bueller HR, Prandoni P. Undiagnosed malignancy in patients with deep vein thrombosis: incidence, risk indicators, and diagnosis. Cancer 1998;83:180–5.

[45] Schulman S, Lindmarker P. Incidence of cancer after prophylaxis with warfarin against recurrent venous thromboembolism: Duration of Anticoagulation Trial. N Engl J Med 2000;342:1953–8.

[46] Warlow C, Ogston D, Douglas AS. Deep venous thrombosis of the legs after stroke. BMJ 1976;1: 1178–81.

[47] Myllynen P, Kammonen M, Rokkananen P, Bostman O, Lalla M, Laasonen E. Deep venous thrombosis and pulmonary embolism in patients with acute spinal cord injury: a comparison with nonparalyzed patients immobilized due to spinal fractures. J Trauma 1985;25: 541–3.

[48] Bromfield EB, Reding MJ. Relative risk of deep venous thrombosis or pulmonary embolism post-stroke based on ambulatory status. Journal of Neurological Rehabilitation 1988;2:51–7.

[49] Merrer J, De Jonghe B, Lefrant J-Y, et al. Complications of femoral and subclavian venous catheterization in critically ill patients: a randomized controlled trial. JAMA 2001;286:700–7.

[50] Danilenko-Dixon DR, Heit JA, Watkins T, et al. Risk factors for deep vein thrombosis and pulmonary embolism during pregnancy or the postpartum period: a population-based case-control study. Am J Obstet Gynecol 2001;184:104–10.

[51] Chasan-Taber L, Stampfer MJ. Epidemiology of oral contraceptives and cardiovascular disease. Ann Intern Med 1998;128:467–77.

[52] Jick H, Kaye JA, Vasilakis-Scaramozza C, Jick SS. Risk of venous thromboembolism among users of third generation oral contraceptives compared with users of oral contraceptives with levonorgestrel before and after 1995: cohort and case-control analysis. BMJ 2000;321: 1190–5.

[53] Kierkegaard A. Incidence and diagnosis of deep vein thrombosis associated with pregnancy. Acta Obstet Gynecol Scand 1983;62:239–43.

[54] Devor M, Barrett-Connor E, Renvall M, Feigal Jr D, Ramsdell J. Estrogen replacement and the risk of venous thrombosis. Am J Med 1992;92:275–82.

[55] Daly E, Vessey MP, Hawkins MM, Carson JL, Gough P, Marsh S. Risk of venous thromboembolism in users of hormone replacement therapy. Lancet 1996;348: 977–80.

[56] Jick H, Derby L, Wald M, Myers MW, Vasilakis C, Newton KM. Risk of hospital admission for idiopathic venous thromboembolism among users of postmenopausal estrogens. Lancet 1996;348:981–3.

[57] Grady D, Hulley SB, Furgerg C. Venous thromboembolism events associated with hormone replacement therapy. JAMA 1997;278:477.

[58] Varas-Lorenzo C, Garcia-Rodriguez LA, Cattaruzzi C, Troncon MG, Agostinis L, Perez-Gutthann S. Hormone replacement and the risk of hospitalization for venous thromboembolism: a population-based study in Southern Europe. Am J Epidemiol 1998;147:387–90.

[59] Meier CR, Jick H. Tamoxifen and the risk of idiopathic venous thromboembolism. Br J Pharmacol 1998;45: 608–12.

[60] Vessey M, Mant D, Smith A, Yeates D. Oral contraceptives and venous thromboembolism: findings in a large prospective study. BMJ 1986;292:526.

[61] World Health Organization. Venous thromboembolic disease and combined oral contraceptives: results of international multicentre case-control study. Lancet 1995;346:1575–82.

[62] Gerstman BB, Piper JM, Tomita DK, Ferguson WJ, Stadel BV, Lundin FE. Oral contraceptive estrogen dose and the risk of deep venous thromboembolitic disease. Am J Epidemiol 1991;133:32–7.

[63] Carr B, Ory H. Estrogen and progestin components of oral contraceptives: relationship to vascular disease. Contraception 1997;55:272.

[64] Böttiger LE, Boman G, Eklund G, Westerholm B. Oral contraceptives and thromboembolic disease: effects of lowering oestrogen content. Lancet 1989;8178: 1097–101.

[65] Bloemenkamp KW, Rosendaal FR, Büller HR, Helmerhorst FM, Colly LP, Vandenbroucke JP. Risk of venous thrombosis with the use of current low-dose oral contraceptives is not explained by diagnostic suspicion and referral bias. Arch Intern Med 1999;159:65–70.

[66] Bloemenkamp KW, Rosendaal FR, Helmerhorst FM, Büller HR, Vandenbrookecke JP. Enhancement by factor V Leiden mutation of risk of deep vein thrombosis associated with oral contraceptives containing a third-generation progestogen. Lancet 1995;346:1593–6.

[67] World Health Organization. Effect of different progestogens in low oestrogen oral contraceptives on venous thromboembolic disease. Lancet 1995;346:1582–8.

[68] Spitzer WO, Lewis MA, Heinemann LAJ, Thorogood M, MacRae KD. Third generation oral contraceptives and the risk of venous thromboembolic disorders: an international case-control study. BMJ 1996;312:83–8.

[69] Kemmeren JM, Algra A, Grobbee DE. Third generation oral contraceptives and risk of venous thrombosis: meta-analysis. BMJ 2001;323:131–4.

[70] McColl MD, Ramsay JE, Tait RC. Risk factors for pregnancy associated venous thromboembolism. Thromb Haemost 1997;78:1183–8.

[71] Middeldorp S, Meinardi JR, Koopman MMW, et al. A prospective study of asymptomatic carriers of the factor V Leiden mutation to determine the incidence of venous thromboembolism. Ann Intern Med 2001; 135:322–7.

[72] HERS Research Group H. Randomized trial of estrogen plus progestin for secondary prevention of coronary heart disease in postmenopausal women: Heart and Estrogen/progestin Replacement Study (HERS) Research Group. JAMA 1998;280:605–13.

[73] Grodstein F, Manson JE, Stampfer MJ. Postmenopausal hormone use and secondary prevention of coronary events in the Nurses' Health Study: a prospective, observational study. Ann Intern Med 2001; 135:1–8.

[74] Grady D, Herrington D, Bittner V, et al. Cardiovascular disease outcomes during 6.8 years of hormone therapy: Heart and Estrogen/progestin Replacement Study follow-up (HERS II). JAMA 2002;288:49–57.

[75] Ray JG, Mamdani M, Tsuyuki RT, Anderson DA, Yeo EL, Laupacis A. Use of statins and the subsequent development of deep vein thrombosis. Arch Intern Med 2001;161:1405–10.

[76] Dangas G, Badimon JJ, Smith DA, et al. Pravastatin therapy in hyperlipidemia: effects of thrombus formation and the systemic hemostatic profile. J Am Coll Cardiol 1999;33:1294–304.

[77] Albert MA, Danielson E, Rifai N, Ridker PM. Effect of statin therapy on C-reactive protein levels. JAMA 2001;286:64–70.

[78] Hiroshi D, Fernández JA, Pabinger I, Heit JA, Griffin JH. Plasma glucosylceramide as a potential risk factor for venous thromboembolism and modulator of anticoagulant protein C pathway. Blood 2001;97: 1907–14.

[79] Goldhaber SZ, Grodstein F, Stampfer MJ, et al. A prospective study of risk factors for pulmonary embolism in women. JAMA 1997;277:642–5.

[80] Khaw FM, Moran CG, Pinder IM, Smith SR. The incidence of fatal pulmonary embolism after knee replacement with no prophylactic anticoagulation. J Bone Joint Surg Br 1993;75:940–1.

[81] Warwick D, Williams MH, Bannister GC. Death and thromboembolic disease after total hip replacement: a series of 1162 cases with no routine chemical prophylaxis. J Bone Joint Surg Br 1995;77:6–10.

[82] Heijboer H, Brandjes DPM, Büller HR, ten Cate JW. Deficiencies of coagulation-inhibiting and fibrinolytic proteins in outpatients with deep vein thrombosis. N Engl J Med 1990;323:1512–6.

[83] Dahlbäck B, Carlsson M, Svensson PJ. Familial thrombophilia due to a previously unrecognized mechanism characterized by poor anticoagulant response to activated protein C: prediction of a cofactor to activated protein C. Proc Natl Acad Sci USA 1993;90:1004–8.

[84] Bertina R, Koeleman B, Koster T, et al. Mutation in blood coagulation factor V associated with resistance to activated protein C. Nature 1994;369:64–7.

[85] Ridker PM, Hennekens CH, Lindpaintner K, Stampfer MJ, Eisenberg PR, Miletich JP. Mutation in the gene coding for coagulation factor V and the risk of myocardial infarction, stroke, and venous thrombosis in apparently healthy men. N Engl J Med 1995;332: 912–7.

[86] Koster T, Rosendaal FR, de Ronde H, Briet E, Vandenbroucke JP, Bertina RM. Venous thrombosis due to poor anticoagulant response to activated protein C. Leiden Thrombophilia Study. Lancet 1993;342: 1503–6.

[87] Rosendaal FR, Koster T, Vandenbroucke JP, Reitsma PH. High risk of thrombosis in patients homozygous for factor V Leiden (activated protein C resistance). Blood 1995;85:1504–8.

[88] van Boven HA, Vandenbroucke JP, Briet E, Rosendaal FR. Gene-gene and gene-environment interactions determine risk of thrombosis in families with inherited antithrombin deficiency. Blood 1999;94:2590–4.

[89] Koeleman B, Reitsma PH, Allaart C, Bertina R. Activated protein C as an additional risk factor for thrombosis in protein C–deficient families. Blood 1994;84: 1031–5.

[90] Zöller B, Berntsdotter A, Carcia de Frutos P, Dahlbäck B. Resistance to activated protein C as an additional genetic risk factor in hereditary deficiency of protein S. Blood 1995;85:3518–23.

[91] Vandenbroucke JP, Koster T, Briet E, Reitsma PH, Bertina RM, Rosendaal FR. Increased risk of venous thrombosis in oral-contraceptive users who are carriers of factor V Leiden mutation. Lancet 1994;344: 1453–7.

[92] Lindahl TL, Lundahl TH, Nilsson L, Andersson CA. APC-resistance is a risk factor for postoperative thromboembolism in elective replacement of the hip or knee–a prospective study. Thromb Haemost 1999;81: 18–21.

[93] Heit JA, Melton III LJ, Lohse CM, Petterson TM, Silverstein MD, Mohr DN, et al. Incidence of venous thromboembolism in hospitalized patients versus community residents. Mayo Clin Proc 2001;76:1102–10.

[94] Heit JA, O'Fallon WM, Petterson TM, et al. Relative impact of risk factors for deep vein thrombosis and pulmonary embolism: a population-based study. Arch Intern Med 2002;162:1245–8.

CLINICS
IN CHEST
MEDICINE

Clin Chest Med 24 (2003) 13–28

Diagnosis of pulmonary embolism: when is imaging needed?

Philip S. Wells, MD, FRCP(C), MSc*,1, Marc Rodger, MD, FRCP(C), MSc2

*Department of Medicine, Ottawa Hospital and the University of Ottawa, Suite F6-47, 1053 Carling Avenue,
Ottawa, Ontario, Canada K1Y 4E9*

Pulmonary embolism is the third leading cause of cardiovascular mortality in North America, with an age- and sex-adjusted estimated incidence rate of 21 to 69 cases per 100,000 population per year in population-based studies [1–3]. Pulmonary embolism is responsible for 5% to 10% of all in-hospital deaths [3–5]. It is an important diagnosis to establish given that undiagnosed pulmonary embolism has a hospital mortality rate as high as 30% that falls to near 8% if diagnosed and treated appropriately [4,6,7]. The mortality rate in ambulatory patients is less than 2% [8].

The diagnosis of pulmonary embolism remains one of the most difficult problems confronting clinicians. Pulmonary embolism is considered in the differential diagnosis of many clinical presentations, including chest pain, hemoptysis, and dyspnea, and in a wide variety of clinical settings, such as emergency departments, obstetric units, surgical wards, and intensive care units. Less than 35% of patients suspected of having pulmonary embolism actually have this condition [9–11]. In most diagnostic studies, less than 25% of suspected patients have pulmonary embolism. Given the potential for death from untreated pulmonary embolism, timely diagnostic testing must be performed to enable the initiation of antithrombotic therapy for patients proven to have this condition while avoiding the risks of anticoagulation

for patients without pulmonary embolism [12]. Many patients without pulmonary embolism are needlessly hospitalized and anticoagulated while awaiting confirmatory testing. Furthermore, many patients who are suspected of having pulmonary embolism in smaller centers without diagnostic imaging are transferred to larger centers for investigation. In larger centers, imaging tests are generally only available during weekdays and daytime hours, complicating the diagnostic approach for patients with suspected pulmonary embolism seen outside these times. Accordingly, multiple researchers interested in the diagnosis of pulmonary embolism have focused on the utility of less expensive, less invasive, and more rapid methods to rule out pulmonary embolism. This article focuses on the use of blood D-dimer measurement in conjunction with clinical assessment to exclude the diagnosis of pulmonary embolism. The accuracy and utility of ventilation–perfusion lung scanning, venous ultrasound imaging of the legs, pulmonary angiography, and spiral CT in patients with suspected pulmonary embolism are reviewed to better understand the need for diagnostic algorithms. Diagnostic management approaches are suggested for patients with suspected pulmonary embolism.

Pulmonary angiography

An intravascular filling defect on pulmonary angiography confirms the presence of pulmonary embolism, whereas the absence of a filling defect refutes its presence [9]. Although it is the gold standard test for the diagnosis of pulmonary embolism, many clinicians choose not to pursue pulmonary angiogra-

* Corresponding author.
E-mail address: pwells@ohri.ca (P.S. Wells).
1 Dr. Wells is a Canada Research Chair in Thromboembolic Diseases.
2 Dr. Rodger holds a New Investigator Award from the Heart and Stroke Foundation of Canada.

0272-5231/03/$ – see front matter © 2003 Elsevier Inc. All rights reserved.
doi:10.1016/S0272-5231(02)00052-7

phy in patients with suspected pulmonary embolism [13–16]. The reasons why clinicians do not use pulmonary angiography include its side effects. Although the procedure is usually well tolerated, arrhythmia, hypotension, and other adverse reactions to contrast dye may be observed. The best data on morbidity and mortality, that is, a death rate of 0.5% and a major nonfatal morbidity rate of 1.0%, were determined before the widespread use of nonionic low-osmolar contrast [17]. Furthermore, three fifths of the deaths occurred in patients with poor cardiopulmonary reserve before angiography; therefore, the procedure is probably safer in patients without poor cardiopulmonary reserve. A more recent single-institution study reported no fatalities in more than 1400 patients and major complications in 0.3% [18]. Nevertheless, the limited availability after hours and in smaller centers and the expense and expertise required to perform pulmonary angiography are the most likely the reasons why a significant number of patients with nondiagnostic ventilation–perfusion scans are managed inappropriately [13]. Pulmonary angiography is also an imperfect test. A patient with a normal pulmonary angiogram can expect a 1.6% rate of a venous thromboembolic event (95% confidence interval [CI], 0.6% to 3.4%) at 1 year follow-up [11]. Although the authors do not suggest that performing angiography in patients with suspected pulmonary embolism is an incorrect approach, the limitations must be appreciated.

Ventilation–perfusion lung scanning

Ventilation–perfusion lung scanning has often been used as the imaging procedure of choice for the evaluation of patients with suspected pulmonary embolism. Two studies have demonstrated that a normal scan essentially excludes the diagnosis of pulmonary embolism, whereas a high-probability scan has an 85% to 90% positive predictive value for pulmonary embolism [9,11]. Using pulmonary angiography as the gold standard, two studies have demonstrated that between 45% and 66% of high-probability lung scans are falsely positive when a skilled clinician deems that the patient's pretest probability for pulmonary embolism is low. Similarly, if the clinical pretest probability is high but the scan is nondiagnostic, further investigation is necessary to exclude or confirm the diagnosis of pulmonary embolism. A further limitation of ventilation–perfusion lung scanning is that most lung scans fit into a nondiagnostic category (neither normal nor high probability) in which the incidence of pulmonary embolism ranges from 10% to 30%.

Venous ultrasound imaging of the legs

Venous ultrasound imaging to detect suspected pulmonary embolism is most useful in patients with a high pretest probability for pulmonary embolism and in patients with risk factors for pulmonary embolism and signs and symptoms of deep vein thrombosis (DVT) [19]. In these groups, ultrasound will be positive in 46% and 15% of patients, respectively [10,19]. The evidence suggesting that venous ultrasound imaging should not be the first diagnostic test in patients with suspected pulmonary embolism, because only 15% of these patients will have evidence of DVT on ultrasonography, does not negate the utility of this test [20]. The authors pooled data from six large diagnostic studies performed on 3399 patients with suspected pulmonary embolism, all of whom underwent ultrasound imaging. A total of 444 of the 870 patients (51%) diagnosed with pulmonary embolism had proximal DVT on ultrasound. The authors have demonstrated that, in the patient with a non–high-probability ventilation–perfusion scan and initial normal ultrasonography, the performance of one additional ultrasound test 1 week later (serial ultrasound testing) is adequate to manage the patient safely without the use of anticoagulants when pulmonary embolism is suspected [21]. The limitations of this approach are that it is inconvenient and cost-ineffective, because relatively few patients undergoing serial testing will actually have pulmonary embolism.

Spiral computed tomography angiography

Over the past decade, contrast-enhanced spiral CT has emerged as a new noninvasive imaging modality for the investigation of patients with suspected pulmonary embolism [22–24]. Spiral CT has made it possible to visualize directly segmental and some subsegmental arteries using a single bolus of contrast while advancing the patient through the x-ray beam. Technical drawbacks of spiral CT include the fact that it requires contrast, greater radiation exposure than with ventilation–perfusion scanning, and a cooperative patient. The evaluation of segmental pulmonary arteries may be suboptimal owing to motion artifact if the patient is unable to hold his or her breath for 15 to 25 seconds. In addition to being a diagnostic test, spiral CT may identify alternative causes for symptoms in patients with suspected pulmonary embolism. Nevertheless, because most parenchymal and pleural changes, including wedge-shaped pleural opacities, are found in patients with and without pulmonary embolism, the rational that an alternative diagnosis can be made by CT is often untrue [25].

A pooled analysis of five comparative studies using pulmonary angiography as the gold standard determined the overall sensitivity and specificity of spiral CT for the diagnosis of pulmonary embolism to be 72% (95% CI, 59% to 83%) and 95% (95% CI, 89% to 98%), respectively [26]. For central pulmonary embolism, that is, a lesion involving the main pulmonary arteries and their segmental branches, the sensitivity of CT increased to 94% (95% CI, 86% to 98%), and the specificity remained high at 94% (95% CI, 88% to 98%). A second systematic review and an accuracy study provide further evidence of the limited accuracy of spiral CT [27,28]. Studies evaluating spiral CT have reported a wide variation in the sensitivity (ranging from 53% to 100%), and most studies have failed to follow basic methodologic principles for evaluating a diagnostic test (eg, consecutive patients, comparison with a gold standard, complete follow-up).

Three small studies have directly compared spiral CT with ventilation–perfusion scanning in cohorts of patients with suspected pulmonary embolism. These studies using pulmonary angiography as the gold standard have consistently favored spiral CT as the more accurate imaging procedure. In a study by Mayo and colleagues [23], among 12 patients in whom there was discordance between the spiral CT and the ventilation–perfusion scan, spiral CT demonstrated the correct diagnosis in 92%. Garg and associates [29] demonstrated in 18 of 21 patients (86%) with intermediate probability ventilation–perfusion scans that the spiral CT concurred with pulmonary angiography findings. Cross [30] performed a randomized crossover study and found that none of 39 patients with negative spiral CT had a high-probability ventilation–perfusion result; however, 2 of 20 patients (10%) with intermediate probability ventilation–perfusion scans had pulmonary embolism detected by spiral CT.

Despite the concerns raised in recent publications about the uncertain sensitivity of spiral CT, and despite the lack of studies evaluating the safety of relying on spiral CT to exclude the diagnosis of pulmonary embolism, its use has been supported strongly in editorials and reviews in the radiology literature [31–34]. In a recent survey of Canadian hospital radiology departments performed by the authors, of the 100 responding hospitals with greater than 200 beds, 91% reported that they performed spiral CT for the diagnosis of pulmonary embolism, whereas 97% reported that they performed ventilation–perfusion scanning. Many of the department heads indi-

cated that spiral CT was the initial test for pulmonary embolism preferred by the clinicians and radiologists in their hospitals (unpublished data; 2000).

Only one study has compared the relative cost-effectiveness of spiral CT and ventilation–perfusion scanning for the evaluation of patients with suspected pulmonary embolism. A spiral CT–based diagnostic algorithm was the most cost-effective regimen ($16,000 per life-year saved) when compared with ventilation–perfusion scanning ($27,000 per life-year saved) [35]. This study based outcome estimates on a literature review that assumed that spiral CT was highly sensitive (97%); the costs were calculated in Dutch currency and in their health care system; and the data were collected in 1996. It is unclear how these costs would compare with the costs in other countries, and how the analysis would change if the lower sensitivities found in the pooled validity studies had been employed.

Despite concerns about the sensitivity of spiral CT, several features make it more attractive than ventilation–perfusion scanning as an imaging procedure for patients with suspected pulmonary embolism. First, the specificity of the test is high (90% to 100%) when compared with ventilation–perfusion scanning (for which a nonhigh nonnormal result has a specificity as low as 10%, although it is over 95% if limited to high-probability scans). Three systematic reviews have verified that a positive spiral CT is sufficient for ruling in a diagnosis of pulmonary embolism in most patients. Second, the sensitivity of spiral CT is high for large central pulmonary emboli (83% to 100% in the systematic reviews), the types of emboli that are most likely to be clinically important. The sensitivity of spiral CT exceeds that of a high-probability lung scan, which was only 41% in the Prospective Investigation of Pulmonary Embolism Diagnosis (PIOPED) study. Most of the discrepancies in the reported sensitivities of spiral CT involve the categorization of small subsegmental pulmonary emboli, which account for 6% to 36% of all pulmonary emboli and are of uncertain clinical significance. In the absence of DVT or ongoing risk factors, these small emboli may be of no significance, but this theory has not been proven in clinical trials. Third, spiral CT may be useful for directly identifying alternative causes for a patient's presentation, in contrast to ventilation–perfusion scanning, which rarely assists in this regard. Fourth, interobserver agreement in interpreting scan results is higher for spiral CT than for ventilation–perfusion scanning [23,36].

Given that spiral CT seems to be a more sensitive and specific test (at least for central pulmonary embolism) than is ventilation–perfusion scanning, it is likely that safe diagnostic management approaches will be developed with spiral CT as the initial diagnostic test. Limitations will be the cost of the test, concerns about the contrast dye in patients with renal dysfunction, indeterminate scan results, and the high dose of radiation.

Spiral CT seems to be a promising tool in the diagnostic management of suspected pulmonary embolism; however, larger trials are required before one can conclude that a negative spiral CT safely excludes pulmonary embolism. Adequately powered randomized trials are required to determine whether diagnostic management approaches based on spiral CT should replace the current standard (ie, diagnostic management approaches based on ventilation–perfusion scanning).

Clinical assessment of suspected pulmonary embolism

The clinical assessment of pulmonary embolism is considered herein by examining the diagnostic value of the individual components (ie, symptoms, signs, risk factors, laboratory tests, electrocardiogram, arterial blood gas levels, and chest radiography), followed by a consideration of the diagnostic value of the overall clinical assessment (ie, the clinician's overall diagnostic impression).

Four groups of researchers have reported on the sensitivity and specificity of individual signs and symptoms [37–40]. Patient age is consistently a statistically significant univariate predictor of pulmonary embolism across these studies. This finding is consistent with population-based epidemiologic data demonstrating an increased incidence of pulmonary embolism with age [1]. Gender is not predictive. Individual presenting symptoms do not reliably differentiate between patients with and without pulmonary embolism. The exceptions in individual studies include pleuritic chest pain and sudden dyspnea. Leg symptoms are consistently more likely in patients with pulmonary embolism. Hemoptysis is a rare presenting symptom in suspected pulmonary embolism; however, in many studies, hemoptysis is consistently more common in patients with pulmonary embolism. Risk factors for venous thromboembolic disease are well characterized in the literature [41]. In a review of 1231 patients treated for confirmed venous thromboembolic disease, one or more risk factors were present in more than 96% of patients. Furthermore, in the PIOPED study, the presence of one or more risk factors was more common in patients with pulmonary embolism.

These risk factors include immobilization, recent surgery, malignancy, and previous venous thromboembolic disease. Patients with pulmonary embolism are more likely to be tachypneic and tachycardic than are patients without pulmonary embolism, but these differences were only statistically significant in one study. In the studies reported to date, there seem to be no differences in blood pressure, in the presence of a pleural rub on auscultation, or in temperature in patients with confirmed and suspected pulmonary embolism. One commonly held misconception is that the presence of chest wall tenderness in patients with pleuritic chest pain excludes pulmonary embolism [42]. The presence of a fourth heart sound (S4), a loud second pulmonary heart sound (P2), and inspiratory crackles on chest auscultation were more common in patients with pulmonary embolism than in patients without pulmonary embolism in one study [38].

A variety of electrocardiographic changes have been suggested to have diagnostic value in patients with suspected pulmonary embolism [37,38,43,44]. Most of these investigations have been limited to patients with confirmed pulmonary embolism. Few studies have reported on the prevalence of electrocardiographic changes in patients with suspected pulmonary embolism. The authors studied unselected patients with suspected pulmonary embolism with gold standard outcome measures. Only tachycardia and incomplete right bundle branch block were significantly more frequent in patients with pulmonary embolism [45]. A normal alveolar–arterial gradient does not exclude pulmonary embolism [46,47]. Two investigators have proposed prediction rules based on arterial blood gas levels, but these rules were not validated in the authors' study [47–49]. Measurement of arterial blood gas levels alone will not rule out pulmonary embolism.

Despite the limitations of the individual clinical predictors described previously, the PIOPED investigators demonstrated that the overall clinical assessment (ie, the clinician's overall diagnostic impression) could be useful in diagnostic management. Experienced clinicians were able to separate a cohort of patients with suspected pulmonary embolism into high-, moderate-, and low-probability groups using clinical assessment alone [9]. More recently, Perrier and colleagues [50] were also able to stratify patients into different risk categories using clinical assessment alone. In both of these studies, patients were stratified into risk categories using the clinical judgment of the individual clinicians based on the overall diagnostic impression alone (ie, not using a predefined clinical decision tool). With empiric assessment, the exact methods that each clinician uses to estimate pretest probably cannot be measured [51]. In addition to the comparison of explicit information such as vital sign data and risk factors, clinicians incorporate many implicit methods to decide whether pulmonary embolism is present. This practice includes determining the discomfort exhibited by the patient, whether the patient has a convincing story for the symptoms that the clinician associates with pulmonary embolism, and whether another diagnosis can explain the patient's complaints. There are several problems with empiric assessment: (1) clinicians often disagree (even for broad categories) on the pretest probability of pulmonary embolism [52]; (2) the clinician's experience level seems to influence the accuracy of his or her pretest assessment [53]; and (3) probability estimates tend to travel a middle road such that fewer patients are categorized in the more useful low- and high-probability groups. Although the empiric method has drawbacks, it is the easiest method to use, because there is no requirement to memorize criteria.

The authors recently published their experience using an explicit clinical model to determine the pretest probability for pulmonary embolism using clinical findings, electrocardiography, and chest radiography [10]. The explicit clinical model consisted of consideration of whether the patient's clinical presentation based on symptoms, signs, and risk factors was typical for pulmonary embolism, and whether there was an alternative diagnosis at least as likely as pulmonary embolism to account for his or her symptoms. More than 1200 inpatients and outpatients with suspected pulmonary embolism were evaluated by clinicians and separated into low-, moderate-, and high-probability subgroups using this explicit clinical model. The prevalences of pulmonary embolism in the low-, moderate-, and high-probability subgroups were 3%, 28%, and 78%, respectively. In an attempt to simplify the explicit clinical model, a logistic regression analysis was performed on the clinical data collected (Table 1) [54]. The authors then validated the simplified explicit clinical model [21]. The simplified explicit clinical model also separated patients into low-, moderate-, and high-risk subgroups, although emergency physicians have a lower threshold for suspecting pulmonary embolism. The overall pulmonary embolism rate was low in the validation study [55]. The main limitation of this model was the need for the physician to consider an alternative diagnosis, which may be dependent on physician expertise. The Kappa value for interobserver variability was reasonable (0.60) despite performing the repeat assessment up to 18 hours after the first assessment.

Table 1
Variables used to determine patient pretest probability[a] for pulmonary embolism

Variable	Points
Clinical signs and symptoms of DVT (minimum of leg swelling and pain with palpation of the deep veins)	3.0
PE as, or more likely than, an alternative diagnosis	3.0
Heart rate greater than 100 beats per min	1.5
Immobilization or surgery in the previous 4 weeks	1.5
Previous DVT/PE	1.5
Hemoptysis	1.0
Malignancy (on treatment, treated in the last 6 months, or palliative)	1.0

Abbreviations: DVT, deep vein thrombosis; PE, pulmonary embolism.

[a] Low probability, < 2.0; moderate probability, $2.0–6.0$; and high probability, > 6.0.

Other clinical assessment and prediction rules have been reported. Miniati and colleagues [56] reported that their combination of clinical predictors (symptoms, electrocardiographic findings, and chest radiography findings) had a negative predictive value of 94%. Pulmonary embolism could be excluded in 42% of patients in their validation set [56]. Nevertheless, their study enrolled a high-prevalence population, did not perform logistic regression to develop a simple rule, had a rate of 10% in the low-risk group, and described criteria for the low-risk group that could apply to any patient with even minimal chest symptoms. Wicki et al [57] devised a model in emergency room patients that could be performed by nonclinicians (Table 2). The disadvantages of their model include the following: it is difficult to memorize; it has not been tested or derived in hospitalized patients; the low probability rate was 10%; there is no consideration of other diagnoses; most of the points are nonspecific; and it has only been tested in one center.

D-dimer assays for diagnosis of venous thromboembolism

D-dimer is a degradation product of a cross-linked fibrin blood clot. Levels of D-dimer are typically elevated in patients with acute venous thromboem-

Table 2
Clinical model described by Wicki et al [57] for assessment
of pretest probability for pulmonary embolism

Criteria	Points[a]
Age 60–79 years	1
Age >79 years	2
Prior DVT/PE	2
Recent surgery	3
Heart rate >100 beats per min	1
$PaCO_2$, mm Hg	
<36	2
36–39	1
PaO_2, mm Hg	
<49	4
49–60	3
>60–71	2
>71–82	1
Chest radiographic findings	
Platelet atelectasis	1
Elevation of hemidiaphragm	1

Abbreviations: DVT, deep vein thrombosis; $PaCO_2$, arterial
partial pressure of carbon dioxide; PaO_2, arterial oxygen
pressure; PE, pulmonary embolism.

[a] Patients with a score from 0 to 4 (49%) had a 10%
mean probability of PE (low risk). Patients with a score from
5 to 8 (44%) had a 38% mean probability of PE (moderate
risk). Patients with a score from 9 to 12 (6%) had an 81%
mean probability of PE (high risk).

bolism. Many different D-dimer assays have been
evaluated for the diagnosis of venous thromboembolism, and the accuracy of these tests varies. The most
sensitive D-dimer tests are the enzyme-linked immu-
nosorbent assays (ELISAs) now available as rapid
fluorescence quantitative assays with test turn around
times of less than 1 hour [58]. Local experience with
these assays reveals that transportation of the spe-
cimen to the laboratory followed by processing
provides results in over 90 minutes.

Two other D-dimer assay methods that have been
evaluated for the diagnosis of pulmonary embolism
are the whole blood agglutination assay (SimpliRED,
Agen Biomedical, Brisbane, Australia) and the automated latex agglutination plasma assay [59,60]. The
whole blood assay is associated with the following
advantages: it is simple to perform; it has a rapid turn
around time if performed at the bedside; and it is
inexpensive. Bedside testing is ideally performed by a
few well-trained personnel. The whole blood and
automated latex assays are less sensitive but more
specific than the ELISA assay [61–63].

Regardless of which assay is used, a positive D-
dimer result is not useful to "rule in" the diagnosis of
venous thromboembolism; rather, the potential value
is for a negative test result to exclude the diagnosis.

Some reports suggest that rapid ELISA tests (eg,
Vidas D-dimer, Biomerieux, France) have 100%
sensitivity, but this assumption may be dangerous,
because few tests consistently have such sensitivity.
The Vidas D-dimer assay had a sensitivity of only
90% in a recent study of patients who underwent
pulmonary angiography [64,65]. The authors pooled
results from several studies of the Vidas D-dimer
assay. The summary data revealed a sensitivity of
97.3% and specificity of 42.6% versus 85% and
75%, respectively, for the SimpliRED and 87% and
71%, respectively, for the IL test (Beckman Coulter,
Lexington, MA) for D-dimer. These values produce
negative likelihood ratios of 0.06, 0.20, and 0.18 for
the Vidas, SimpliRED, and IL tests, respectively. The
importance of these figures is described in a later
section of this article. The negative predictive value
of the D-dimer increases proportionally depending
on the sensitivity of the assay but is inversely related
to the prevalence of venous thromboembolism in the
population under study; therefore, the specificity of
the particular D-dimer assay and the population
under study influence the utility of the assay to
exclude the diagnosis of venous thromboembolism.
The use of ELISA assays in ill hospitalized patients
would be predicted to be of lower value owing to the
expected high false-positive rates, and this finding
has been demonstrated in at least one study [58].
Conversely, the higher specificity assays may be
more useful as recently demonstrated in a study of
hospitalized medical and surgical patients. The SimpliRED D-dimer assay was negative in 47% of the
patients, and the negative predictive value was 100%.
Similarly, the Vidas and other ELISA assays have
poor specificity in elderly patients, a problem that
may not exist with the SimpliRED assay [66,67].

In general, the SimpliRED and other assays with
lower sensitivity than ELISA tests should be considered as exclusionary tests in patient populations
identified to have a lower prevalence of venous
thromboembolism, or used in conjunction with other
diagnostic tests [68]. The validity of this recommendation was demonstrated in a recent study evaluating the SimpliRED D-dimer assay in a cohort of
1177 inpatients and outpatients with suspected pulmonary embolism [60]. The D-dimer assay had a
sensitivity of 85%, a specificity of 68%, and a
negative predictive value of 96%. The negative
predictive value of the D-dimer test varied depending
on the clinical probability, ranging from 99.0% (95%
CI, 97.8% to 99.7%) in patients at low pretest
probability to 87.9% (95% CI, 81.9% to 92.4%) in
moderate probability patients to 64.3% (95% CI,
35.1% to 87.2%) in high probability patients.

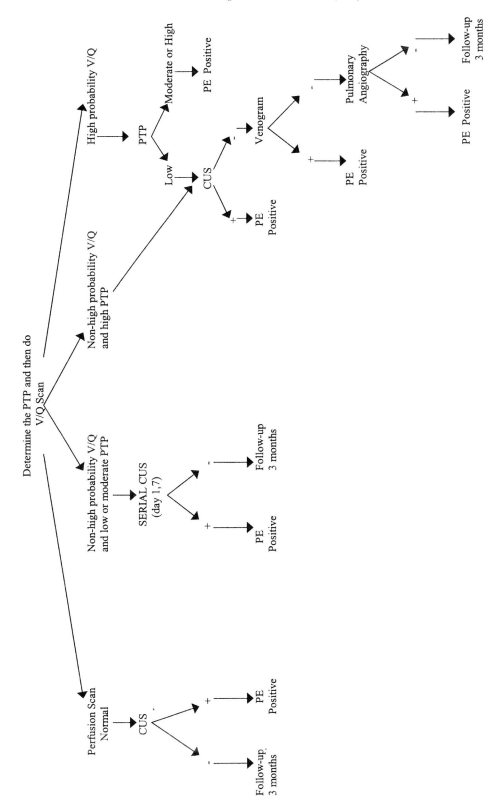

Fig. 1. Diagnostic strategy in which clinical probability is used in patients with suspected pulmonary embolism. CUS, compression ultrasound; PE, pulmonary embolism; PTP, pretest probability; V/Q, ventilation–perfusion lung scan.

Diagnostic management of patients with suspected pulmonary embolism: selecting patients in whom diagnostic imaging is not needed or can be decreased

The safety of a protocol for the diagnosis of pulmonary embolism is primarily defined by the rate of pulmonary embolism in patients in whom the protocol excludes pulmonary embolism after performing the indicated investigations, that is, the false-negative rate. It is unlikely that the protocol will produce a 0% posttest probability. Instead, one must settle on a low threshold of about 1% to 2%, comparable with the reference standard of pulmonary angiography. Accepted methods to rule out pulmonary embolism are the ventilation–perfusion scan with a normal perfusion pattern or pulmonary angiography with no evidence of pulmonary embolism. On follow-up, approximately 1% of patients with a normal ventilation–perfusion scan or a negative pulmonary angiography are diagnosed with pulmonary embolism in the subsequent year [69–72]. Furthermore, studies [11,73,74] suggest that the rate of pulmonary embolism discovered in a composite population of hospitalized patients and outpatients without recognized signs or symptoms of pulmonary embolism but who undergo contrast-enhanced CT scanning of the chest is approximately 1% [75]. If a posttest probability of less than 1% were sought, this quest would lead to an unacceptable trade-off in increased pulmonary vascular imaging and increased false-positive diagnosis of pulmonary embolism [76].

The posttest probability is derived from the pretest probability and the sensitivity and specificity of the objective test. The D-dimer assay can be considered the first objective test used in addition to clinical assessment with the goal of determining which patients require diagnostic imaging. Selection of patients with a relatively low pretest probability comprises the single most important factor in the derivation of a protocol to rule out pulmonary embolism safely. The most studied clinical prediction rule has been described by the authors, but it is likely that the rule described by Wicki et al will also be effective [21,77]. Selection of the rule depends on which D-dimer assay is employed. In the choice of the D-dimer test, sensitivity and specificity are important. Patients can die if the test is frequently negative when the patient has a pulmonary embolism, but a safe protocol must also have reasonably high specificity for two reasons. First, the isolated use of a very sensitive test can reduce the posttest probability to 1%, but only in a relatively small subset of patients with suspected pulmonary embolism if the specificity is very poor. Second, a test

with low specificity will lead to increased use of imaging tests in relatively low-risk patients owing to the high false-positive rate. A D-dimer–based protocol may lead to an increase in testing for pulmonary embolism in a relatively low-risk patient population that would probably not be studied if the clinician were forced to order a ventilation–perfusion or CT scan as the first objective test. If clinicians order a screening test that is often positive in patients who do not have pulmonary embolism, most of these patients will be sent for imaging tests. CT and ventilation–perfusion scans show evidence of a diagnostic "positive" result in approximately 5% and 10% of patients without pulmonary embolism, respectively [26,27,78–80]. Such findings result in at least 6 months of unnecessary oral anticoagulation therapy with the risk of major hemorrhage and effects on the patient's personal expenditure on health and life insurance. From a probabilistic standpoint, the chance of this impropriety will increase in proportion to the number of low-risk patients that are imaged. The primary benchmark for a safe protocol is for 1% to 2% of patients with a negative result to really have the disease. In an attempt to avoid an increase in the rate of false-positive diagnoses of pulmonary embolism, a safe protocol should also be engineered to prevent a significant increase in ventilation–perfusion or CT scan use.

Three approaches can be used for the diagnosis of pulmonary embolism in which ventilation perfusion lung scanning or spiral CT with contrast is the primary diagnostic test. In the first approach (Fig. 1), patients should have a pretest probability assigned by clinical assessment (by the overall diagnostic impression or, ideally, an explicit clinical model), followed by the performance of a ventilation–perfusion scan. A normal scan safely excludes the diagnosis of pulmonary embolism. If the lung scan result is high probability, the diagnosis of pulmonary embolism can be made with greater than 90% certainty as long as the clinical suspicion for pulmonary embolism is moderate or high. If the clinical likelihood of pulmonary embolism is low, patients with high-probability lung scans should undergo confirmatory testing with pulmonary angiography or spiral CT. If the lung scan is non–high probability, additional diagnostic testing is required to confirm or exclude the diagnosis of pulmonary embolism. Historically, it has been recommended that patients with non–high-probability lung scans undergo pulmonary angiography. Although this recommendation is an effective way to confirm or exclude pulmonary embolism, as discussed previously, this approach is not practical in many centers and has other limitations. In recent years, much attention has focused on the use of ultrasound imaging to

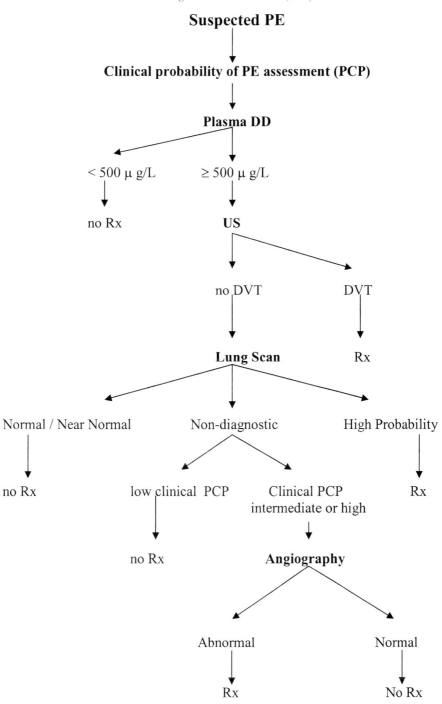

Fig. 2. Diagnostic algorithm in patients with suspected pulmonary embolism that uses D-dimer as the first diagnostic test. DD, Vidas D-dimer; DVT, deep vein thrombosis; PCP, pretest clinical probability; PE, pulmonary embolism; Rx, anticoagulant therapy; US, ultrasound.

detect DVT in patients with suspected pulmonary embolism who have non–high-probability lung scans. The rationale for this approach is that the current therapeutic management of DVT and pulmonary embolism is similar. If ultrasound confirms the presence of DVT, appropriate antithrombotic therapy can be initiated without the need to demonstrate conclusively by angiography that pulmonary embolism is present. On the other hand, if noninvasive testing for proximal DVT is negative, it is reasonable to withhold antithrombotic therapy, because such patients will potentially be at relatively low risk for additional pulmonary emboli (Fig. 1). The safety of using serial ultrasound imaging was recently demonstrated in a study performed by the authors [10]. Patients at a low or moderate clinical pretest probability for pulmonary embolism who had a non–high-probability lung scan and an initial negative ultrasound could be observed safely with serial ultrasonography without the need to institute anticoagulant therapy or perform pulmonary angiography. A total of 665 patients who had two or three negative ultrasounds performed over a 2-week period following their initial evaluation had no greater risk (0.5%; 95% CI, 0.1% to 1.3%) for venous thromboembolic complications over a 3-month period than did 334 patients whose initial lung scan was normal (0.6%; 95% CI, 0.1% to 1.8%).

An alternative approach for the management of patients with non–high-probability lung scans is to incorporate clinical probability and D-dimer assays into the diagnostic management algorithm. Perrier et al [50] studied 444 patients with suspected pulmonary embolism presenting at the emergency department or outpatient clinics. First, the clinical probability of pulmonary embolism was determined using the principles described herein (ie, looking at risk factors, signs and symptoms, and an alternative diagnosis) but not using an explicit model. A rapid ELISA D-dimer test (Vidas) was performed next. If negative, pulmonary embolism was considered excluded. Patients with a positive D-dimer test had venous ultrasound imaging performed. If abnormal, pulmonary embolism was diagnosed. If the ultrasound was normal, a ventilation–perfusion scan was performed. If the ventilation–perfusion scan was normal or near normal, pulmonary embolism was excluded. If the scan was high probability, pulmonary embolism was diagnosed. The remaining patients had non–high-probability ventilation–perfusion scans. If the clinical probability was low, pulmonary embolism was excluded; otherwise, pulmonary angiography was performed. Only 11% of patients required angiography, and follow-up event rates were low (Fig. 2). The authors do not recommend this approach, because the pooled sensitivity of the Vidas D-dimer test is 97.3%, and pulmonary embolism will be missed. Furthermore, initial reliance on a laboratory test runs the risk of indiscriminant screening of patients for pulmonary embolism and of ordering more imaging tests then would have been performed if D-dimer assays had not been used.

The authors recommend that physicians use the clinical model described herein or the model described by Wicki et al to categorize patients' pretest probabilities as low, moderate, or high. If the authors' model is used, the SimpliRED or IL test D-dimer assay should be performed next. If Wicki's rule is used, the Vidas D-dimer or a higher sensitivity D-dimer assay can be performed next. Patients with a low pretest probability and a negative D-dimer assay using the SimpliRED, IL test, or Vidas method need no further work-up and are considered to have a diagnosis of pulmonary embolism excluded. Because the negative likelihood ratio with the IL test and SimpliRED assay is about 0.20, the patient's pretest probability of pulmonary embolism must be 5% to 10% to rule out pulmonary embolism with a negative D-dimer assay. If the pretest probability is 5%, the posttest probability is about 1%. If the pretest probability is 10%, the posttest probability is just over 2%. This fact is derived from Bayes' theorem and the following formulas:

Pretest Probability$/1$ – Pretest Probability =

   Pretest Odds

LR × Pretest Odds = Posttest Odds

Posttest odds$/1$ + Posttest Odds =

   Posttest Probability

Negative LR = 1 – SN$/$SP

where *LR* is the likelihood ratio, *SN* is sensitivity, and *SP* is specificity. In general, sensitivity and specificity are constant for a diagnostic test.

Fig. 3. Algorithm combining D-dimer and clinical probability for patients with suspected pulmonary embolism. CT, computed tomography; DVT, deep vein thrombosis; LMWH, low molecular weight heparins; PE, pulmonary embolism; VQ, ventilation–perfusion lung scan.

Determine Pretest Probability

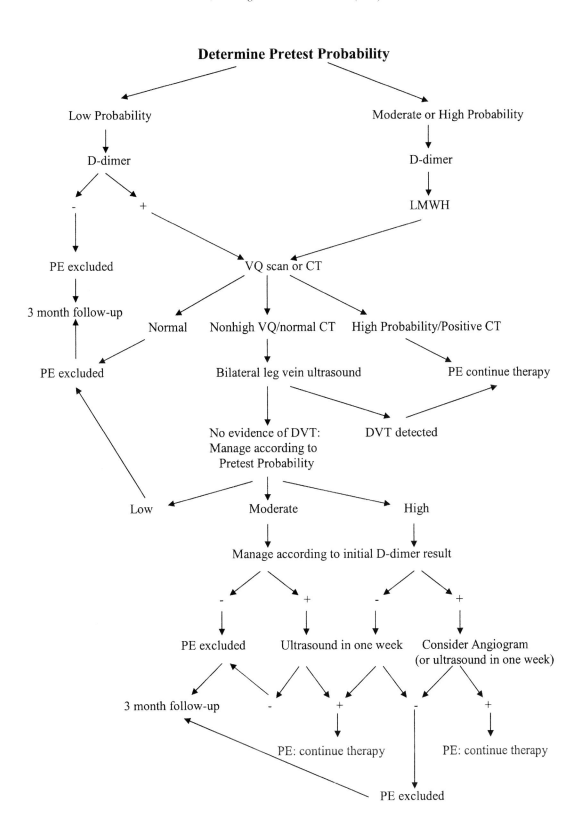

All other patients should undergo ventilation–perfusion lung scans or high-resolution spiral CT with contrast as outlined in Fig. 3. Bilateral deep vein ultrasound is performed if the ventilation–perfusion scan is nondiagnostic or the CT scan is normal. High-probability ventilation–perfusion results or positive results on the CT scan should be considered diagnostic of pulmonary embolism in most cases. Further testing by serial ultrasound or angiography depends on the pretest probability as outlined in Fig. 3. In general, negative D-dimer results in moderate- or high-probability patients negate the need for serial testing with ultrasound or angiography. This strategy should result in less than 1% of patients considered to have pulmonary embolism ruled out experiencing venous thromboembolic events during 3-month follow-up. Incorporation of the D-dimer assay into the diagnostic algorithm with pretest probability significantly and safely decreases the need for diagnostic tests [81].

If the Vidas D-dimer assay is performed in patients who are considered unlikely to have pulmonary embolism using the authors' revised model [54] or considered low probability using the Wicki clinical model, the physician can avoid the need for diagnostic imaging when the D-dimer assay is negative. The likelihood ratio of 0.06 with the Vidas test implies patients can have a pretest probability of 15%, and a negative D-dimer assay will negate the need for diagnostic imaging. The Vidas test is limited by very low specificity in elderly and hospitalized patients; therefore, imaging tests are often required in these groups. Negative results in a patient with a pretest probability of 15% or less rule out the need for imaging tests.

Improvements in care by using diagnostic management algorithms have recently been confirmed outside of the research setting by Berghout et al [82]. Before the use of an algorithm, 55% of patients with abnormal perfusion scans were treated with anticoagulants without a confirmed diagnosis, and only 11% of patients had adequate confirmation of pulmonary embolism when the scan was abnormal. These rates decreased to 13% and increased to 59%, respectively, after the use of a diagnostic management algorithm. Further improvement occurred after another year of observation.

The use of these diagnostic algorithms will most likely increase the numbers of patients in whom a diagnosis of pulmonary embolism is considered, thereby increasing the total time spent in the emergency department by patients undergoing pulmonary embolism evaluation. With implementation of the algorithm, physicians will probably increase the rate

of evaluation, that is, they will "screen" patients for pulmonary embolism. Such an effect was demonstrated in the authors' recent study by the lower prevalence of pulmonary embolism in the patient population enrolled. The increase in the number of patients considered for a possible diagnosis of pulmonary embolism may increase the overall number of imaging tests performed. Goldstein et al [83] implemented a D-dimer–based screening system for hospitalized patients and found a 40% increase in the rate of ventilation–perfusion scanning. Although this finding suggests that algorithms do not improve efficiency, algorithms do have a positive effect. With implementation of the screening system, the diagnosis of pulmonary embolism will be made in more patients. In fact, in the study by Goldstein et al, although the D-dimer protocol led to an increase in the rate of ventilation–perfusion scanning of inpatients, the percentage of scans that were ultimately read as positive for pulmonary embolism actually increased [83]. Furthermore, the number of patients in whom pulmonary embolism was diagnosed almost doubled in the centers using the D-dimer algorithm. At a hospital where pulmonary vascular imaging is not available at night, algorithms may offer a rational method to decide which patients should receive temporary anticoagulation until pulmonary vascular imaging is available. Emergency physicians faced with a requirement to understand so many diseases welcome protocols that simplify care in a safe manner.

The prognostic significance of diagnostic tests

It is logical to assume that pulmonary embolism and DVT are different manifestations of the same disease, because as many as 80% of patients with pulmonary embolism have DVT demonstrated by venography. A series of six studies demonstrated that 48% of patients with DVT had high-probability ventilation–perfusion scans despite a lack of symptoms in the majority. Douketis et al [84] demonstrated that the probability of death was higher in patients who presented with symptoms of pulmonary embolism rather than just DVT. Another investigator demonstrated similar findings [85]. The reasons for these differences are unclear, and it would be helpful to develop tools to prognosticate. It has been suggested that right ventricular hypokinesis detected by echocardiography at the time of diagnosis portends a higher risk of death [86]. Other investigators have reported similar findings [87,88]. Recently, Giannitsis et al [89] identified cardiac troponin T as an independent predictor of 30-day mortality. The level of cardiac troponin T may be related to an acute increase in right ventricular afterload and consequent severe myocardial ischemia, the latter not caused by coronary artery disease, because most of the patients had insignificant coronary disease on angiography. Although it may be possible to identify higher risk patients with other imaging tests, it is not clear this will affect outcome, and all of the studies assessing prognosis have limitations. Nonetheless, in patients with pre-existing cardiopulmonary disease or any degree of hemodynamic instability, it is probably worthwhile to perform echocardiography to assess right ventricular function to help select those patients who warrant close observation. These patients may be at higher risk if outpatient therapy is performed, and it is possible, but not yet proven, that they may benefit from more aggressive therapy, such as thrombolytic agents or inferior vena caval filters.

Summary

Recent advances in the management of patients with suspected pulmonary embolism have improved diagnostic accuracy and made management algorithms safer and more accessible. Ongoing clinical trials are evaluating whether these diagnostic processes can be made even simpler and less expensive. It is now possible to identify low-risk patients with suspected pulmonary embolism in whom imaging procedures can be avoided altogether.

References

[1] Anderson Jr FA, Wheeler HB, Goldberg RJ, Hosmer DW, Patwardhan NA, Jovanovic B, et al. A population-based perspective of the hospital incidence and case-fatality rates of deep vein thrombosis and pulmonary embolism: the Worcester study. Arch Intern Med 1991;151:933–8.

[2] Silverstein MD, Heit JA, Mohr DN, Petterson TM, O'Fallon WM, Melton III LJ. Trends in the incidence of deep vein thrombosis and pulmonary embolism: a 25-year population-based study. Arch Intern Med 1998;158:585–93.

[3] Nordstrom M, Lindblad B. Autopsy-verified venous thromboembolism within a defined urban population–the city of Malmo, Sweden. APMIS 1998;106: 378–84.

[4] Dalen JE, Alpert JS. Natural history of pulmonary embolism. Prog Cardiovasc Dis 1975;17:259–70.

[5] Dismuke SE. Pulmonary embolism as a cause of death. JAMA 1986;255:2039–42.

[6] Carson JL, Kelley MA, Duff A, Weg JG, Fulkerson WJ, Palevsky HI, et al. The clinical course of pulmonary embolism. N Engl J Med 1992;326:1240–5.

[7] Alpert JS, Smith R, Carlson CJ, Ockene IS, Dexter L, Dalen JE. Mortality in patients treated for pulmonary embolism. JAMA 1976;236:1477–80.

[8] Hirsh J, Bates SM. Prognosis in acute pulmonary embolism. Lancet 1999;353:1375–6.

[9] The PIOPED Investigators. Value of the ventilation/perfusion scan in acute pulmonary embolism: results of the Prospective Investigation of Pulmonary Embolism Diagnosis (PIOPED). JAMA 1990;263:2753–9.

[10] Wells PS, Ginsberg JS, Anderson DR, Kearon C, Gent M, Turpie AG, et al. Use of a clinical model for safe management of patients with suspected pulmonary embolism. Ann Intern Med 1998;129:997–1005.

[11] Hull RD, Hirsh J, Carter CJ, Jay RM, Dodd PE, Ockelford PA, et al. Pulmonary angiography, ventilation lung scanning, and venography for clinically suspected pulmonary embolism with abnormal perfusion lung scan. Ann Intern Med 1983;98:891–9.

[12] Hyers TM, Agnelli G, Hull RD, Morris TA, Samama M, Tapson V, et al. Antithrombotic therapy for venous thromboembolic disease. Chest 2001;119(1 Suppl): 176S–93S.

[13] Schluger N, Henschke C, King T, Russo R, Binkert B, Rackson M, et al. Diagnosis of pulmonary embolism at a large teaching hospital. J Thorac Imaging 1994;9: 180–4.

[14] van Beek EJ, Buller HR, Brandjes DP, Rutten GC, ten Cate JW. Diagnosis of clinically suspected pulmonary embolism: a survey of current practice in a teaching hospital. Neth J Med 1994;44:50–5.

[15] Egermayer P, Town GI. The mortality of untreated pulmonary embolism in patients with intermediate probability lung scans. Chest 1998;114:1497.

[16] Egermayer P, Town GI. The clinical significance of pulmonary embolism: uncertainties and implications for treatment–a debate. J Intern Med 1997;241:5–10.

[17] Stein PD, Athanasoulis C, Alavi A, Greenspan RH, Hales CA, Saltzman HA, et al. Complications and validity of pulmonary angiography in acute pulmonary embolism. Circulation 1992;85:462–8.

[18] Hudson ER, Smith TP, McDermott VG, Newman GE, Suhocki PV, Payne CS, et al. Pulmonary angiography performed with iopamidol: complications in 1434 patients. Radiology 1996;198:61–5.

[19] Wells PS, Ginsberg JS, Anderson DR, Kearon C, Gent M, Weitz J, et al. Utility of ultrasound imaging of the lower extremities in the diagnostic approach in patients with suspected pulmonary embolism. J Intern Med 2001;250:262–4.

[20] Turkstra F, Kuijer PMM, van Beek EJR, Brandjes DPM, ten Cate JW, Buller HR. Diagnostic utility of ultrasonography of leg veins in patients suspected of having pulmonary embolism. Ann Intern Med 1997; 126:775–81.

[21] Wells PS, Anderson DR, Rodger MA, Stiell I, Dreyer JF, Barnes D, et al. Excluding pulmonary embolism at the bedside without diagnostic imaging: management

of patients with suspected pulmonary embolism presenting to the emergency department by using a simple clinical model and D-dimer. Ann Intern Med 2001; 135:98–107.

[22] Remy-Jardin M, Remy J. Spiral CT angiography of the pulmonary circulation. Radiology 1999;212:615–36.

[23] Mayo JR, Remy-Jardin M, Muller NL, Remy J, Worsley DF, Hossein-Foucher C, et al. Pulmonary embolism: prospective comparison of spiral CT with ventilation-perfusion scintigraphy. Radiology 1997; 205:447–52.

[24] Birdwell BG, Raskob GE, Whitsett TL, Durica SS, Comp PC, George JN, et al. Predictive value of compression ultrasonography for deep vein thrombosis in symptomatic outpatients: clinical implications of the site of vein noncompressibility. Arch Intern Med 2000;160:309–13.

[25] Shah AA, Davis SD, Gamsu G, Intriere L. Parenchymal and pleural findings in patients with and patients without acute pulmonary embolism detected at spiral CT. Radiology 1999;211:147–53.

[26] Rathbun SW, Raskob G, Whitsett TL. Sensitivity and specificity of helical computed tomography in the diagnosis of pulmonary embolism: a systematic review. Ann Intern Med 2000;132:227–32.

[27] Mullins MD, Becker DM, Hagspiel KD, Philbrick JT. The role of spiral volumetric computed tomography in the diagnosis of pulmonary embolism. Arch Intern Med 2000;160:293–8.

[28] Perrier A, Howarth N, Didier D, Loubeyre P, Unger PF, de Moerloose P, et al. Performance of helical computed tomography in unselected outpatients with suspected pulmonary embolism. Ann Intern Med 2001;135: 88–97.

[29] Garg K, Welsh CH, Feyerabend AJ, Subber SW, Russ PD, Johnston RJ, et al. Pulmonary embolism: diagnosis with spiral CT and ventilation-perfusion scanning— correlation with pulmonary angiographic results or clinical outcome. Radiology 1998;208:201–8.

[30] Cross JL. Spiral CT and ventilation perfusion scintigraphy for the diagnosis of pulmonary embolism—reply. Clin Radiol 1998;53:784.

[31] Greaves MS, Hart EM, Aberle DR. CT of pulmonary thromboembolism. Semin Ultrasound CT MR 1997; 18:323–37.

[32] Goodman LR. Helical CT for initial imaging of pulmonary embolus. AJR Am J Roentgenol 1998;171: 1153–4.

[33] Goodman LR. CT of acute pulmonary emboli: where does it fit? Radiographics 1997;17:1037–42.

[34] Remy-Jardin M, Remy J, Artraud D, Fribourg M, Beregi JP. Spiral CT of pulmonary embolism: diagnostic approach, interpretive pitfalls and current indications. Eur Radiol 1998;8:1376–90.

[35] van Erkle AR, van Rossum AB, Bloem JL, Kievit J, Pattynama PMT. Spiral CT angiography for suspected pulmonary embolism: a cost-effective analysis. Radiology 1996;201:29–36.

[36] Chartrand-Lefebvre C, Howarth N, Lucidarme O, Bei-

gelman C, Cluzel P, Mourey-Gerosa I, et al. Contrast-enhanced helical CT for pulmonary embolism detection: inter- and intraobserver agreement among radiologists with variable experience. AJR Am J Roentgenol 1999; 172:107–12.

[37] Stein PD, Saltzman HA, Weg JG. Clinical characteristics of patients with acute pulmonary embolism. Am J Cardiol 1991;68:1723–4.

[38] Stein PD, Terrin ML, Hales CA, Palevsky HI, Saltzman HA, Thompson BT, et al. Clinical, laboratory, roentgenographic, and electrocardiographic findings in patients with acute pulmonary embolism and no pre-existing cardiac or pulmonary disease. Chest 1991; 100:598–603.

[39] Susec O, Boudrow D, Kline JA. The clinical features of acute pulmonary embolism in ambulatory patients. Acad Emerg Med 1997;4:891–7.

[40] Manganelli D, Palla A, Donnamaria V, Giuntini C. Clinical features of pulmonary embolism: doubts and certainties. Chest 1996;107(1 Suppl):25S–32S.

[41] Anderson Jr FA, Wheeler HB. Venous thromboembolism: risk factors and prophylaxis. Clin Chest Med 1995;16:235–51.

[42] Hull RD, Raskob G, Carter CJ, Coates G, Gill GJ, Sackett DL, et al. Pulmonary embolism in outpatients with pleuritic chest pain. Arch Intern Med 1988;148: 838–44.

[43] Stein PD, Dalen JE, McIntyre KM, Sasahara AA, Wenger NK, Willis III PW. The electrocardiogram in acute pulmonary embolism. Prog Cardiovasc Dis 1975;17:247–57.

[44] Ferrari E, Imbert A, Chevalier T, Mihoubi A, Morand P, Baudouy M. The ECG in pulmonary embolism: predictive value of negative T waves in precordial leads–80 case reports. Chest 1997;111:537–43.

[45] Rodger MA, Makropoulos D, Turek M, Quevillon J, Raymond F, Rasuli P, et al. Diagnostic value of the electrocardiogram in suspected pulmonary embolism. Am J Cardiol 2000;86:807–9.

[46] McFarlane MJ, Imperiale TF. Use of the alveolar–arterial oxygen gradient in the diagnosis of pulmonary embolism. Am J Med 1994;96:57–62.

[47] Stein PD, Goldhaber SZ, Henry JW. Alveolar-arterial oxygen gradient in the assessment of acute pulmonary embolism. Chest 1995;107:139–43.

[48] Stein PD, Goldhaber SZ, Henry JW, Miller AC. Arterial blood gas analysis in the assessment of suspected acute pulmonary embolism. Chest 1996;109:78–81.

[49] Rodger MA, Carrier MC, Jones GN, Rasuli P, Raymond F, Djunaedi H, et al. Diagnostic value of arterial blood gas measurement in suspected pulmonary embolism. Am J Respir Crit Care Med 2000;162:2105–8.

[50] Perrier A, Desmarais S, Miron MJ, de Moerioose P, Lepage R, Slosman D, et al. Non-invasive diagnosis of venous thromboembolism in outpatients. Lancet 1999; 353:190–5.

[51] Richardson WS. Where do pretest probabilities come from? ACP J Club 1999;4:68–9.

[52] Jackson RE, Rudoni RR, Pascual R. Emergency physi-

cian assessment of the pretest probability of pulmonary embolism. Acad Emerg Med 1999;4:891–7.

[53] Rosen MP, Sands DZ, Morris J, Drake W, Davis RB. Does a physician's ability to accurately assess the likelihood of pulmonary embolism increase with training? Acad Med 2000;75:1199–205.

[54] Wells PS, Anderson DR, Rodger MA, Ginsberg JS, Kearon C, Gent M, et al. Derivation of a simple clinical model to categorize patients probability of pulmonary embolism: increasing the models utility with the SimpliRED D-dimer. Thromb Haemost 2000;83:416–20.

[55] Furlong W, Feeny D, Torrance GW, Horsman J. Guide to design and development of health state utility instrumentation. Hamilton, Ontario: McMaster University Centre for Health Economics and Policy Analysis; 1990.

[56] Miniati M, Prediletto R, Formichi B, Marini C, DiRicco C, Tonelli L, et al. Accuracy of clinical assessment in the diagnosis of pulmonary embolism. Am J Respir Crit Care Med 1999;159:864–71.

[57] Wicki J, Perrier A, Perneger TV, Bounameaux H, Junod AF. Predicting adverse outcome in patients with acute pulmonary embolism: a risk score. Thromb Haemost 2000;84:548–52.

[58] Freyburger G, Trillaud H, Labrouche S, Gauthier P, Javorschi S, Grenier N. Rapid ELISA D-dimer testing in the exclusion of venous thromboembolism in hospitalized patients. Clin Appl Thrombosis / Haemostasis 2000;6:77–81.

[59] Kovacs MJ, MacKinnon KM, Anderson D, O'Rourke K, Keeney M, Kearon C, et al. A comparison of three rapid D-dimer methods for the diagnosis of venous thromboembolism. Br J Haematol 2001;115:140–4.

[60] Ginsberg JS, Wells PS, Kearon C, Anderson DR, Crowther M, Weitz JI, et al. Sensitivity and specificity of a D-dimer in the diagnosis of pulmonary embolism. Ann Intern Med 1998;129:1006–11.

[61] Dempfle C-E. Use of D-dimer assays in the diagnosis of venous thrombosis. Semin Thromb Hemost 2000;26:631–41.

[62] Freyburger G, Trillaud H, Labrouche S, Gauthier P, Javorschi S, Bernard P, et al. D-dimer strategy in thrombosis exclusion: a gold standard study in 100 patients suspected of deep vein thrombosis or pulmonary embolism. Eight DD methods compared. Thromb Haemost 1998;79:32–7.

[63] Brill-Edwards P, Lee A. D-dimer testing in the diagnosis of acute venous thromboembolism. Thromb Haemost 1999;82:688–94.

[64] Sijens PE, van Ingen HE, van Beek EJR, Berghout A, Oudkerk M. Rapid ELISA assay for plasma D-dimer in the diagnosis of segmental and subsegmental pulmonary embolism: a comparison with pulmonary angiography. Thromb Haemost 2000;84:156–9.

[65] Hoch JR. Management of the complications of long-term venous access. Semin Vasc Surg 1997;10:135–43.

[66] Tardy B, Tardy-Poncet B, Viallon A, Lafond P, Page Y,

Venet C, et al. Evaluation of D-dimer ELISA test in elderly patients with suspected pulmonary embolism. Thromb Haemost 1998;79:38–41.

[67] van der Graaf F, van den BH, van der KM, de Wild PJ, Janssen GW, van Uum SH. Exclusion of deep venous thrombosis with D-dimer testing—comparison of 13 D-dimer methods in 99 outpatients suspected of deep venous thrombosis using venography as reference standard. Thromb Haemost 2000;83:191–8.

[68] Owings JT, Gosselin RC, Battistella FD, Anderson JT, Petrich M, Larkin E. Whole blood D-dimer assay: an effective noninvasive method to rule out pulmonary embolism. J Trauma Injury Infect Crit Care 2000;48:795–800.

[69] Henry JW, Relyea B, Stein PD. Continuing risk of thromboemboli among patients with normal pulmonary angiograms. Chest 1995;107:1375–8.

[70] Hull RD, Raskob GE, Coates G, Panju AA. Clinical validity of a normal perfusion lung scan on patients with suspected pulmonary embolism. Chest 1990;97:23–6.

[71] van Beek EJR, Kuyer PMM, Schenk BE, Brandjes DPM, ten Cate JW, Büller HR. A normal perfusion lung scan in patients with clinically suspected pulmonary embolism: frequency and clinical validity. Chest 1995;108:170–3.

[72] Kipper MS, Moser KM, Kortman KE, Ashburn WL. Long-term follow-up of patients with suspected pulmonary embolism and a normal lung scan: perfusion scans in embolic suspects. Chest 1982;82:411–5.

[73] Hillarp A, Svensson P, Dahlback B. Prothrombin gene mutation and venous thrombosis in unselected outpatients [abstract]. Thromb Haemost Supplement 1997; OC-1545:378–9.

[74] Rock G, Wells PS. New concepts in coagulation. Crit Rev Clin Lab Sci 1997;34:475–501.

[75] Gosselin MV, Rubin GD, Leung AN, Huang J, Rizk NW. Unsuspected pulmonary embolism: prospective detection on routine helical CT scans. Radiology 1998;208:209–15.

[76] Feinstein AR. "Clinical judgment" revisited: the distraction of quantitative models. Ann Intern Med 1994;120:799–805.

[77] Wicki J, Perneger TV, Junod AF, Bounameaux H, Perrier A. Assessing clinical probability of pulmonary embolism in the emergency ward: a simple score. Arch Intern Med 2001;161:92–7.

[78] Farmer RDT, Lawrenson RA, Thompson CR, Kennedy JG, Hambleton IR. Population-based study of risk of venous thromboembolism associated with various oral contraceptives. Lancet 1997;349:83–8.

[79] Worsley DF, Alavi A. Comprehensive analysis of the results of the PIOPED study: Prospective Investigation of Pulmonary Embolism Diagnosis. J Nucl Med 1995;36:2380–7.

[80] Cohen J. Statistical power analysis for the behavioural sciences. 2nd edition. Hillsdale (NJ): Lawrence Erlbaum; 1988.

[81] Wells PS, Anderson DR, Burton E. Management of patients with suspected pulmonary embolism (PE) pre-

senting to the emergency department (ED) using clinical probability and D-dimer [abstract]. Blood 1999; 94(10 Suppl 1):25.

[82] Berghout A, Oudkerk M, Hicks SG, Teng TH, Pillay M, Buller HR. Active implementation of a consensus strategy improves diagnosis and management in suspected pulmonary embolism. Q J Med 2000;93:335–40.

[83] Goldstein NM, Kollef MH, Ward S, Gage BF. The impact of the introduction of a rapid D-dimer assay on the diagnostic evaluation of suspected pulmonary embolism. Arch Intern Med 2001;161:567–71.

[84] Douketis JD, Kearon C, Bates S, Duku EK, Ginsberg JS. Risk of fatal pulmonary embolism in patients with treated venous thromboembolism. JAMA 1998; 279:458–62.

[85] Heit J, Silverstein MD, Mohr DN, Petterson TM, O'Fallon WM, Melton III LM. Predictors of survival after deep vein thrombosis and pulmonary embolism. Arch Intern Med 1999;159:445–53.

[86] Goldhaber SZ, Visani L, De Rosa M. Acute pulmonary embolism: clinical outcomes in the International Cooperative Pulmonary Embolism Registry (ICOPER). Lancet 1999;353:1386–9.

[87] Kasper W, Konstantinides S, Geibel A, Tiede N, Krause T, et al. Prognostic significance of right ventricular afterload stress detected by echocardiography in patients with clinically suspected pulmonary embolism. Heart 1997;77:346–9.

[88] Ribeiro A, Lindmarker P, Juhlin-Dannfelt A, Johnsson H, Jorfeldt L. Echocardiography Doppler in pulmonary embolism: right ventricular dysfunction as a predictor of mortality rate. Am Heart J 1997;134:479–87.

[89] Giannitsis E, Mueller-Bardorff M, Kurowski V, Weidtmann B, Wiegand U, Kampmann M, et al. Independent prognostic value of cardiac troponin T in patients with confirmed pulmonary embolism. Circulation 2000; 102:211–7.

CLINICS
IN CHEST
MEDICINE

Clin Chest Med 24 (2003) 29–38

Imaging of acute pulmonary thromboembolism: should spiral computed tomography replace the ventilation–perfusion scan?

Tom Powell, FFR (RCSI), Nestor L. Müller, MD, PhD*

Department of Radiology, University of British Columbia, Vancouver General Hospital, 899 West 12th Avenue, Vancouver, BC, V5Z 1M9, Canada

For several decades, ventilation–perfusion (V/Q) scintigraphy has been the main imaging modality used in the evaluation of patients with suspected acute pulmonary embolism (PE) [1,2]. A high-probability V/Q scan provides sufficient certainty to confirm the diagnosis of PE, whereas a normal or near-normal scan reliably excludes the diagnosis [2]. In the Prospective Investigation of Pulmonary Embolism Diagnosis (PIOPED) study, indeterminate scans present in 39% of patients (364 of 931) showed a 30% incidence of PE, and low-probability scans seen in 34% of patients (312 of 931) showed a 14% incidence. Based on these data, it was concluded that indeterminate and low-probability lung scans (ie, two-thirds of V/Q scans in the PIOPED study) were not useful in establishing or excluding a diagnosis of acute PE [2]. Furthermore, although there was good interobserver agreement for high-probability and normal V/Q scans, there was a 25% to 30% disagreement between observers in the interpretation of intermediate and low-probability scans [2].

Pulmonary angiography has traditionally been considered the gold standard for diagnosing PE [1]. Pulmonary angiography allows direct visualization of the pulmonary arterial tree and the detection of filling defects that are typically seen in acute PE. Nevertheless, it is an invasive test with associated morbidity (6%) and mortality (0%–0.5%) and is underused [3]. It has been estimated that, even in academic centers,

only 12% to 14% of patients with a nondiagnostic V/Q scan undergo pulmonary angiography [3,4].

The introduction of spiral CT in the late 1980s made it possible to image the entire chest in a short period of time and to analyze the pulmonary arteries during the peak of contrast enhancement. Several studies have shown a high sensitivity and specificity of spiral CT in the diagnosis of PE [5–18]. The accuracy has been improved further with the recent introduction of multidetector CT [18,19]. In an increasing number of centers, spiral CT has become the imaging modality of choice in the evaluation of patients with a clinical suspicion of acute PE.

This article discusses the role of the various imaging modalities in the diagnosis of acute PE and suggests a diagnostic imaging algorithm based on current evidence in the literature.

Chest radiography

Chest radiography is of limited value in the diagnosis of PE (Box 1). Its major importance lies in excluding other disease processes that can mimic PE, such as pneumonia and pneumothorax [20–22].

The chest radiographs of 1063 patients who were suspected of having acute PE and who were part of the PIOPED study were interpreted independently by two radiologists [20]. Of these patients, 383 had angiographically proven PE and 680 a normal pulmonary angiogram. The prevalence of the most common findings, such as atelectasis and focal areas of increased opacity, was not significantly different

---

* Corresponding author.
E-mail address: nmuller@vanhosp.bc.ca (N.L. Müller).

Box 1. Value of chest radiography in the diagnosis of acute pulmonary embolism

Limited value in diagnosis
Performed mainly to exclude other
    diseases that may mimic PE clinically
Findings with low sensitivity and
    relatively high specificity
    Peripheral oligemia (Westermark
    sign)
    Enlargement of central pulmonary
    artery (Fleischner's sign)
    Pleural-based opacity (Hampton's
    hump)
    Elevated hemidiaphragm
Nonspecific findings
    Air–space consolidation
    Linear atelectasis
    Pleural effusion
Radiograph normal in 10% to 15% of
    cases with proven diagnosis

from that in patients who did not have embolism. Overall, atelectasis had a sensitivity of 20% and a specificity of 85%, and pleural-based areas of increased opacity (Hampton's hump) had a sensitivity of 22% and a specificity of 82% in the diagnosis of acute PE. Similarly, oligemia (Westermark sign), a prominent central pulmonary artery (Fleischner's sign), vascular redistribution, and pleural effusion were poor predictors of PE. The chest radiograph was interpreted as normal in 12% of patients who had PE and in 18% of patients in whom PE was absent at angiography.

In another study, chest radiographs of 152 patients who were suspected of having acute PE were randomized and presented for interpretation to nine readers (seven of whom were subspecialty chest radiologists) [21]. Only 108 of the 152 patients proved to have PE at pulmonary angiography. The readers were asked to answer the question, "Does this patient have PE?" The average true-positive ratio (sensitivity) was 0.33 (range, 0.08–0.52) and the average true-negative ratio (specificity), 0.59 (range, 0.31–0.80).

Most episodes of PE produce no symptoms or detectable changes at chest radiography. Even if the diagnosis is suspected clinically and confirmed angiographically, no abnormalities are seen on radiographs in approximately 10% to 15% of cases (see Box 1).

Ventilation–perfusion scintigraphy

In a random sample of 931 patients who underwent scintigraphy in the PIOPED study, 13% had high-probability scans, 39% had intermediate-probability scans, 34% had low-probability scans, and 14% had normal or near-normal scans [2]. There was good agreement for classifying V/Q scans as high probability (95%) or as normal (94%); however, there was a 25% to 75% disagreement in interpreting intermediate-probability and low-probability scans [2]. Of the 931 patients, 755 underwent pulmonary angiography. Of patients who had high-probability scans and a definitive diagnosis at angiography, 88% had emboli compared with 33% of patients who had intermediate-probability scans, 16% who had low-probability scans, and 9% who had near-normal or normal scans. The diagnostic value was not significantly different between men and women and among patients of different ages [23,24].

Diagnostic utility was similar among patients who had pre-existing cardiac or pulmonary disease when compared with patients who had no such disease. In a subset of patients who had chronic obstructive pulmonary disease (COPD), the sensitivity of a high-probability scan was significantly lower than in patients who had no pre-existing cardiopulmonary disease [25]; however, the positive predictive value of a high-probability scan was 100% and the negative predictive value of a low-probability or very low–probability scan, 94%.

Although clinical assessment of patients who have suspected acute PE does not lead to a definitive diagnosis in most instances, the results from the PIOPED study emphasize the importance of incorporating the pretest clinical likelihood of PE in the overall diagnostic evaluation. In patients who had low-probability or very low-probability V/Q scans and no history of immobilization, recent surgery, trauma to the lower extremities, or central venous instrumentation, the prevalence of PE was 4.5% [26]. In patients who had low-probability or very low-probability V/Q scan interpretations and one risk factor, the prevalence of PE was 12%; in patients who had two or more risk factors, the prevalence was 21%. Most patients had intermediate-probability or low-probability V/Q scans and an intermediate clinical likelihood of PE. For these patients, the combination of clinical assessment and V/Q scans did not provide adequate information to direct patient management accurately, and further investigation with peripheral venous studies, spiral CT, or pulmonary angiography was required.

The value of V/Q scans in patients who have COPD is controversial. In one combined V/Q-angiographic study of 83 patients who had COPD and suspected PE, the overall sensitivity and specificity of V/Q imaging were 0.83 and 0.92, respectively [27]. False-negative interpretations occurred in 3 of the 16 patients who showed ventilation abnormalities in more than 50% of the lungs, whereas in the 67 patients who had ventilation abnormalities affecting 50% or less of the lungs, the sensitivity (0.95) and specificity (0.94) for detecting PE were high. The researchers concluded that V/Q imaging was a reliable method for detecting PE in patients who had regions of V/Q-matched defects as long as ventilation abnormalities were limited in extent.

In a later study performed to assess the accuracy of chest radiographs in predicting the extent of airway disease in patients with suspected PE, investigators found that V/Q scans were indeterminate in all 21 patients who had radiographic evidence of widespread COPD, in 35% of patients who had focal obstructive disease, and in 18% of patients whose chest radiographs revealed no evidence of COPD [28]. The investigators concluded that ventilation imaging probably was not warranted in patients who had radiographic evidence of widespread COPD.

When an attempt is made to distinguish V/Q matching that is compatible with PE from that caused by COPD, a computation of the actual V/Q ratio may be useful. In one study in which a V/Q ratio of 1.25 or higher was used to define an area of mismatch, the percentage of patients classified correctly as having PE or COPD increased from 56% to 88%, based simply on a consideration of the matched or mismatched character of perfusion [29].

In another study of 108 patients who had COPD and who were suspected of having PE (21 of whom had the diagnosis confirmed by angiography), it was not possible to distinguish between patients who had and did not have emboli by clinical assessment alone [25]. Among the 108 patients, high-probability, intermediate-probability, low-probability, and normal-probability scan results were present in 5%, 60%, 30%, and 5%, respectively. The frequency of PE in these categories was 100%, 22%, 2%, and 0%, respectively. Although high-probability and low-probability V/Q scan results have good predictive values, most patients who have COPD have intermediate-probability scans and require further investigation, which may include spiral CT and angiography.

Approximately 15% of patients who have PE have high-probability V/Q scan results, 40% have intermediate-probability scans, 30% have low-probability scans, and 15% have normal or near-normal scan results [2]. Approximately 90% of patients who have high-probability scan results have PE compared with 30% of patients who have intermediate-probability scans, 15% who have low-probability scan results, and 9% who have normal or near-normal scans [2,30].

The diagnostic accuracy can be improved by combining the results of V/Q scanning with the clinical impression. In the PIOPED study, a pretest clinical probability of PE was estimated before lung scanning [2]. Three probabilities were considered: low (0% to 19%), intermediate (20% to 79%), and high (80% to 100%). A low-probability scan result paired with a low clinical index of suspicion had a negative predictive value of 96%. Conversely, a concordant high-probability V/Q scan result paired with a high clinical index of suspicion had a positive predictive value of 96%. Only 25% of patients fit into these clinicoscintigraphic categories, with 75% of patients having an uncertain diagnosis [2]. Even under optimal circumstances of excellent clinical assessment and expert interpretation of V/Q scans, further investigation is often required to establish the presence or absence of emboli.

Spiral computed tomography

The introduction of spiral CT in the late 1980s made it possible to image large portions of the chest during a single breath hold and to image the pulmonary arteries during peak enhancement with intravenous contrast. Several studies have shown that spiral CT has a high sensitivity and specificity in the diagnosis of emboli in the central and segmental pulmonary arteries. These studies, performed in the 1990s, were based on the use of single-detector CT scanners. Recently, a new generation of CT scanners has been introduced. These scanners have multiple detector rows (4, 8, and, since 2002, 16 rows) (multidetector CT) and greater rotation speeds. Multidetector CT scanners allow imaging of the entire chest during a single breath hold with thinner sections. The improved spatial resolution allows assessment of subsegmental vessels while the greater rotation speeds of the CT gantry result in reduced artifacts from cardiac and respiratory motion. Multidetector CT with 1.25mm-thick sections allows accurate analysis of peripheral pulmonary arteries down to the fifth order [19].

The diagnosis of acute PE on contrast-enhanced CT scan is based on the presence of partial or complete filling defects within the pulmonary arteries (Box 2) [5,31]. A partial filling defect is defined as an

Box 2. Acute pulmonary embolism—spiral CT findings

Vascular findings
    Intravascular filling defect
    Acute angles with vessel wall
    Complete cutoff of vascular
        opacification
    Increased diameter of occluded
        vessel
Helpful parenchymal findings
    Wedge-shaped nonenhancing,
        pleural-based opacities
    Linear atelectasis
Sensitivity of spiral CT, 90%; specificity, 90%
False-negative interpretation mainly
    owing to subsegmental emboli
False-positive interpretation owing to
    hilar nodes and technical pitfalls

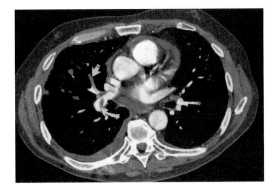

Fig. 2. Acute PE. Multidetector spiral CT image shows a complete filling defect in the medial segmental artery of the right middle lobe (*straight arrow*) and a partial filling defect in the right lower lobe artery (*curved arrow*).

intravascular central or marginal area of low attenuation surrounded by variable amounts of contrast material (Figs. 1, 2). A complete filling defect is defined as an intraluminal area of low attenuation that occupies the entire arterial section, as evidenced by the abrupt termination of the contrast column within a visible vessel (Fig. 2) [5,6]. The most reliable sign of an acute embolus is a filling defect forming an acute angle with the vessel wall and outlined by contrast material (Fig. 3). Although filling defects that form a

smooth obtuse angle with the vessel wall or a complete cutoff of contrast opacification of a vessel may be caused by acute emboli, they also may be seen with chronic emboli.

The diagnosis of acute PE requires an assessment of vascular and parenchymal findings. An assessment of the lung windows will not only help to identify the segmental and subsegmental pulmonary arteries by their proximity to the bronchi but will also assess for the presence of ancillary signs that may be helpful in suggesting the presence of PE [32].

The most helpful ancillary sign is the presence of a nonenhancing pleural-based, wedge-shaped pul-

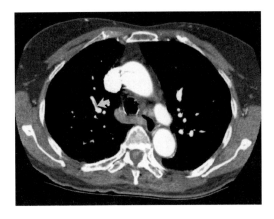

Fig. 1. Acute PE. Multidetector spiral CT image shows a partial filling defect in the anterior segmental artery of the right upper lobe (*arrow*).

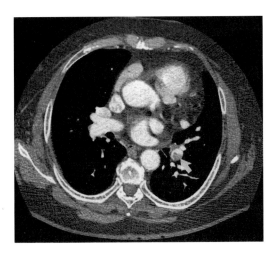

Fig. 3. Acute PE. Multidetector spiral CT image shows a partial filling defect in left lower lobe pulmonary artery (*arrow*), outlined by contrast and forming an acute angle with the vessel wall.

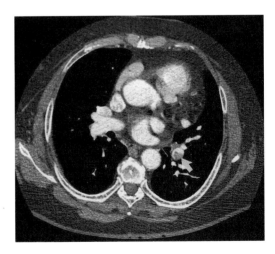

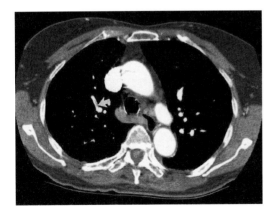

monary opacity [32]. Linear (platelike) atelectasis is also seen with increased frequency on CT in patients with acute PE [32]. Other findings, such as areas of decreased attenuation and pleural effusion, are not helpful in distinguishing patients with and without acute PE [32].

In a study of 88 patients who had suspected PE [32], the findings that were seen most commonly in patients who had PE included wedge-shaped, pleural-based opacities (present in 62% of patients who had emboli compared with 27% of patients who did not) and linear opacities (present in 46% with emboli and 21% without). Areas of oligemia were seen in 3 of 26 patients (11%) who had acute PE but also in 6 of 62 patients (10%) who did not have emboli.

In a second investigation of 92 patients, the only parenchymal abnormality significantly associated with acute PE was the presence of a peripheral wedge-shaped opacity [33]. This abnormality was seen in 7 of 28 patients (25%) who had PE compared with 3 of 64 patients (5%) who did not. As a manifestation of PE, a wedge-shaped pulmonary opacity abutting the pleural surface is seen more commonly on CT scan than on the chest radiograph [34]. The opacities may have the configuration of a full triangle or a truncated cone with a concave or convex apex (Fig. 4). It has been postulated that the latter appearance may be related to sparing of the apex of the cone from infarction as a result of collateral circulation from bronchial arteries [34].

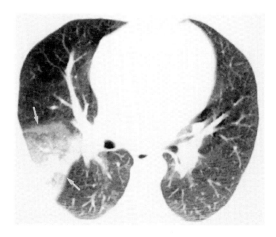

Fig. 4. Multidetector spiral CT image shows a wedge-shaped pulmonary opacity abutting the pleural surface in the posterior segment of the right upper lung lobe (*arrows*). Occlusive thrombus was present in the posterior segmental artery to the right upper lobe.

On CT, most infarcts appear to be reabsorbed partially or completely after 1 month, sometimes being manifested only as a scar [34].

Pitfalls and artifacts of computed tomography

Several technical, anatomic, and patient-related pitfalls may lead to misinterpretation of the CT images. Technical failures occur in 1% to 5% of scans and are usually caused by motion artifacts in dyspneic patients or insufficient vascular enhancement [9]. In patients with severe dyspnea, motion artifacts can produce respiratory misregistration and inadequate sampling of the pulmonary vessels, resulting in focal areas of decreased attenuation that can mimic a clot.

The lymphatic and connective tissue located adjacent to the pulmonary arteries may mimic the appearance of PE. This pitfall is minimized by careful review of the images and the use of additional imaging-rendering tools, such as cineviewing and multiplanar reconstruction.

Diagnostic accuracy of spiral computed tomography

The reported diagnostic accuracy of spiral CT has varied depending on the technique used, the patient population, and whether investigators have limited the analysis to the central pulmonary arteries down the level of the segmental vessels or have included subsegmental arteries (Table 1) [6,8,9,11,14,15,18]. Overall, these studies have shown a sensitivity of spiral CT of approximately 90%, a specificity of 90%, a positive predictive value of 93%, and a negative predictive value of 94% for emboli down to and including the level of the segmental pulmonary arteries [35]. The results of the various studies in the literature indicate that, although single-detector spiral CT has a high sensitivity in the detection of central emboli, it is of limited value in the diagnosis of subsegmental emboli. The clinical significance of isolated subsegmental emboli, especially in patients with no underlying disease, is controversial. Furthermore, it has been shown that, even though pulmonary angiography is considered the gold standard for the diagnosis of PE, the interobserver agreement for the diagnosis of subsegmental emboli on angiography is only 66% [3]. Experimental work in a porcine model has shown that single-detector spiral CT using thin collimation (3 mm or less) is comparable with pul-

Table 1
Accuracy of spiral computed tomography in the diagnosis of acute pulmonary embolism

| Study | Year | Number of patients in study | CT protocols | | Sensitivity (%) | Specificity (%) | κ value |
			Collimation (mm)	Lower anatomic level of interpretation			
Remy-Jardin, et al [5]	1992	42	5	Segmental	100	96	NC
Goodman, et al [6]	1995	20	5	Segmental	86	92	NC
Senac, et al [7]	1995	45	5	Segmental	86	100	NC
van Rossum, et al [8]	1996	149	5	Segmental	82–90	93–96	0.774
Remy-Jardin, et al [9]	1996	75	5, 3	Segmental	91	78	NC
Ferretti, et al [10]	1997	164	5	Segmental	NC	NC	NC
Mayo, et al [11]	1997	142	3	Segmental	87	95	0.85
van Rossum, et al [12]	1998	123	5	Segmental	75	90	NC
Drucker, et al [13]	1998	47	5	Segmental	53–60	81–97	NC
Herold, et al [14]	1998	401	3	Subsegmental	88	94	0.72
Garg, et al [15]	1998	54	3	Subsegmental	67	100	NC
Baghaie, et al [16]	1998	370	3, 2	Subsegmental	96	100	0.87
Kim, et al [17]	1999	110	3	Segmental	92	96	NC
Qanadli, et al [18]	2000	157	2.5 (dual section)	Subsegmental	90	94	0.86

Abbreviations: k, kappa statistic; NC, not calculated.

monary angiography in the diagnosis of segmental and subsegmental PE [36].

Technique for spiral computed tomography

Optimal assessment of the pulmonary vessels on spiral CT requires careful attention to several parameters, including scan collimation, imaging volume, and contrast enhancement.

The imaging protocol depends on whether single-detector or multidetector CT is used. On single-detector CT, the following protocol is recommended: spiral CT during a 20- to 30-second breath hold using 3-mm collimation, a table speed of 5 to 6 mm/second, a pitch of 1.7 to 2.0, 120 kVp, and 180 to 320 mA. Images are reconstructed at 1.5-mm intervals and a field of view appropriate for the size of the patient.

Multiple detector row spiral CT scanners allow the acquisition of contiguous 0.7- to 2.5-mm thick slices through the entire chest during a single breath hold. The authors recommend use of the narrowest possible detector aperture within the constraints imposed by

the duration of the contrast material bolus and the breath-holding capability of the patient. In patients who cannot hold their breath for the duration of the scan, good quality images can usually be obtained during quiet breathing.

The lung volume that is scanned should be large enough to include all segmental and subsegmental pulmonary arteries. This goal can be achieved by scanning from the top of the aortic arch to the dome of the diaphragm. Although the scans can be performed in the craniocaudal direction, scanning caudocranially helps to minimize motion artifacts, particularly in patients unable to hold their breath for the duration of the scan [37,38].

Nonionic iodinated contrast material is administered through an antecubital venous access or a central line using a power injector [37,38]. Injection rates ranging from 2 to 7 mL/second have been reported. The authors use 120 to 150 mL of 30% nonionic iodinated contrast material injected at a rate of 4 mL/second. In hemodynamically stable patients, a 10- to 15-second scan delay usually provides optimal contrast enhancement of the pulmonary arteries.

This delay may need to be increased in patients with severe pulmonary hypertension or right-sided heart failure. To determine the optimal time delay, a test injection can be performed to assess the circulation time. A total of 20 mL of contrast material is injected at a rate of 4 mL/second and serial scans performed at 3- to 5-second intervals for 20 seconds at the level of the main pulmonary artery. To ensure opacification of the peripheral arteries during the diagnostic study, 5 seconds are added to the time to peak enhancement of the main pulmonary artery [37,38].

Images are viewed at the workstation at settings appropriate for visualization of pulmonary vasculature (window width, 400 Hu; window level, 35 Hu) and lung parenchyma (window width, 1500 Hu; window level, −700 Hu). In selected cases, multiplanar reformatting may be helpful in demonstrating the extent of the PE [37] (Figs. 5, 6).

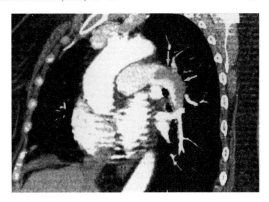

Fig. 6. Sagittal-oblique reformatted multislice CT image shows extent of thrombus narrowing the left lower lobe pulmonary artery as it curves posterolaterally and inferiorly (arrow).

Outcome studies

Traditionally, pulmonary angiography has been considered the gold standard in the diagnosis of acute PE. Nevertheless, it has two main limitations: (1) it is seldom performed, even when indicated [3,4]; and (2) it is associated with considerable interobserver disagreement, particularly for the diagnosis of subsegmental emboli [39]. In the PIOPED study [2], interobserver agreement was 92% for pulmonary angiography showing the presence of PE and 83% for studies showing the absence of PE.

Interobserver agreement is even lower when confined to angiography showing the presence of PE limited to the subsegmental pulmonary arteries [40]. Stein et al [40] reviewed data from patients partici-

pating in PIOPED. The copositivity of readings of PE in subsegmental branches (66%) was significantly lower than the copositivity of 98% for readings of PE in the main or lobar pulmonary arteries ($P < 0.001$) and the copositivity of 90% for readings of PE in the segmental arteries ($P < 0.05$) [40]. It has been proposed that the gold standard in the diagnosis of PE should be patient outcome and not pulmonary angiography [39].

Patients with suspected acute PE and negative CT results have an excellent outcome without anticoagulation [41]. The outcomes are similar to those reported after withholding anticoagulation after a normal or low-probability V/Q scan or a negative angiogram [41–43]. Swensen et al reviewed the records of 1512 consecutive patients who were referred for CT with clinically suspected acute PE [41]. A total of 993 of these patients received no anticoagulation and had CT scans interpreted as negative for acute PE. A 3-month probability of venous thromboembolism of 0.5% was identified in these patients. This finding compares well with the reported incidence of venous thromboembolism in untreated patients with negative angiograms [44] and negative V/Q scintigraphy results [45]. Hull et al [45] found a 3-month cumulative incidence of 0.2% for nonfatal PE in 515 untreated patients with negative perfusion lung scan results.

Another clinical outcome study compared 198 patients with negative spiral CT findings with 350 patients with a negative V/Q scan (normal or low probability) [42]. During 3-month follow-up, subsequent PE was observed in 1% of the spiral CT group compared with 1.5% of the V/Q group (not statistically significant).

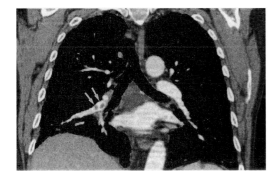

Fig. 5. Multislice spiral CT angiogram, reformatted in the coronal plane, shows nonocclusive emboli in the right lower lobe artery (arrows).

In a third investigation, the risk for PE was assessed in a group of 185 patients who had negative CT pulmonary angiograms, who had not received anticoagulation, and who were followed up clinically at 3 months, 6 months, and 1 year. A total of 135 of these patients had underlying lung disease, and 50 patients had no history of respiratory disorder [46]. No significant difference was seen between the 98% (132 of 135) negative predictive value of spiral CT angiography in patients with underlying lung disease and the 100% (50 of 50) negative predictive value in patients who had no history of respiratory disorder.

Based on the results of outcome studies, it seems safe to withhold anticoagulation in patients who have a negative spiral CT and no clinical evidence of deep vein thrombosis.

Should spiral computed tomography replace the ventilation–perfusion scan?

Several groups of investigators have shown that CT angiography is superior to V/Q scintigraphy in the diagnosis of acute PE [9,11,47]. In one prospective comparison of spiral CT and V/Q scintigraphy in 142 patients, two experienced observers assessed the results of both procedures independently [11]. The combination of a high-probability V/Q scan result and a spiral CT finding of PE was considered diagnostic, and no further imaging studies were performed. The combination of a normal, very low–probability, or low-probability V/Q scan and a negative spiral CT in a patient with a low clinical suspicion of PE was considered sufficient to exclude the disease. All other patients underwent pulmonary angiography. Twelve patients had discordant spiral CT and V/Q scans. Using angiographic results as the gold standard, the spiral CT interpretation was correct in 11 patients and the V/Q scan in 1 patient. Overall, CT angiography had a sensitivity of 87% and a specificity of 98% in the diagnosis of acute PE compared with a sensitivity of 65% and a specificity of 94% for a high-probability V/Q scan. There was better interobserver agreement in the interpretation of the spiral CT scans than the V/Q scans.

In a second investigation, spiral CT angiography was compared with V/Q scintigraphy in 179 patients [48]. CT angiography had a sensitivity of 94% and a specificity of 94%, whereas scintigraphy had a sensitivity of 81% and a specificity of 74% in the diagnosis of acute PE. Interobserver agreement was much better for interpretation of CT angiography (κ statistic = 0.72) than for scintigraphy (κ = 0.22) [48].

In a prospective randomized trial of 78 patients who had suspected PE, spiral CT or V/Q scans were performed as part of the initial investigation [47]. A confident diagnosis of PE was made in 35 of 39 patients (90%) who underwent spiral CT compared with 21 of 39 patients (54%) who underwent scintigraphy first. The main reason for this difference was the ability of CT to show lesions other than PE that were considered to be responsible for the symptoms of 13 of 39 patients (33%).

In another prospective study of 110 patients, spiral CT helped identify correctly 23 of 25 patients who had PE (sensitivity, 92%). In 57 of the 85 patients (67%) who did not have PE, spiral CT provided additional information that suggested or confirmed the alternate clinical diagnosis [17]. In this series, the most common diagnoses in patients with an abnormal CT scan who did not have PE were pneumonia, cardiovascular disease, interstitial lung disease, trauma-related chest abnormalities, and pulmonary or pleural malignancy.

Analysis of a decision model based on the published data has shown that the use of spiral CT is likely to improve cost-effectiveness in the work-up of PTE and to be associated with decreased mortality [49]. Various diagnostic algorithms have been assessed, including various combinations of V/Q scintigraphy, ultrasound, D-dimer assay, spiral CT, and conventional angiography for all realistic values of the pretest probability of PTE and coexisting DVT and of the diagnostic accuracy of spiral CT. All of the best diagnostic strategies include CT angiography [49].

Initially, spiral CT was only recommended in patients who had indeterminate or low-probability V/Q scans and a high clinical index of suspicion for PE [5,8,11]. Subsequently, it was suggested that spiral CT should be used instead of scintigraphy in the assessment of patients with underlying cardiopulmonary disease and an abnormal chest radiograph [47]. More recently, various investigators have suggested that spiral CT should replace scintigraphy in the assessment of patients whose symptoms are suggestive of acute PE [12,15,39,41].

Based on the data in the literature demonstrating a higher diagnostic accuracy of spiral CT when compared with scintigraphy in the diagnosis of acute PE, a better interobserver agreement, and the ability to suggest an alternate diagnosis in patients without PE, the authors believe that spiral CT should replace scintigraphy in the assessment of patients with clinically suspected acute PE.

Recommended imaging algorithm in patients with suspected acute pulmonary embolism

Given the data in the literature, the following imaging algorithm is recommended for the evaluation of patients suspected of having acute PE:

All patients should have a chest radiograph, the main role of which is to exclude abnormalities such as acute pneumonia that may mimic PE clinically.

Patients with symptoms or signs of deep vein thrombosis should undergo evaluation of the leg veins, the most commonly recommended technique being Doppler ultrasound. If the Doppler study is positive, the patient can be considered to have acute PE and usually does not require further investigation.

Patients with clinically suspected acute PE and no signs or symptoms of deep vein thrombosis should undergo spiral CT pulmonary angiography. Spiral CT angiography requires the use of iodinated contrast material. Patients with a contraindication to the use of iodinated contrast material should undergo V/Q scintigraphy.

Patients in whom the CT scans are suboptimal and patients in whom the CT scan results are negative but who have a high clinical index of suspicion for acute PE should undergo pulmonary angiography.

References

[1] Matsumoto AH, Tegtmeyer CJ. Contemporary diagnostic approaches to acute pulmonary emboli. Radiol Clin North Am 1995;33:167–83.

[2] Value of the ventilation/perfusion scan in acute pulmonary embolism: results of the Prospective Investigation of Pulmonary Embolism Diagnosis (PIOPED). JAMA 1990;263:2753–9.

[3] Stein PD, Athanasoulis C, Alavi A, Greenspan RH, Hales CA, Saltzman HA, et al. Complications and validity of pulmonary angiography in acute pulmonary embolism. Circulation 1992;85:462–8.

[4] Khorasani R, Gudas TF, Nikpoor N, et al. Treatment of patients with suspected pulmonary embolism and intermediate-probability lung scans: is diagnostic imaging underused? AJR Am J Roentgenol 1997;169:1355–7.

[5] Remy-Jardin M, Remy J, Wattinne L, Giraud F. Central pulmonary thromboembolism: diagnosis with spiral volumetric CT with the single-breath-hold technique. Comparison with pulmonary angiography. Radiology 1992;185:381–7.

[6] Goodman LR, Curtin JJ, Mewissen MW, et al. Detection of pulmonary embolism in patients with unresolved clinical and scintigraphic diagnosis: helical CT versus angiography. AJR Am J Roentgenol 1995; 164:1369–74.

[7] Senac JP, Verhnet H, Bousquet C, et al. Embolie pulmonaire: apport de la tomodensitometrie helicoïdale. J Radiol 1995;76:339–45.

[8] van Rossum AB, Pattynama PM, Ton ER, Treurniet FE, Arndt JW, van Eck B, et al. Pulmonary embolism: validation of spiral CT angiography in 149 patients. Radiology 1996;201:467–70.

[9] Remy-Jardin M, Remy J, Deschildre F, Artaud D, Beregi JP, Hossein-Foucher C, et al. Diagnosis of pulmonary embolism with spiral CT: comparison with pulmonary angiography and scintigraphy. Radiology 1996;200: 699–706.

[10] Ferretti GR, Bosson J-L, Buffaz P-D, Ayanian D, Pison C, Blanc F, et al. Acute pulmonary embolism: role of helical CT in 164 patients with intermediate probability at ventilation-perfusion scintigraphy and normal results at duplex US of the legs. Radiology 1997;205:453–8.

[11] Mayo JR, Remy-Jardin M, Müller NL, Remy J, Worsley DF, Hossein-Foucher C, et al. Pulmonary embolism: prospective comparison of spiral CT with ventilation-perfusion scintigraphy. Radiology 1997; 205(2):447–52.

[12] van Rossum AB, Pattynama PM, Mallens WM, Hermans J, Heijerman HG. Can helical CT replace scintigraphy in the diagnostic process in suspected pulmonary embolism? A retrospective-prospective cohort study focusing on total diagnostic yield. Eur Radiol 1998; 8:90–6.

[13] Drucker EA, Rivitz SM, Shepard JO, Boiselle PM, Trotman-Dickenson B, Welch TJ, et al. Acute pulmonary embolism: assessment of helical CT for diagnosis. Radiology 1998;209(1):235–41.

[14] Herold C, Remy-Jardin M, Grenier PH, et al. Prospective evaluation of pulmonary embolism: initial results of the European Multicenter Trial (ESTIPEP) [abstract]. Radiology 1998;209(P):299.

[15] Garg K, Welsh CH, Feyerabend AJ, et al. Pulmonary embolism: diagnosis with spiral CT and ventilation-perfusion scanning. Correlation with pulmonary angiographic results or clinical outcome. Radiology 1998; 208:201–8.

[16] Baghaie F, Remy-Jardin M, Remy J, Artaud D, Fribourg M, Duhamel A. Diagnosis of peripheral acute pulmonary emboli: optimization of the spiral CT acquisition protocol [abstract]. Radiology 1998; 209(P):299.

[17] Kim K-I, Müller NL, Mayo JR. Clinically suspected pulmonary embolism: utility of spiral CT. Radiology 1999;210:693–7.

[18] Qanadli SD, Hajjam ME, Mesurolle B, Barre O, Bruckert F, Joseph T, et al. Pulmonary embolism detection: prospective evaluation of dual section helical CT versus selective pulmonary arteriography in 157 patients. Radiology 2000;217:447–55.

[19] Ghaye B, Szapiro D, Mastora I, Delannoy V, Duhamel A, Remy J, et al. Peripheral pulmonary arteries: how far in the lung does multidetector row spiral CT allow analysis? Radiology 2001;219(3):629–36.

[20] Worsley DF, Alavi A, Aronchick JM, et al. Chest radiographic findings in patients with acute pulmonary embolism: observations from the PIOPED study. Radiology 1993;189:133–6.

[21] Greenspan RH, Ravin CE, Polansky SM, McLoud TC. Accuracy of the chest radiograph in the diagnosis of pulmonary embolism. Invest Radiol 1982;17(6): 539–43.

[22] Alderson P, Martin EC. Pulmonary embolism: diagnosis with multiple imaging modalities. Radiology 1987; 164:297–312.

[23] Quinn DA, Thompson BT, Terrin ML, Thrall JH, Athanasoulis CA, McKusick KA, et al. A prospective investigation of pulmonary embolism in women and men. JAMA 1992;268(13):1689–96.

[24] Worsley DF, Alavi A, Palevsky H, Kundel HL. Comparison of the diagnostic performance of ventilation/ perfusion lung scanning in different patient populations. Radiology 1996;199:481–3.

[25] Lesser BA, Leeper Jr KV, Stein PD, Saltzman HA, Chen J, Thompson BT, et al. The diagnosis of acute pulmonary embolism in patients with chronic obstructive pulmonary disease. Chest 1992;102(1):17–22.

[26] Worsley DF, Palevsky HI, Alavi A. Clinical characteristic of patients with pulmonary embolism and low or very low probability lung scan interpretations. Arch Intern Med 1994;154:2737–41.

[27] Alderson P, Biello DR, Sachariah KG, Siegel BA. Scintigraphic detection of pulmonary embolism in patients with obstructive pulmonary disease. Radiology 1981; 138(3):661–6.

[28] Smith R, Ellis K, Alderson P. Role of chest radiography in predicting the extent of airway disease in patients with suspected pulmonary embolism. Radiology 1986;159(2):391–4.

[29] Meignan M, Simonneau G, Oliveira L, Harf A, Cinotti L, Cavellier JF, et al. Computation of ventilation-perfusion ratio with Kr-81m in pulmonary embolism. J Nucl Med 1984;25(2):149–55.

[30] Ralph DD. Pulmonary embolism: the implications of prospective investigation of pulmonary embolism diagnosis. Radiol Clin North Am 1994;32:679–87.

[31] Teigen CL, Maus TP, Sheedy PF, Johnson CM, Stanson AW, Welch TJ. Pulmonary embolism: diagnosis with electron-beam CT. Radiology 1993;188:839–45.

[32] Coche EE, Müller NL, Kim W, Wiggs BR, Mayo JR. Acute pulmonary embolism: ancillary findings at spiral CT. Radiology 1998;207:753–8.

[33] Shah AA, Davis SD, Gamsu G, Intriere L. Parenchymal and pleural findings in patients with and patients without acute pulmonary embolism detected at spiral CT. Radiology 1999;211:147–53.

[34] Sinner WN. Computed tomographic patterns of pulmonary thromboembolism and infarction. J Comput Assist Tomogr 1978;2:395–9.

[35] Maki DD, Gefter WB, Alavi A. Recent advances in pulmonary imaging. Chest 1999;116:1388–402.

[36] Baile EM, King GG, Müller N, D'Yachkova Y, Coche E, Paré PD, et al. Spiral computed tomography is comparable to angiography for the diagnosis of pulmonary embolism. Am J Respir Crit Care Med 2000;161: 1010–5.

[37] Remy-Jardin M, Remy J, Baghaie F, Artaud D, Fribourg M. CT angiography of pulmonary embolism. RSNA Categorical Course in Vascular Imaging. Oakbrook (IL): RSNA; 1998. p. 157–69.

[38] Kuzo RS, Goodman L. CT evaluation of pulmonary embolism: technique and interpretation. AJR Am J Roentgenol 1997;169:959–65.

[39] Ryu JH, Swensen SJ, Olson EJ, Pellikka PA. Diagnosis of pulmonary embolism with use of computed tomographic angiography. Mayo Clin Proc 2001;76:59–65.

[40] Stein PD, Henry JW, Gottschalk A. Reassessment of pulmonary angiography for the diagnosis of pulmonary embolism. Radiology 1999;210:689–91.

[41] Swensen SJ, Sheedy PF, Ryu JH, Pickett DD, Schleck DM, Ilstrup DM, et al. Outcomes after withholding anticoagulation from patients with suspected acute pulmonary embolism and negative computed tomographic findings: a cohort study. Mayo Clin Proc 2002;77: 130–8.

[42] Goodman LR, Lipchik RJ, Kuzo RS, Liu Y, McAuliffe TL, O'Brien DJ. Subsequent pulmonary embolism: risk after a negative helical CT pulmonary angiogram—prospective comparison with scintigraphy. Radiology 2000;215:535–42.

[43] Gottsäter A, Berg A, Centergard J, Frennby B, Nirhov N, Nyman U. Clinically suspected pulmonary embolism: is it safe to withhold anticoagulation after a negative spiral CT? Eur Radiol 2001;11:65–72.

[44] Henry JW, Relyea B, Stein PD. Continuing risk of thromboemboli among patients with normal pulmonary angiograms. Chest 1995;107:1375–8.

[45] Hull RD, Raskob GE, Coates G, Panju AA. Clinical validity of a normal perfusion lung scan in patients with suspected pulmonary embolism. Chest 1990;97: 23–6.

[46] Tillie-Leblond I, Mastora I, Radenne F, Paillard S, Tonnel A-B, Remy J, et al. Risk of pulmonary embolism after a negative spiral CT angiogram in patients with pulmonary disease: 1-year clinical follow-up study. Radiology 2002;223:461–7.

[47] Cross JJL, Kemp PM, Walsh CG, Flower CDR, Dixon AK. A randomized trial of spiral CT and ventilation perfusion scintigraphy for the diagnosis of pulmonary embolism. Clin Radiol 1998;53:177–82.

[48] Blachere H, Latrabe V, Montaudon M, et al. Pulmonary embolism revealed on helical CT angiography: comparison with ventilation-perfusion radionuclide lung scanning. AJR Am J Roentgenol 2000;174:1041–7.

[49] van Erkel AR, van Rossum AB, Bloem JL, Kievit J, Pattynama PM. Spiral CT angiography for suspected pulmonary embolism: a cost-effectiveness analysis. Radiology 1996;201(1):29–36.

Clin Chest Med 24 (2003) 39–47

Heparin and low molecular weight heparin: background and pharmacology

Timothy A. Morris, MD

Division of Pulmonary and Critical Care Medicine, University of California, San Diego Medical Center, 200 West Arbor Drive, San Diego, CA 92103-8378, USA

All heparins and low molecular weight heparins (LMWHs) are heterogeneous mixtures of modified polysaccharides (glycosaminoglycans) derived from animal products that catalyze the blood enzyme antithrombin (AT), also referred to as antithrombin III, to neutralize activated clotting factors [1,2]. The various LMWHs are produced by chemical or enzymatic cleavage of unfractionated heparin (UH), yielding similarly heterogeneous mixtures of smaller molecules. Each LMWH has its own spectrum of biologic properties, determined by the characteristics of the parent UH and by the effects of the cleavage process on the structures and functions of the lower molecular weight fragments generated [3–5]. The relative therapeutic superiority of the LMWHs, when compared with one another and with UH, is a topic of considerable controversy. This controversy stems in large part from a poor understanding of the mechanisms by which each agent exerts its antithrombotic activity (the ability to inhibit the formation and enlargement of blood clots in the body) and of their adverse effects.

Heparin was discovered by McLean in 1916 and has been used clinically as an antithrombotic agent for several decades [6]. UH is an inexpensive and highly effective drug for the prophylaxis and treatment of various thrombotic disorders, for which it is therapeutic in at least a partially dose-dependent fashion [7]. The therapeutic benefits of heparin are limited by an increased risk of bleeding, which is also at least partially a dose-dependent phenomena [8]. To optimize the balance between efficacy and bleeding, clinicians have adopted two dosing practices: (1) frequent estimation of UH plasma levels using an in vivo marker of anticoagulant activity, the activated partial thromboplastin time (aPTT); and (2) continuous intravenous administration of UH in an attempt to allow multiple rapid dosage adjustments guided by aPTT values. Although the cost of the aPTT test is minimal, the requirement for repeated blood tests and dose adjustments and the need for maintenance of an intravenous catheter make this method of managing UH so laborious that hospitalization is nearly always required [9]. As a consequence, the cost of therapy is greatly increased [10]. Although both of these strategies have been widely adopted, clinical trials using UH for the treatment of venous thromboembolism (VTE) have not shown a consistent benefit for either aPTT monitoring [11] or intravenous (versus subcutaneous) administration [12].

Low molecular weight heparins were developed for clinical use with the intention of overcoming the therapeutic limitations of UH [13]. Encouraging preclinical data suggested that LMWH was superior to UH from biologic and pharmacokinetic standpoints. Biologically, animal experiments suggested that the therapeutic window would be larger for LMWH, resulting in a lower risk of bleeding than an equally effective dose of UH [14]. Unfortunately, clinical trials of VTE treatment have not demonstrated statistically significant differences in bleeding rates with the use of LMWH or UH [15]. From a pharmacokinetic perspective, at least one assay of blood anticoagulant potency, that is, the ability to catalyze the neutralization of activated factor X (anti-Xa activity),

E-mail address: tlmorris@ucsd.edu

doi:10.1016/S 0 2 7 2 - 5 2 3 1 (0 2)0 0 0 5 3 - 9

suggests that LMWH has a more predictable and favorable pharmacokinetic profile than UH [16,17]. Nevertheless, the clinical relevance of this finding depends in large part on the importance of anti-Xa activity in the therapeutic and adverse effects of LMWH and UH.

Pharmacokinetics

Comparing the pharmacokinetics of LMWH and UH is conceptually complex. Ordinarily, pharmacokinetic calculations such as clearance and half-life describe the rise and fall in concentration of a specific molecular entity in the body. The concentration of UH or LMWH is difficult to define even before administration, because both agents are composed of mixtures of glycosaminoglycan molecules of various lengths, chemical compositions, and biologic activities [3]. Absolute drug levels (ie, molecular concentrations) are virtually irrelevant to the therapeutic and toxic effects of either drug.

Pharmaceutical preparations of UH and LMWH are measured in terms of their biologic activities in in vitro models of anticoagulation. The activity of heparin, which exerts its anticoagulant effect by inactivating thrombin and factor Xa, is measured in terms of the United States Pharmacopoeia unit, defined as the quantity of drug that prevents 1 mL of sheep plasma from clotting for 1 hour under defined conditions [18]. The activity of LMWH, which exerts its anticoagulant effect primarily by inactivating factor Xa, is more difficult to measure by clotting tests, because these methods tend to be more sensitive to the inhibition of thrombin activity. LMWH is quantified in terms of anti-Xa activity concentration [18] in assays performed by incubating the drug with an excess of AT, purified (unbound) factor Xa, and a chromogenic factor Xa substrate. Anti-Xa activity is defined as the potency of the drug for causing AT-mediated factor Xa inactivation (and thereby preventing a color change in the Xa substrate). Although clotting and factor Xa activity assays are widely used to standardize the manufacture and administration of UH and LMWH, the relationship between either of these types of assay and the actual pharmacologic activity of the drugs in vivo is unclear [7,19]. The clinical relevance of this paradox is that the recommended therapeutic doses measured using these anticoagulation indexes are different among the individual LMWHs and, of course, between any of them and UH.

Unfortunately, no method is available to quantitate reliably the in vivo antithrombotic activities of anticoagulants in humans. Although clinical indicators of antithrombotic efficacy, such as repeated imaging studies or symptomatic follow-up, provide useful data for patient care, they are inappropriate for use in pharmacokinetic calculations. Anticoagulation tests that employ various in vitro models of thrombosis to measure the concentration of some aspect of enzymatic activity thought to be relevant to inhibiting thrombosis are often used as surrogate markers of antithrombotic activity. No single test can be used to compare the concentrations of two distinct medications, and anticoagulation tests, in general, have serious limitations in their ability to quantitate the amount of antithrombotic activity in the blood after the administration of LMWH or UH. Different UH and LMWH preparations have markedly distinct potencies of activity with regard to the values measured by different anticoagulation tests [20]. Similarly, when administered to patients, therapeutic doses of various LMWHs (and of UH) yield disparate results from each other on different anticoagulation assays [21]. Furthermore, depending on the parameter measured, the same drug may demonstrate different comparative bioavailibilities, clearances, and half-lives [20]. For example, in normal volunteers, the half-life of anti-Xa activity is much longer for subcutaneous enoxaparin (40 mg, 4000 anti-Xa U) than for UH (5000 U); however, in the same patients, the half-life of activity against thrombin (anti-IIa activity) of both drugs is roughly equivalent [22]. In addition, the variably sized molecules that make up UH and LMWH preparations are cleared from the circulation at different rates, and the range of fragment lengths (and the spectrum of activities) of the drugs before administration is different from what is found in the plasma [20]. No single anticoagulation test result is equally applicable to the various LMWHs and to UH for predicting clinical efficacy or bleeding. For these reasons, the dogma that LMWHs inherently have longer half-lives, higher bioavailabilities, and more predictable responses than UH should be re-examined in light of the limitations of the tests used to compare the two drug types.

Measuring the biologic effects of low molecular weight heparin

The biologic and the pharmacokinetic arguments in favor of using LMWH over UH (and of using one LMWH over another) depend in large part on the degree of understanding regarding the differences in mechanisms of action between the two drugs. This differentiation is confounded by the many similarities that exist among the various mechanisms of action through which the heparins, as a single class of antithrombotic agents, exert their anticoagulant effects. Although UH and the respective LMWHs have their own particular spectrum of potencies for these various mechanisms, the relative importance of each mechanism to antithrombotic efficacy and the risk of bleeding is fundamental to the question of the clinical superiority of one drug over another. A brief review of several key biologic mechanisms highlights the complexity of measuring and comparing the activities of different LMWH preparations and UH. An exhaustive list of the full spectrum of activities is beyond the scope of this article, and excellent descriptions have been published elsewhere [13,23,24].

Effects mediated by antithrombin

A major portion of the clinical effects of UH and LMWH occurs through enhancement of the antithrombotic action of AT, an important endogenous inhibitor of coagulation that acts primarily by inactivating factor IIa (thrombin) and factor Xa [1]. The fundamental biologic difference between UH and LMWH stems from the relative potency of the drug to accelerate the basal rate of AT-mediated thrombin and factor Xa inactivation [13]. UH preparations enhance the inactivation of thrombin and factor Xa, whereas LMWHs catalyze factor Xa inactivation predominantly.

Antithrombin, a serine protease inhibitor, inactivates thrombin and factor Xa via a similar mechanism of action by binding irreversibly to the serine proteases' respective active sites in a process poetically referred to as "suicide inhibition" [25]. AT inactivates thrombin and factor Xa slowly while natural anticoagulant molecules, heparan sulfates that line the vascular endothelium, act as cofactors to enhance dramatically the low basal rate of inactivation. UH and LMWHs are the therapeutic form of these natural anticoagulant molecules, acting to catalyze AT-mediated inhibition of thrombin and factor Xa activity.

The structure and the size of individual UH or LMWH molecules determine the specificity for enhancement of AT-mediated thrombin inhibition, factor Xa inhibition, or both [26]. A specific pentasaccharide sequence must be present on the UH or LMWH molecule to bind AT and thereby enhance its basal inhibitory activity, and molecules of UH or LMWH that lack this particular structure have no significant potentiating effect [27]. Only about one third of the molecules in UH preparations contain the

specific pentasaccharide sequence, and this proportion is even lower for LMWHs [28,29].

In addition to the pentasaccharide structural requirement, the size of the UH or LMWH molecule influences the specificity of the AT-mediated reaction that is catalyzed. Heparin molecules that contain the pentasaccharide sequence and that are smaller than 5.4 kd can only catalyze AT-mediated factor Xa inactivation. Larger pentasaccharide-containing molecules can induce AT to inactive factor Xa and thrombin. With increasing size of the heparin molecule, the activity of AT increases against thrombin but remains relatively stable against factor Xa. The molecular weight range of heparin molecules contained within UH or any particular LMWH preparation largely determines the drug's relative activities against thrombin and factor Xa [30]. UH has a mean molecular weight between 12 and 15 kd (range, 5–30 kd) and has, by definition, equal activities against thrombin and factor Xa. The LMWHs such as enoxaparin (mean molecular weight, 4.5 kd; range, 3–8 kd), dalteparin (mean, 5 kd; range, 2–9 kd), and logiparin (mean, 4.5 kd; range, 3–6 kd) have, to varying degrees, relatively more anti-Xa activity than anti-IIa (thrombin) activity [13].

Less well characterized are the effects on AT specificity of other properties of the heparin molecules, including their degree of sulfation, charge distribution, and characteristics of the terminal saccharide residues. All of these properties differ among UH and LMWH products [5] and contribute to each drug's particular spectrum of relative activity against thrombin and factor Xa. The optimal spectrum of activity is unclear.

Activity against free factor Xa

The activation of factor X to factor Xa represents the first step in the final common pathway of the intrinsic and extrinsic arms of the coagulation cascade. Factor Xa in its free circulating form slowly converts prothrombin to the active enzyme, thrombin. When factor Xa is bound to a phospholipid membrane along with factor Va and calcium (the prothrombinase complex), the reaction proceeds at a much faster rate and accounts for the majority of thrombin production in vivo [31]. In addition, factor Xa within the prothrombinase complex, as distinct from free factor Xa, is much less vulnerable to inactivation by AT, regardless of whether AT activity is enhanced by UH or LMWH [32]. Perhaps for this reason, the plasma assay of anti-Xa activity, which measures the ability to inactivate free (purified) factor Xa, does not predict the antithrombotic activity of different LMWHs and UH in animal models of thrombosis.

The inhibition of free factor Xa is not solely responsible for the anticoagulant action of LMWH. In an experimental group of animals, the pentasaccharide molecule (the minimum sequence in heparin chains required for AT binding and enhancement of factor Xa inactivation but not large enough for enhancement of thrombin inactivation) arrested thrombosis only when the plasma anti-Xa activity was several times higher than that in a similar group given LMWH [33]. Likewise, the profile of plasma anti-Xa activities in LMWH clinical trials did not correlate well with therapeutic efficacy or complication rates of patients treated with UH or a variety of LMWHs [19,21,34].

Activity against free thrombin

Thrombin is responsible for several reactions in the coagulation cascade. The most straightforward function is to convert soluble fibrinogen to fibrin, which spontaneously polymerizes to form the structural framework of the blood clot. Thrombin also is involved in numerous positive and negative feedback steps within the coagulation cascade and has a major role in controlling the rate of thrombosis. In a striking example of thrombin's positive feedback role, the thrombin-mediated activation of factor V to form factor Va, a fundamental constituent of the prothrombinase complex, may be the rate-limiting step in the ongoing production of thrombin during the initiation and propagation of blood clotting [35]. For many reasons, thrombin activity is essential to thrombus enlargement.

An understanding of the importance of thrombin in the control of coagulation is fundamental when making comparisons between LMWH and UH; the higher-molecular weight constituents of both drug types enable thrombin inactivation [16]. Platelet factor 4, a protein released from activated platelets, binds to and clears higher molecular weight heparin molecules from the circulation, eliminating some of the anti-IIa activity of LMWH and UH [36]. This interaction forms one of the antigens responsible for the heparin-induced thrombocytopenia that complicates treatment with both medications [37]. Perhaps for this reason, the pharmacokinetics of anti-IIa activity in subcutaneous injections of UH (5000 U) and the LMWH enoxaparin (40 mg, 4000 anti-Xa U) in healthy volunteers are remarkably similar [22].

As is true for factor Xa, thrombin exists in a bound form where its activity is retained but no longer susceptible to inactivation by AT. As a thrombus develops, thrombin binds to sites on the fibrin polymer, where it continues to activate the coagulation cascade [38]. UH and LMWH enable AT to inactivate thrombin in its free state, whereas fibrin-bound thrombin is no longer susceptible to the effects of either drug [38]. The relative importance of free and fibrin-bound thrombin to the overall kinetics of clot propagation in clinical situations is unknown.

All LMWHs have a high ratio of anti-Xa activity to anti-IIa activity, although the ratio varies widely among different specific drugs. Anti-Xa activity also varies according to different assays [39–41], and the more commonly used ones may overestimate the actual activity of the drugs [39]. The ideal anti-Xa activity to anti-IIa activity ratio is currently unknown. Recently completed phase III trials of VTE prophylaxis evaluating novel drugs that specifically inhibit factor Xa [42–44] or thrombin [45,46] may help to determine the relative importance of inactivating these two coagulation enzymes [47]. Currently available assays used for pharmacokinetic comparisons measure only the inhibition of free factor Xa (or, less commonly, of free thrombin), and the mechanisms of action of UH and LMWH are much more complicated [39]. It is unknown whether actual AT-mediated antithrombotic activity parallels the results of either one of these two assays or some combination of both. Because UH and LMWH preparations are heterogeneous in terms of the size, composition, and clearance of their constituent molecules, it is plausible that the molecules tracked by any particular assay are not identical to the ones causing the greatest AT-mediated thrombus inhibition [48].

Effects not mediated by antithrombin

Unfractionated heparin and LMWH also exert antithrombotic effects through mechanisms that are independent of AT. The release of tissue factor pathway inhibitor (TFPI) by LMWH and UH is increasingly recognized as an important example [22,49]. When the extrinsic pathway of coagulation is triggered by vascular injury, tissue factor binds to factor VII, and the tissue factor–factor VIIa complex activates factor X [50]. TFPI is an important regulator of this coagulation step based on its ability to bind to the tissue factor–factor VII complex and neutralize it, leading to the suppression of factor X activation and the inhibition of thrombin generation and inhibiting clot formation [51]. TFPI is stored in high quantities on the surface of vascular endothelium. After the administration of LMWH or UH, TFPI is released into the circulation [52]. Although UH and LMWH cause TFPI release in a dose-dependent fashion, plasma TFPI concentrations do not necessarily parallel the pharmacokinetics of other measurements of heparin activity, such as the aPTT or anti-Xa, AT, or Heptest (Haemachem, Inc., St. Louis, MO) assays [22]. It is even possible that the heparin constituents of LMWH and UH that cause TFPI release have no interaction with AT [48] and would be undetectable by traditional testing. Furthermore, because the antithrombotic mechanism of TFPI release is a "post-drug" effect active even after the elimination of the drug from the plasma, the pharmacodynamics of the biologic effects of LMWH and UH may not match their pharmacokinetics (as is true for corticosteroids) [53].

Recent in vitro experiments have disclosed another possible AT-independent antithrombotic mechanism of LMWH and UH, that is, the enhancement of protein C inactivation of factor Va. Activated protein C inhibits thrombosis by cleaving factor Va, an essential element of the prothrombinase complex, into an inactive form [54]. LMWHs and UH augment this antithrombotic property of protein C [55,56]. Although firm evidence supports the vital role of protein C in the control of coagulation, the clinical importance of UH- and LMWH-mediated enhancement of factor Va inactivation by protein C is currently unknown.

The complexity of the interaction between the heparin family of drugs and numerous coagulation cascade enzymes makes it unlikely that any particular anticoagulation assay will enable a valid comparison of the efficacy and pharmacokinetics of LMWH and UH.

Antithrombotic activity

Although LMWHs may have different potencies relative to their multiple mechanisms of action, the ultimate biochemical goal is the same, that is, to prevent thrombin-mediated conversion of fibrinogen to fibrin and to stop thrombus propagation (antithrombosis). Unfortunately, the anticoagulant potencies of these medications as measured by in vitro tests of activity, such as the aPTT and plasma anti-Xa activity, do not reliably predict their antithrombotic effects in animal models [33,57,58].

The antithrombotic activity of different LMWHs and UH regimens has been compared directly in animal experiments. Virtually all of these experiments have employed some measurement of thrombus propagation on pre-existing thrombi, on sites of vascular injury, or on a thrombotic substance introduced into the vasculature. Different anticoagulants are then administered and the ability to suppress thrombus propagation directly measured. Fig. 1 describes the results of experiments using a radiolabeled antifibrin antibodies that binds only to newly formed subunits on the fibrin network, measuring the rate of fibrin deposition on preformed thrombi [58]. This technique disclosed differences in the antithrombotic activity of the drug regimens employed that were not evident on simultaneous plasma measurements of anti-Xa or anti-IIa (thrombin) activity.

Although animal models may disclose substantial differences in antithrombotic activity, their relevance to human therapy is limited by several factors. There may be considerable species-specific

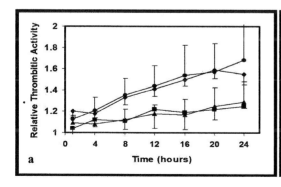
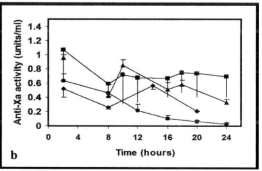

Fig. 1. Plasma anticoagulation assays do not predict the ability of distinct anticoagulants to suppress thrombus propagation. (a) Propagation of preformed in situ thrombi is estimated by the accumulation of radiolabeled anti-$\beta_{15\text{-}22}$. By 24 hours, the thrombosed femoral area in the enoxaparin group (diamonds) emitted 1.71 ± 0.06 times the counts in the contralateral (no clot) area. For the dalteparin group (circles), the ratio was 1.68 ± 0.36. The ratio was less for the subcutaneous UH group (triangles) and for the intravenous UH group (squares). (b) Plasma anti-Xa activities did not correlate with the antithrombotic activities.

differences in physiologic aspects in humans, such as drug absorption and clearance; thrombus formation, composition, and dissolution; and the sensitivity of thrombus propagation to the action of anticoagulants. In addition, particular characteristics of the model, including the thrombotic stimulus and the method of measuring clot propagation, may affect the relevance to the clinical situation. For example, clot induction by laceration of the jugular vein and insertion of thrombogenic wires may have important pathophysiologic differences with clinical deep vein thrombosis.

Measuring the antithrombotic effects of anticoagulants in humans with VTE is difficult. The most commonly used noninvasive tests for the diagnosis of deep vein thrombosis (compression ultrasonography, impedance plethysmography, and MR imaging) and pulmonary embolism (ventilation–perfusion scanning and helical CT scanning) do not provide sufficiently detailed anatomic information to measure reliably the enlargement of thromboemboli during acute treatment [59]. Invasive studies such as contrast venography and angiography, although better at demonstrating gross changes in thrombus size [60], can be painful and are often impractical for follow-up. Furthermore, they may not be able to detect subtle increases in clot dimensions owing to ongoing thrombosis. All of the anatomic tests described previously share the limitation of being unable to differentiate the effects of anticoagulation (preventing clot enlargement) from the effects of the intrinsic fibrinolytic system (reducing clot size).

Attempts to measure the antithrombotic activity of LMWHs and UH directly in humans have focused on the ability of these drugs to suppress the formation of serologic markers of thrombosis [61]. The popular D-dimer plasma test is actually a marker of plasmin-mediated dissolution of thrombi. Although it is useful to rule out the presence of a thrombus, because the level of D-dimer remains elevated even during anticoagulation, it is not a valid marker of antithrombotic activity [62]. Potential thrombosis markers are for the most part biologic byproducts of coagulation that have been released into the circulation, such as prothrombin fragment $1 + 2$ (F1 + 2) (released as prothrombin is converted to thrombin), thrombin–AT complexes (TAT) (reflecting thrombin formation, because nearly all free thrombin is eventually inactivated into this complex), and fibrinopeptide A (FPA)(released as thrombin cleaves soluble fibrinogen into fibrin) [63]. The analytes in the first two assays, F1 + 2 and TAT, are serum markers of thrombin generation, whereas FPA is a marker of thrombin activation [64].

Although levels of these and other hemostatic markers are often used as an index of the effectiveness of an antithrombotic agent, the reliability of such measurements can be questioned on several grounds. First, anticoagulants with different spectra of activity against factor Xa and thrombin whose mechanism of action involves the inhibition of thrombin generation (the factor Xa–selective synthetic pentasaccharide fondaparinux), the inhibition of thrombin activity (the direct thrombin-specific inhibitor hirudin), or some degree of both (UH, LMWH) would be expected to result in differences in circulating levels of these markers, even if the antithrombotic effects of the drugs in vivo were the same. Second, although FPA is primarily released from fibrinogen by thrombin during the formation of fibrin clots and should theoretically represent an accurate measure of the rate and extent of fibrin formation/propagation occurring during in vivo thrombosis [65], artifactually elevated plasma FPA levels are a common confounding problem. FPA is so easily cleaved from fibrinogen that even when collection tubes are supplemented with proteolytic inhibitors, the sampling procedure can cause FPA release [66]. Falsely elevated FPA levels have been associated with factors such as venipuncture techniques [63] and phlebotomy through indwelling catheters [67]. Moreover, FPA may not be the most accurate marker of fibrin formation in vivo, because des-FPA fibrin represents an intermediate molecule whose fate is determined based on whether its subsequent interaction is with plasmin, resulting in degradation, or with thrombin, resulting in release of fibrinopeptide B (FPB) and the formation of "mature" (des-FPA–des-FPB fibrin) [68].

The assays currently available for the quantitation of thrombosis markers have limitations that prevent their routine use for the direct measurement of thrombotic activity to compare the antithrombotic potency of LMWHs with each other and with UH. Large clinical trials have not confirmed an association between the suppression of these markers and clinical outcome in patients treated with LMWH for thrombotic disorders [64].

Summary

The various LMWHs available for therapeutic use have multiple mechanisms of action, most of which are similar to the mechanisms of UH. The relative potencies of expression of the mechanisms differ between LMWH and UH and among specific LMWHs. The pharmacokinetics of LMWHs and UH are often measured according to the results of anti-Xa assays, although the correlation between anti-Xa levels and the antithrombotic activities of the drugs is questionable. Animal models of thrombosis give some information regarding the antithrombotic efficacy of different LMWHs when compared with UH and with other LMWHs, but the results are not directly applicable to human thrombosis. Unfortunately, no single measure of antithrombosis has been developed in humans whereby the potencies of LMWHs, UH, and other new anticoagulants can be directly compared.

Large clinical outcome studies are expensive and difficult to carry out. Perhaps for this reason, different subcutaneous LMWHs have not been compared with each other in this format. Various LMWHs have demonstrated equivalent efficacy and safety when compared with intravenous UH and high-dose subcutaneous UH, and it is reasonable to assume that there would not be large differences in efficacy and safety among different agents. The superiority of one subcutaneous regimen over another can be confirmed (or refuted) only by the performance of well-planned clinical studies.

References

[1] Rosenberg RD, Damus PS. The purification and mechanism of action of human antithrombin-heparin cofactor. J Biol Chem 1973;248:6490–505.

[2] Rosenberg RD. Actions and interactions of antithrombin and heparin. N Engl J Med 1975;292:146–51.

[3] Linhardt RJ, Gunay NS. Production and chemical processing of low molecular weight heparins. Semin Thromb Hemost 1999;25(Suppl 3):5–16.

[4] Casu B, Torri G. Structural characterization of low molecular weight heparins. Semin Thromb Hemost 1999;25(Suppl 3):17–25.

[5] Jeske W, Fareed J. In vitro studies on the biochemistry and pharmacology of low molecular weight heparins. Semin Thromb Hemost 1999;25(Suppl 3):27–33.

[6] Crafoord C, Jovanovic B. Heparin as a prophylactic against thrombosis. JAMA 1941;116:2831.

[7] Anand S, Ginsberg JS, Kearon C, Gent M, Hirsh J. The relation between the activated partial thromboplastin time response and recurrence in patients with venous thrombosis treated with continuous intravenous heparin. Arch Intern Med 1996;156:1677–81.

[8] Wester JP, de Valk HW, Nieuwenhuis HK, et al. Risk factors for bleeding during treatment of acute venous thromboembolism. Thromb Haemost 1996;76:682–8.

[9] Hirsch DR, Lee TH, Morrison RB, Carlson W, Goldhaber SZ. Shortened hospitalization by means of adjusted-dose subcutaneous heparin for deep venous thrombosis. Am Heart J 1996;131:276–80.

[10] Gould MK, Dembitzer AD, Sanders GD, Garber AM. Low-molecular-weight heparins compared with unfractionated heparin for treatment of acute deep venous thrombosis: a cost-effectiveness analysis [see comments]. Ann Intern Med 1999;130:789–99.

[11] Anand SS, Bates S, Ginsberg JS, et al. Recurrent venous thrombosis and heparin therapy: an evaluation of the importance of early activated partial thromboplastin times. Arch Intern Med 1999;159:2029–32.

[12] Hommes DW, Bura A, Mazzolai L, Buller HR, ten Cate JW. Subcutaneous heparin compared with continuous intravenous heparin administration in the initial treatment of deep vein thrombosis: a meta-analysis [see comments]. Ann Intern Med 1992;116:279–84.

[13] Hirsh J, Levine MN. Low molecular weight heparin. Blood 1992;79:1–17.

[14] Carter CJ, Kelton JG, Hirsh J, Cerskus A, Santos AV, Gent M. The relationship between the hemorrhagic and antithrombotic properties of low molecular weight heparin in rabbits. Blood 1982;59:1239–45.

[15] Dolovich LR, Ginsberg JS, Dpiletos JD, Holbrook AM, Cheah G. A meta-analysis comparing low-molecular-weight heparin with unfractionated heparin in the treatment of venous thromboembolism. Arch Intern Med 2000;160:181–8.

[16] Bendetowicz AV, Beguin S, Caplain H, Hemker HC. Pharmacokinetics and pharmacodynamics of a low molecular weight heparin (enoxaparin) after subcutaneous injection, comparison with unfractionated heparin–a three way cross over study in human volunteers. Thromb Haemost 1994;71:305–13.

[17] Frydman AM, Bara L, Le Roux Y, Woler M, Chauliac F, Samama MM. The antithrombotic activity and pharmacokinetics of enoxaparin, a low molecular weight heparin, in humans given single subcutaneous doses of 20 to 80 mg. J Clin Pharmacol 1988;28:609–18.

[18] Majerus PW, Broze GJ, Miletich JP, Tollefsen DM. Anticoagulant, thrombolytic and antiplatelet drugs. In: Gilman AG, Rall TW, Nies AS, Taylor P, editors. Goodman and Gilman's the pharmacological basis of therapeutics. New York: Pergamon Press; 1990. p. 1311–31.

[19] Leizorovicz A, Bara L, Samama MM, Haugh MC. Factor Xa inhibition: correlation between the plasma levels of anti-Xa activity and occurrence of thrombosis and haemorrhage. Haemostasis 1993;23(Suppl 1):89–98.

[20] Brieger D, Dawes J. Production method affects the pharmacokinetic and ex vivo biological properties of low molecular weight heparins. Thromb Haemost 1997;77:317–22.

[21] Lindhoff-Last E, Mosch G, Breddin HK. Treatment doses of different low molecular weight heparins and unfractionated heparins differ in their anticoagulating effects in respect to aPTT, Heptest, anti-IIa- and anti-Xa activity. Lab Med 1992;16:174–7.

[22] Bara L, Bloch MF, Zitoun D, et al. Comparative effects of enoxaparin and unfractionated heparin in healthy volunteers on prothrombin consumption in whole blood during coagulation, and release of tissue factor pathway inhibitor. Thromb Res 1993;69:443–52.

[23] Hirsh J. Heparin. N Engl J Med 1991;324:1565–74.

[24] Hirsh J, Fuster V. Guide to anticoagulant therapy. Part 1. Heparin: American Heart Association. Circulation 1994;89:1449–68.

[25] Carrell RW, Evans DL, Stein PE. Mobile reactive centre of serpins and the control of thrombosis. Nature 1991;353:576–8.

[26] Danielsson A, Raub E, Lindahl U, Bjork I. Role of ternary complexes, in which heparin binds both anti-thrombin and proteinase, in the acceleration of the re-actions between antithrombin and thrombin or factor Xa. J Biol Chem 1986;261:15467–73.

[27] Olson ST, Bjork I, Sheffer R, Craig PA, Shore JD, Choay J. Role of the antithrombin-binding pentasac-charide in heparin acceleration of antithrombin-pro-teinase reactions: resolution of the antithrombin conformational change contribution to heparin rate en-hancement. J Biol Chem 1992;267:12528–38.

[28] Lam LH, Silbert JE, Rosenberg RD. The separation of active and inactive forms of heparin. Biochem Biophys Res Commun 1976;69:570–7.

[29] Andersson G, Fagrell B, Holmgren K, et al. Subcuta-neous administration of heparin: a randomised compar-ison with intravenous administration of heparin to patients with deep vein thrombosis. Thromb Res 1982;27:631–9.

[30] Bendetowicz AV, Pacaud E, Baeguin S, Uzan A, Hemker HC. On the relationship between molecular mass and anticoagulant activity in a low molecular weight heparin (enoxaparin). Thromb Haemost 1992; 67:556–62.

[31] Tracy PB, Eide LL, Mann KG. Human prothrom-binase complex assembly and function on isolated peripheral blood cell populations. J Biol Chem 1985; 260:2119–24.

[32] Bendetowicz AV, Bara L, Samama MM. The inhibition of intrinsic prothrombinase and its generation by hep-arin and four derivatives in prothrombin poor plasma. Thromb Res 1990;58:445–54.

[33] Carrie D, Caranobe C, Boneu B. A comparison of the antithrombotic effects of heparin and of low molecular weight heparins with increasing antifactor Xa / antifac-tor IIa ratio in the rabbit. Br J Haematol 1993;83:622–6.

[34] Harenberg J, Stehle G, Blauth M, Huck K, Mall K, Heene DL. Dosage, anticoagulant, and antithrombotic effects of heparin and low-molecular-weight heparin in the treatment of deep vein thrombosis. Semin Thromb Hemost 1997;23:83–90.

[35] Mann KG. Biochemistry and physiology of blood co-agulation. Thromb Haemost 1999;82:165–74.

[36] Padilla A, Gray E, Pepper DS, Barrowcliffe TW. In-hibition of thrombin generation by heparin and low molecular weight (LMW) heparins in the absence and presence of platelet factor 4 (PF4). Br J Haematol 1992;82:406–13.

[37] Suh JS, Aster RH, Visentin GP. Antibodies from pa-tients with heparin-induced thrombocytopenia/throm-bosis recognize different epitopes on heparin: platelet factor 4. Blood 1998;91:916–22.

[38] Weitz JI, Hudoba M, Massel D, Maraganore J, Hirsh J. Clot-bound thrombin is protected from inhibition by heparin-antithrombin III but is susceptible to inactiva-tion by antithrombin III-independent inhibitors. J Clin Invest 1990;86:385–91.

[39] Beguin S, Welzel D, Al Dieri R, Hemker HC. Con-jectures and refutations on the mode of action of hep-arins: the limited importance of anti-factor Xa activity as a pharmaceutical mechanism and a yardstick for therapy. Haemostasis 1999;29:170–8.

[40] Kitchen S, Iampietro R, Woolley AM, Preston FE. Anti Xa monitoring during treatment with low molecular weight heparin or danaparoid: interassay variability. Thromb Haemost 1999;82:1289–93.

[41] Kovacs MJ, Keeney M, MacKinnon K, Boyle E. Three different chromogenic methods do not give equivalent anti-Xa levels for patients on therapeutic low molec-ular weight heparin (dalteparin) or unfractionated hep-arin. Clin Lab Haematol 1999;21:55–60.

[42] Turpie AG, Bauer KA, Eriksson BI, Lassen MR. Post-operative fondaparinux versus postoperative enoxapar-in for prevention of venous thromboembolism after elective hip-replacement surgery: a randomised dou-ble-blind trial. Lancet 2002;359:1721–6.

[43] Lassen MR, Bauer KA, Eriksson BI, Turpie AG. Post-operative fondaparinux versus preoperative enoxaparin for prevention of venous thromboembolism in elective hip-replacement surgery: a randomised double-blind comparison. Lancet 2002;359:1715–20.

[44] Bauer KA, Eriksson BI, Lassen MR, Turpie AG. Fon-daparinux compared with enoxaparin for the preven-tion of venous thromboembolism after elective major knee surgery. N Engl J Med 2001;345:1305–10.

[45] Colwell CW, Berkowitz SD, Davidson BL. Random-ized, double-blind, comparison of ximelagatran, an oral direct thrombin inhibitor, and enoxaparin to pre-vent venous thromboembolism (VTE) after total hip arthroplasty (THA). Blood 2001;98:706a.

[46] Francis CW, Davidson BL, Berkowitz SD, et al. Xi-melagatran versus warfarin for the prevention of ve-nous thromboembolism after total knee arthroplasty. A randomized, double-blind trial. Ann Intern Med 2002;137(8):648–55.

[47] Prager NA, Abendschein DR, McKenzie CR, Eisen-berg PR. Role of thrombin compared with factor Xa in the procoagulant activity of whole blood clots. Cir-culation 1995;92:962–7.

[48] Barrow RT, Parker ET, Krishnaswamy S, Lollar P. In-hibition by heparin of the human blood coagulation intrinsic pathway factor X activator. J Biol Chem 1994;269:26796–800.

[49] Fareed J, Jeske W, Hoppensteadt D, Clarizio R, Wa-lenga JM. Are the available low-molecular-weight hep-arin preparations the same? Semin Thromb Hemost 1996;22:77–91.

[50] Nemerson Y. Tissue factor and hemostasis. Blood 1988;71:1–8.

[51] Broze GJJ, Warren LA, Novotny WF, Higuchi DA, Gir-ard JJ, Miletich JP. The lipoprotein-associated coagula-

tion inhibitor that inhibits the factor VII–tissue factor complex also inhibits factor Xa: insight into its possible mechanism of action. Blood 1988;71:335–43.

[52] Hoppensteadt DA, Walenga JM, Fasanella A, Jeske W, Fareed J. TFPI antigen levels in normal human volunteers after intravenous and subcutaneous administration of unfractionated heparin and a low molecular weight heparin. Thromb Res 1995;77:175–85.

[53] Kong AN, Ludwig EA, Slaughter RL, et al. Pharmacokinetics and pharmacodynamic modeling of direct suppression effects of methylprednisolone on serum cortisol and blood histamine in human subjects. Clin Pharmacol Ther 1989;46:616–28.

[54] Esmon CT. The regulation of natural anticoagulant pathways. Science 1987;235:1348–52.

[55] Petaja J, Fernandez JA, Gruber A, Griffin JH. Anticoagulant synergism of heparin and activated protein C in vitro: role of a novel anticoagulant mechanism of heparin, enhancement of inactivation of factor V by activated protein C. J Clin Invest 1997;99:2655–63.

[56] Fernandez JA, Petaja J, Griffin JH. Dermatan sulfate and LMW heparin enhance the anticoagulant action of activated protein C. Thromb Haemost 1999;82:1462–8.

[57] Carrie D, Caranobe C, Gabaig AM, Larroche M, Boneu B. Effects of heparin, dermatan sulfate and of their association on the inhibition of venous thrombosis growth in the rabbit. Thromb Haemost 1992;68:637–41.

[58] Morris TA, Marsh JJ, Konopka R, Pedersen CA, Chiles PG. Antithrombotic efficacies of enoxaparin, dalteparin, and unfractionated heparin in venous thromboembolism. Thromb Res 2000;100:185–94.

[59] Tapson VF, Carroll BA, Davidson BL, et al. The diagnostic approach to acute venous thromboembolism: clinical practice guideline. American Thoracic Society. Am J Respir Crit Care Med 1999;160:1043–66.

[60] Fiessinger JN, Lopez-Fernandez M, Gatterer E, et al. Once-daily subcutaneous dalteparin, a low molecular weight heparin, for the initial treatment of acute deep vein thrombosis. Thromb Haemost 1996;76:195–9.

[61] Ofosu FA, Levine M, Craven S, Dewar L, Shafai S, Blajchman MA. Prophylactically equivalent doses of enoxaparin and unfractionated heparin inhibit in vivo coagulation to the same extent. Br J Haematol 1992;82:400–5.

[62] Becker DM, Philbrick JT, Bachhuber TL, Humphries JE. D-dimer testing and acute venous thromboembolism: a shortcut to accurate diagnosis? Arch Intern Med 1996;156:939–46.

[63] Miller GJ, Bauer KA, Barzegar S, et al. The effects of quality and timing of venipuncture on markers of blood coagulation in healthy middle-aged men. Thromb Haemost 1995;73:82–6.

[64] Markers of hemostatic system activation in acute deep venous thrombosis—evolution during the first days of heparin treatment: the DVTENOX Study Group. Thromb Haemost 1993;70:909–14.

[65] Gando S, Tedo I. Diagnostic and prognostic value of fibrinopeptides in patients with clinically suspected pulmonary embolism. Thromb Res 1994;75:195–202.

[66] van Hulsteijn H, Briet E, Koch C, Hermans J, Bertina R. Diagnostic value of fibrinopeptide A and beta-thromboglobulin in acute deep venous thrombosis and pulmonary embolism. Acta Med Scand 1982;211:323–30.

[67] Yung GL, Marsh JJ, Berstein RJ, Hirsh AM, Channick RN, Moser KM. Fibrinopeptide A levels in primary pulmonary hypertension [abstract]. Am J Respir Crit Care Med 1998;157:A592.

[68] Nossel HL. Relative proteolysis of the fibrinogen B beta chain by thrombin and plasmin as a determinant of thrombosis. Nature 1981;291:165–7.

Clin Chest Med 24 (2003) 49–61

CLINICS IN CHEST MEDICINE

Outpatient treatment of acute venous thromboembolic disease

Roger D. Yusen, MD, MPH[a,b,*], Brian F. Gage, MD, MSc[b]

[a]Division of Pulmonary and Critical Care Medicine, Washington University School of Medicine and Barnes-Jewish Hospital, Box 8052, 660 South Euclid Avenue, St. Louis, MO, 63110, USA
[b]Division of General Medical Sciences, Washington University School of Medicine and Barnes-Jewish Hospital, Box 8005, 660 South Euclid Avenue, St. Louis, MO, 63110, USA

Traditionally, clinicians have treated patients with venous thromboembolism (VTE), deep venous thrombosis (DVT) or pulmonary embolism (PE), in the hospital. Use of intravenous unfractionated heparin (UFH) and monitoring of the partial thromboplastin time made outpatient therapy impractical. While receiving UFH for at least 5 days, patients remained hospitalized until an oral vitamin K antagonist (a coumarin) reached a therapeutic threshold (ie, international normalized ratio [INR] of ≥2.0 for 2 consecutive days) [1].

The higher bioavailability and more rapid antithrombotic effect after subcutaneous administration of the low molecular weight heparins (LMWHs), when compared with the UFHs, have facilitated outpatient VTE therapy (see the article by Morris elsewhere in this issue). In most patients, LMWHs have a predictable dose–response and do not require laboratory monitoring. Nevertheless, the dose–response is less predictable in patients who have renal insufficiency, morbid

obesity, or pregnancy. The long elimination half-life of the LMWHs allows for once- or twice-daily dosing.

Recently, clinical trials have analyzed the efficacy, safety, and costs of full or partial outpatient LMWH therapy for uncomplicated proximal lower-extremity DVT [2–6]. Outpatient LMWH therapy for PE has received less attention [7,8]. This article addresses outpatient therapy for DVT and PE.

Goals of therapy for venous thromboembolism

The goals of treatment of VTE are (1) to prevent VTE extension, embolism, recurrence, and death; (2) to diminish postthrombotic complications of postphlebitic syndrome from DVT and pulmonary hypertension and hypoxemia from PE; and (3) to avoid bleeding and heparin-induced thrombocytopenia and its sequelae. In addition to being efficacious and safe, treatment should be affordable.

Pharmacologic agents for secondary prophylaxis of venous thromboembolism

The most commonly used agents to treat VTE are UFH, LMWH, and vitamin K antagonists (see the articles by Morris and Kearon elsewhere in this issue). Newer agents, such as long-acting pentasaccharides (eg, fondaparinux and idraparinux) and oral direct thrombin inhibitors (eg, ximelagatran), are being evaluated in clinical trials.

Dr. Yusen has been an investigator in clinical trials sponsored by Aventis Pharmaceuticals, Inc. (Bridgewater, NJ), Organon, Inc. (West Orange, NJ) and Sanofi-Synthelabo, Inc. (Malvern, PA). Dr. Yusen has also been a consultant for Aventis and has served on the speaker's bureau for Aventis and Dupont Pharmaceuticals (Wilmington, DE).

* Corresponding author. Washington University School of Medicine, Box 8052, 660 S. Euclid Avenue, St. Louis, MO 63110.

E-mail address: yusenr@msnotes.wustl.edu (R.D. Yusen).

doi:10.1016/S0272-5231(02)00071-0

Unless contraindicated, UFH or LMWH should be prescribed for the initial treatment of VTE [1]. In a randomized controlled trial, treatment of patients with proximal lower-extremity DVT with an oral coumarin alone increased the risk for clot extension and recurrence of VTE when compared with treatment with UFH combined with an oral coumarin [9]. Typically, patients receive an oral vitamin K antagonist for long-term therapy (see the article by Kearon elsewhere in this issue). UFH or LMWH may be discontinued after 4 to 7 days once the INR is 2 or greater for 2 consecutive days [10,11]. Patients with massive VTE may benefit from a longer duration of heparin therapy [1].

For patients with VTE who have contraindications to anticoagulation, placement of an inferior vena cava filter protects against PE [12]. Because these filters predispose the patient to DVT formation, patients may benefit from long-term anticoagulant therapy if their initial contraindication to such therapy resolves.

Inferior vena cava filters are also used in combination with anticoagulation in patients who have a VTE recurrence despite adequate anticoagulation [1]. Inferior vena cava filters, in combination with anticoagulation, may decrease the risk of death from recurrent PE in patients with impaired cardiopulmonary reserve, although limited data support this assertion. Thrombolysis or embolectomy does not pertain to the outpatient setting, and the reader is referred to the article by Arcasoy for further discussion of these therapies.

Clinical trials of low molecular weight heparins for the initial inpatient treatment of venous thromboembolism

Over the past 2 decades, multiple clinical trials have demonstrated the equivalent or superior efficacy and safety of LMWHs when compared with UFHs

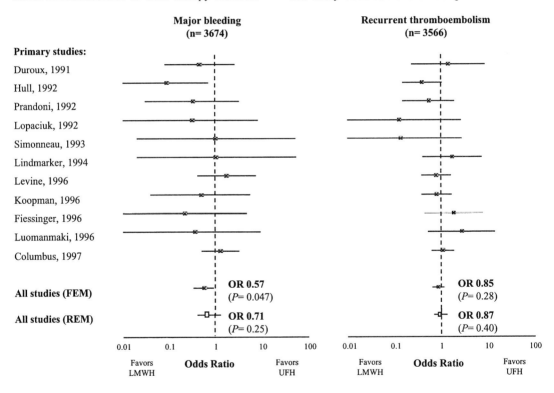

Fig. 1. Primary study and summary ORs for major bleeding and recurrent VTE in patients with acute VTE randomized to LMWH or UFH. ORs are indicated by boxes. Horizontal lines represent 95% CI. ORs less than 1 favor LMWH; ORs greater than 1 favor UFH. The summary OR for major bleeding favors LMWHs, but this finding is not statistically significant under the assumptions of the REM. The CI for the summary OR for recurrent VTE also crosses 1, indicating no statistically significant difference between the treatments. CI, confidence interval; FEM, fixed-effects model; LMWH, low molecular weight heparin; OR, odds ratio; REM, random-effects model; UFH, unfractionated heparin; VTE, venous thromboembolism. (*Adapted from* Gould M, Dembitzer A, Doyle R, Hastie T, Garber A. Low-molecular-weight heparins compared with unfractionated heparin for treatment of acute deep venous thrombosis: a meta-analysis of randomized, controlled trials. Ann Intern Med 1999;130:800–9; with permission.)

for the inpatient treatment of acute DVT [12–27] and PE [4,28]. Recent meta-analyses [29–31] have suggested that LMWHs are at least as safe and effective as UFH for the treatment of DVT, with a trend favoring improved outcomes in patients receiving LMWHs. The methodologically sound meta-analysis by Gould and colleagues [29] compared the safety and efficacy of various LMWHs with UFHs based on randomized controlled trials of the treatment of acute DVT. LMWHs and UFHs were associated with equivalent VTE recurrence and major bleeding rates (Fig. 1). Although only 1 [17] of the 11 studies in the meta-analysis found a significant reduction in mortality, the combined studies revealed a 29% relative

risk reduction in mortality with the use of LMWH versus UFH (Fig. 2).

Clinical trials of low molecular weight heparins for the outpatient treatment of venous thromboembolism

Two large randomized controlled trials of the treatment of acute proximal lower-extremity DVT have compared outpatient subcutaneous LMWH to inpatient therapy with intravenous UFH [2,3]. A third large randomized study of LMWH versus UFH therapy in patients with VTE allowed home therapy

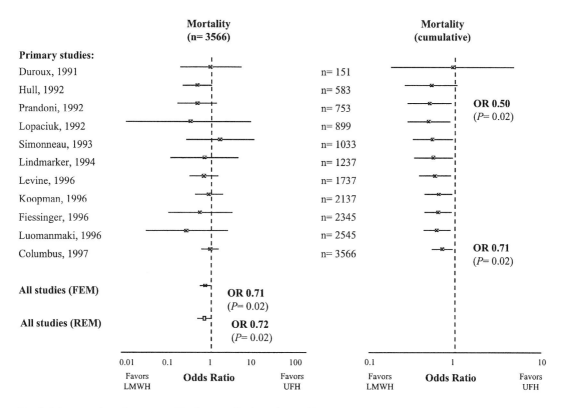

Fig. 2. Primary study and summary ORs for mortality in patients with acute VTE randomized to LMWH or UFH. ORs are indicated by boxes. Horizontal lines represent 95% CI. ORs less than 1 favor LMWH; ORs greater than 1 favor UFH. The left portion illustrates conventional meta-analysis results showing a statistically significant benefit for LMWH treatment. The right portion illustrates the results of cumulative meta-analysis in which the summary OR is recalculated after individual studies are added one at a time by year of publication. A statistically significant benefit for LMWH is apparent after the addition of the third study. The direction and statistical significance of the treatment effect remain constant with the addition of each new study, although the magnitude of the effect lessens slightly over time. CI, confidence interval; FEM, fixed-effects model; LMWH, low molecular weight heparin; OR, odds ratio; REM, random-effects model; UFH, unfractionated heparin; VTE, venous thromboembolism. (*Adapted from* Gould M, Dembitzer A, Doyle R, Hastie T, Garber A. Low-molecular-weight heparins compared with unfractionated heparin for treatment of acute deep venous thrombosis: a meta-analysis of randomized, controlled trials. Ann Intern Med 1999;130:800–9;with permission.)

Table 1
Outcomes in trials of outpatient deep vein thrombosis treatment

Outcome measure	Koopman et al, 1996 [3]		Levine et al, 1996 [2]		Columbus Investigators, 1997 [4]	
	Nadroparin (n = 202)	UFH (n = 198)	Enoxaparin (n = 247)	UFH (n = 253)	Reviparin (n = 510)	UFH (n = 511)
Recurrence (%)	6.9	8.6	5.3	6.7	5.3	4.9
Major bleeding (%)	0.5	1.0	2.0	1.2	2.0	1.6
Death (%)	6.9	8.1	4.5	6.7	7.1	7.6
Hospital LOS (d)	2.7	8.1	1.1	6.5	6.4	9.4

Major bleeding assessed during initial treatment with LMWH or UFH plus 48 hours in the Koopman and Levine studies, or during the first 14 days of treatment in the Columbus study. Recurrence and death rates were assessed during 3 months of follow-up in the Levine and Columbus studies and during 6 months of follow-up in the Koopman study.

Abbreviations: LOS, length of stay; UFH, unfractionated heparin.

in a subgroup of patients with DVT receiving LMWH [4]. These three well-conducted, large randomized controlled trials (Tables 1, 2) and two smaller trials of home therapy are discussed in detail herein. A Medline search of the literature did not identify any randomized controlled trials of outpatient versus inpatient therapy for PE.

For their multicenter Canadian treatment trial, Levine and colleagues [2] screened 2230 consecutive outpatients with acute proximal lower-extremity DVT. Among the 1491 excluded patients, the most common reasons for exclusion were comorbidity (41%), symptomatic PE (15%), previous treatment with UFH for more than 48 hours (9%), geographic inaccessibility (8%), and two or more previous episodes of VTE (7%) (Table 2). A total of 739 patients (33%) were eligible for study participation, and 500 (68% of the eligible) consented and were randomized to receive either enoxaparin (1 mg/kg) injected subcutaneously twice daily or intravenous nomogram-adjusted UFH. Oral coumarin was initiated on the second day of treatment. After at least 5 days of UFH or LMWH and 2 consecutive days of a therapeutic INR, UFH or LMWH was discontinued and coumarin continued long-term. Patients randomized to receive LMWH were eligible for full or partial home therapy; 120 of 247 patients (48.6%) received LMWH completely at home, whereas 29 of 247 (11.7%) had partial home therapy. Sixty percent of the patients randomized to LMWH received partial or full home therapy. Over the 3 months of follow-up, the efficacy and safety of the two regimens were not significantly different (see Table 1). Nevertheless, the allowance for home therapy with LMWH significantly decreased the average length of stay by an average of 5.4 days and halved the associated costs when compared with inpatient therapy with UFH.

For their multicenter treatment trial in Europe, Australia, and New Zealand, Koopman and colleagues [3] screened 692 consecutive patients with acute symptomatic proximal lower-extremity DVT. Among the 216 ineligible patients, the most common reasons for exclusion were recent VTE (18%), suspected PE (15%), previous use of anticoagulant drugs for more than 48 hours (12%), geographic inaccessibility (15%), short life expectancy (6%), and post-thrombotic syndrome (4%) (Table 2). The feasibility of home therapy was not considered in the determination of eligibility, although only outpatients were recruited. A total of 476 patients (69%) were eligible for study participation; 400 patients (84% of the eligible) consented and were randomized to receive either weight-based nadroparin (total daily doses of 8200 International Factor Xa Inhibitory Units [IU]/L for weight < 50 kg, 12,300 IU/L for weight 50–70 kg, and 18,400 IU/L for weight > 70 kg) injected subcutaneously twice daily versus intravenous-adjusted UFH. Oral coumarin was initiated on the first day of treatment. After at least 5 days of UFH or LMWH and 2 consecutive days of a therapeutic INR, the heparin was discontinued and coumarin continued long-term. Patients randomized to receive LMWH were eligible for full or partial home therapy; 72 of 202 patients (35.6%) received LMWH completely at home, and 80 of 202 patients (39.6%) had partial home therapy. Seventy-five percent of patients randomized to LMWH received partial or full home therapy. Only two patients in each group did not complete the 6-month follow-up. The efficacy and safety of the two randomized regimens were not statistically significantly different (see Table 1); however, the use of LMWH at home decreased the average length of stay by 67% when compared to inpatient therapy with UFH. Patients who received LMWH had better health-related quality of life in the domains of social

Table 2
Criteria for outpatient management of proximal lower-extremity deep venous thrombosis

Criteria	Yusen et al [57]	Koopman et al [3]	Levine et al [2]	Columbus Investigators [4]
Inclusion criteria				
Adult age	+	+	+[a]	+
Acute proximal lower-extremity DVT documented by ultrasonography or venogram	+	+	+	+[b]
Exclusion criteria				
General				
Hospital admission for illness other than DVT	+	−[c]	+[b]	−
Known allergy to UFH or LMWH	+	+[a]	+[a]	+[a]
Pregnancy	+	+	+	+
Potential high complication risk				
Related to recurrent clotting or bleeding				
Advanced age	+	−	−	−
Obesity	−	−	−	+[a]
History of heparin-induced thrombocytopenia	+	+[a]	+[a]	+[a]
High risk of noncompliance or inaccessibility that would affect follow-up	+	+[d]	+	+[d]
Related to recurrent clotting				
High risk for VTE recurrence: previous VTE recurrence, hereditary clotting disorder	−	+[e]	+	−
Related to bleeding				
Marked anemia	+	−	−	+[a]
Active bleeding/ high risk of hemorrhage[f]	+	+[a]	+	+
Significant renal dysfunction	+	−	+[a]	+[a]
Signs of symptoms of PE or limited cardiopulmonary reserve				
Confirmed or suspected symptomatic PE	+	+	+	−
Abnormal vital signs	+	+[a]	+[a]	+[a]
Other				
Overt postthrombotic syndrome	−	+	−	−

Other protocol-specific criteria from the published studies, not used for reasons related to patient care, have been excluded from this table (eg, exclusion of patients using heparin for $\geq 24-48$ hours before study enrollment).

Abbreviations: DVT, deep venous thrombosis; LMWH, low molecular weight heparin; PE, pulmonary embolism; UFH, unfractionated heparin; VTE, venous thromboembolism; +, criterion used in the study; −, criterion not used in the study.

Adapted from Yusen R, Haraden B, Gage B, Woodward R, Rubin B, Botney M. Criteria for outpatient management of proximal lower extremity deep venous thrombosis. Chest 1999;115:972–9; with permission.

[a] Criterion not explicitly stated in the same manner in the cited publication was confirmed by phone conversation with the primary author.

[b] Used as a criterion for a subset of patients in the study.

[c] Only outpatients were eligible for enrollment.

[d] Only geographic factors taken into account; other factors related to feasibility of home therapy were not used as exclusion criteria.

[e] Only previous DVT was used as an exclusion criterion from this category of exclusions.

[f] High risk of hemorrhage refers to patients who have had recent surgery, stroke, trauma, peptic ulcer disease, angiodysplasia of the colon, thrombocytopenia, among other events.

functioning and physical activity when compared with patients who received UFH. Other domains showed no significant differences. The health-related quality of life differences were most apparent after 1 to 2 weeks of therapy.

For their international (Europe, Canada, New Zealand, and Australia) trial, the Columbus investigators [4] screened 1745 patients with acute symptomatic VTE (proximal or distal lower-extremity DVT or PE). Among the 424 ineligible patients, the most common reasons for exclusion were previous use of therapeutic doses of anticoagulant drugs for more than 24 hours (47%), contraindications to anticoagulant therapy (16%), and difficulty with follow-up because of geographic location (14%) (Table 2). The feasibility of home therapy was not considered in the determination of eligibility. A total of 1320 patients (76%) were eligible for study participation, and 1021 of the eligible patients (77%) consented and were enrolled. Ten percent had calf DVT alone, 63.5% had proximal DVT, and 26.5% had PE. Patients were randomized to receive either weight-based reviparin (3500 anti–factor Xa IU for weight 35–45 kg, 4200 IU for weight 46–60 kg, and 6300 IU for weight >60 kg) injected subcutaneously twice daily or intravenous nomogram-adjusted UFH. Oral coumarin was initiated on the first or second day of treatment. After at least 5 days of UFH or LMWH and 2 consecutive days of a therapeutic INR, the heparin was discontinued and coumarin continued long-term. Patients randomized to LMWH were eligible for full or partial home therapy. Of the 372 patients with DVT randomized to receive LMWH, 100 patients (27%) received LMWH completely at home, and 56 of 372 (15%) had partial home therapy. Forty-two percent of participants with DVT randomized to LMWH received partial or full home therapy. No patients were lost during the 3-month follow-up. The efficacy and safety of the two randomized regimens were not statistically significantly different (see Table 1). Event rates were not provided in the subgroup of patients with DVT who were eligible for home therapy; however, the allowance for home therapy with LMWH significantly decreased the average length of stay by one third when compared with inpatient therapy with UFH.

For their multicenter treatment trial in France, Boccalon and colleagues [6] screened patients with acute proximal lower-extremity or pelvic DVT for enrollment. Reasons for exclusion were thrombus in the inferior vena cava, floating thrombus, a history of DVT within the preceding 6 months, symptomatic PE, a clinical context needing hospitalization, a contraindication to anticoagulation, treatment with therapeutic doses of UFH within the previous 48 hours, pregnancy, or unfeasibility of home therapy. A total of 201 (approximately 12% of eligible) patients consented for participation in the study and were randomized to outpatient or 10 days of inpatient therapy. All of the patients received one of the LMWHs available in France and oral coumarin therapy. After an average of 8.6 days of nadroparin, enoxaparin, or dalteparin, the LMWH was discontinued while warfarin was continued long-term. Most patients (73.4%) received LMWH completely at home or for no more than 24 hours in the hospital. Thirty-eight of 201 patients (18.9%) did not complete the 6 months of follow-up. The efficacy and safety of therapy in the two groups were not statistically significantly different. The rates of recurrence, major bleeding, and death in the inpatient group were each 2%, whereas the rates of recurrence (1%), major bleeding (2%), and death (0%) in the outpatient group were similar. The allowance for home therapy decreased the average length of stay from 9.6 to 1.0 days, but the protocol mandated much of this difference; therefore, the cost reduction of 56% may not be generalizable.

Belcaro and colleagues [5] screened 589 consecutive patients with acute proximal lower-extremity or pelvic DVT. Among the 264 ineligible patients, the most common reasons for exclusion were comorbidity, an inability to receive outpatient therapy, geographic inaccessibility, previous use of anticoagulant drugs for more than 48 hours, a history of recurrent VTE, and concurrent PE. A total of 379 patients (64%) were eligible for study participation; 325 patients (86% of the eligible) consented and were randomized to receive (1) weight-based nadroparin (100 anti–factor Xa IU/kg, rounded to the dose closest to one of three available prepackaged syringe doses of 6150, 8200, or 10,250 anti–factor Xa IU) injected subcutaneously twice daily, (2) intravenous-adjusted UFH therapy, or (3) fixed-dose UFH (12,500 IU) injected subcutaneously twice daily. The subcutaneous UFH group remained on UFH during the entire study period. The intravenous UFH and LMWH groups used coumarin long-term. In these two groups, oral coumarin was initiated on the second day of treatment. After at least 4 days of UFH or LMWH and 2 consecutive days of a therapeutic INR, heparin was discontinued and coumarin continued long-term. Patients randomized to receive subcutaneous LMWH were eligible for full or partial home therapy; 33 of 98 patients (34%) received LMWH completely at home. The proportion of patients who received partial home therapy was not described. All of the patients randomized to subcutaneous UFH were treated at home. Ten percent of patients did not complete the 3-month follow-up. The efficacy and safety of the three randomized regimens were not statistically significantly different, with DVT recurrence rates ranging from 6.1% to 7.1%, 0% major bleeding, and an overall death rate of 1.8%. Surprisingly, the use of LMWH did not significantly decrease the average length of stay when compared with mandated inpatient therapy with UFH.

Observational studies of low molecular weight heparins for the outpatient treatment of venous thromboembolism

Cohort studies and case series have supported the findings of the randomized controlled trials and have demonstrated the feasibility of outpatient LMWH therapy for the treatment of proximal and distal lower-extremity DVT [7,32–43]. These relatively small observational studies have found that most outpatients with DVT undergo initial treatment at home. Selection, reporting, publication, and other biases may skew such estimates. A recent prospective multicenter registry study of approximately 5000 patients at 150 various size hospitals in the United States suggested that clinicians treated the minority of patients diagnosed with acute DVT by compression ultrasound with LMWH in the outpatient setting (Vic Tapson, MD, personal communication, September 2002).

In a Canadian, two-center, prospective cohort study, Wells and colleagues [7] assessed expanded eligibility criteria for the outpatient treatment of VTE. Of the 233 consecutive outpatients with VTE who were screened, 39 (17%) were not eligible for home treatment. Exclusion criteria consisted of massive PE, active bleeding or a high risk for bleeding, phlegmasia cerulea dolens, or the need for hospitalization for other reasons. Initially, the study excluded patients with PE, but the investigators removed this exclusion criterion in the latter half of the study. Of the 194 patients treated fully or partially at home, 184 (95%) were treated entirely at home, supervised by experienced nurses. Patients received once-daily subcutaneous dalteparin (200 IU/kg) or twice-daily subcutaneous dalteparin (100 IU/kg; only used in the first 38 patients). Oral coumarin therapy was initiated on the first or second day of treatment. After at least 5 days of LMWH and 2 consecutive days of an INR greater than 1.9, LMWH was discontinued and coumarin continued long-term. Thirty-four of 194 patients (18%) in the study had PE. Patients had a recurrent VTE rate of 3.6%, a major hemorrhage rate of 2.1%, and a death rate of 7.2% during the 3-month follow-up. Wells concluded that most patients evaluated at a tertiary care hospital could undergo safe and effective nurse-supervised home therapy for DVT or nonmassive PE.

Kovacs and colleagues [8] assessed the outpatient treatment of PE with LMWH in a prospective cohort study in three Canadian teaching hospitals. Exclusion criteria for outpatient treatment of PE included age less than 18 years, the need for hospitalization for another reason, active bleeding or a high risk of major bleeding, hemodynamic instability (presumably due to PE), pain requiring parenteral narcotics, the requirement of supplemental oxygen therapy, and the likelihood of poor compliance. Of the 158 eligible patients with PE, 108 (68.4%) were treated partly or fully at home with a once-daily subcutaneous injection of dalteparin (200 IU/kg). Oral coumarin therapy was initiated on the first day of treatment. After a minimum of 5 days of LMWH and 2 consecutive days of an INR greater than1.9, the LMWH was discontinued and warfarin continued long-term. Approximately half of the patients (81 of 158) received LMWH completely at home, and an additional 17.1% (27 of 158) had partial home therapy. Two thirds of patients treated with LMWH received partial or complete home therapy. None of the 108 outpatients required readmission to the hospital during the LMWH therapy, but the study did not report the number of missing patients over 3 months of follow-up. Of the 108 patients treated at home, 5 had a recurrent PE, 1 had a recurrent DVT, and 2 had a major bleed. Four additional patients died of a cause unrelated to PE or bleeding. Kovacs concluded that the study demonstrated the feasibility and safety of partial or complete outpatient LMWH treatment for patients with nonmassive PE; however, the risk of adverse events was approximately 11% (12 of 108).

These studies by Wells et al [7] and Kovacs et al [8] of home therapy with LMWH evaluated fewer than 150 patients with PE; therefore, the confidence intervals around the estimated rates of VTE recurrence, major bleeding, and death were wide. Although the studies did not explicitly exclude patients with poor cardiopulmonary reserve, the increased risk of VTE recurrence [44] and the increased risk of death from recurrent PE in such patients might preclude home therapy. Home therapy for PE requires further evaluation before it can be recommended outside of a trial or other supervised setting.

Pharmacoeconomic and health-related quality of life studies of outpatient therapy for deep vein thrombosis with low molecular weight heparin

Low molecular weight heparins have a higher acquisition cost when compared with UFHs. Nevertheless, in a study that assumed similar outcomes with both treatments, the use of LMWHs for inpatients with acute proximal lower-extremity DVT did not significantly increase medical expenditure [45]. Because of the lower incidence of adverse events when compared with UFHs, LMWHs seem to be cost-effective when prescribed to inpatients. The incremental cost-effectiveness of prescribing inpatient LMWH therapy versus inpatient UFH therapy is approximately $7820 per quality-adjusted life year gained [46]. In studies that have allowed for outpatient care of DVT, LMWHs have been cost neutral [47] or have produced cost savings when compared with inpatient care with UFH [6,32,48–52]. Greater cost savings occur as the proportion of patients treated in the outpatient setting increases [46,53].

Home therapy for acute symptomatic DVT with LMWH may improve health-related quality of life and satisfaction of patients [34,50,54,55]. O'Brien et al [50] performed an evaluation of a subset of patients from the study by Levine et al [2] of outpatient therapy with LMWH versus inpatient therapy with UFH. O'Brien and colleagues analyzed data from the subgroup of 300 patients who presented as outpatients with proximal lower-extremity acute DVT. When compared with inpatient therapy with UFH, treatment at home with LMWH did not compromise outcomes or general health-related quality of life. Inpatients treated with UFH had a significantly greater decrement in social functioning when compared with outpatients treated with LMWH as measured by the Medical Outcomes Study 36-item Short Form (SF-36) questionnaire on day 0 and day 7. Other changes in general health-related quality of life were similar between the two groups. The subgroup analysis did not preserve the randomization, and bias may have affected the conclusions. A prospective cohort study in Canada demonstrated that most patients with DVT who were treated with LMWH at home were pleased with home treatment, felt comfortable self-injecting the LMWH, and were satisfied with the support and instruction they received [34].

Criteria for outpatient venous thromboembolism therapy

Clinical trials have demonstrated that most patients with acute DVT can be treated safely at home, and that outpatient treatment can reduce medical expenditure. The salient clinical issue is how to select patients who can be treated safely at home. Clinical trials that have demonstrated the safety and efficacy of outpatient therapy for VTE using LMWH have typically excluded patients with the following characteristics: suspected or documented acute PE, other illness requiring inpatient care, a high risk of recurrent thrombosis, active or a high risk of bleeding, significant renal dysfunction, pregnancy, and a low likelihood of compliance with medication administration or follow-up (Table 2). The determination of eligibility for home therapy with LMWH depends on historical information, physical examination findings, and diagnostic test results.

Absolute exclusion criteria for initial outpatient treatment of VTE with LMWH are the need for hospitalization for sequelae or comorbidity, an allergy to LMWH, a history of heparin-induced thrombocytopenia, severe coagulopathy, and active bleeding. Weighing the risks and benefits of outpatient initial VTE therapy includes consideration of additional exclusion criteria. During a 3- to 6-month course of therapy for VTE, the highest rates of major bleeding [44] and VTE recurrence [5,7,28,44,56] occur during the first few weeks of therapy. Home therapy might not be preferable for patients with severe acute systemic hypertension, endocarditis, pericarditis, recent major surgery, recent stroke, and recent spinal or epidural procedures because of their increased risk of bleeding. Home therapy for patients with a hypercoagulable state and a history of previous VTE might not be preferable because of the high risk for recurrence.

Even if adverse events occur at home, the outcomes of patients treated at home might not be different than if the adverse events occurred in the hospital. Home therapy might avoid some of the iatrogenic complications associated with hospitalizations. Patient and physician preferences should determine candidacy for home treatment. Home therapy might be appropriate in a patient with end-stage malignancy at high-risk for bleeding and VTE recurrence who prefers to spend his or her remaining days alive at home.

Assuming the major goal of home therapy is the avoidance of adverse events, exclusion criteria should include the following: the need for hospitalization for sequelae or comorbidity, active bleeding or a high bleeding risk (Table 3), a high risk for recurrent VTE, suspected or known PE, and poor cardiopulmonary reserve. One study validated these criteria outside of the setting of a clinical trial [57]. Researchers at Washington University retrospectively applied explicit criteria (see Table 2) to 195 consecutive inpatients with newly diagnosed proximal lower-extremity DVT. Outpatient DVT therapy was rarely used during the study period. Patients were classified as eligible, possibly eligible, or ineligible for home treatment based on the selection criteria. The frequency of complications during initial therapy, including major bleeding, symptomatic VTE, and death, was assessed. None of the 18 inpatients (9%) classified as eligible and none of the 18 (9%) classified as possibly eligible for outpatient therapy experienced complications. Of the 159 inpatients (82%) classified

Table 3
Clinical risk factors for coumarin-related hemorrhage

Factor	Relative risk[a]
Chronic renal disease	2.2
Other antithrombotic therapy	1.6
Uncontrolled blood pressure	1.7
Malignancy	1.6
Alcoholism	2.1
Rebleeding	2.1
Increased age	1.6
Neuropsychiatric or physical impairment	1.4
Stroke	1.9

[a] Estimated from Beyth RJ, Milligan PE, Gage BF. Risk factors for bleeding in patients taking coumarins. Curr Hem Reports 2002; I:41–9.

as ineligible, 13 (8.2%; 95% confidence interval, 4% to 12%) died or experienced serious complications. It was concluded that explicit selection criteria can identify a subset of patients with acute proximal lower-extremity DVT who can be treated safely at home. The study did not assess patients with distal lower extremity, pelvic, or upper-extremity DVT. Because the study was conducted at a large tertiary care referral center where patients had a high level of acuity, the eligibility rates for home therapy are likely to be greater in community settings.

Expanded criteria, such as those proposed by Wells et al [7], may lead to a greater number of patients receiving home therapy without necessarily worsening outcomes. Although patients with non-massive or uncomplicated PE may do well with home therapy, their risk for recurrent fatal PE is greater than in patients with DVT [44,56].

Practical aspects of initiating home low molecular weight heparin therapy for venous thromboembolism

The medical staff and the patient should determine the feasibility of home therapy, including reimbursement issues and willingness and ability to perform the required tasks. Once a patient is deemed eligible for home therapy, he or she should be educated and have appropriate follow-up arranged. The LMWH can be injected by the patient, by his or her relatives, or by visiting nurses at home, or the outpatient can travel to an office, clinic, or hospital to receive injections.

Health care workers should educate patients about the risks and benefits of home anticoagulant therapy

for VTE and about the mechanics of self-injection. Patients should receive verbal and written instructions regarding the symptoms or signs of bleeding (including pink urine and black stools) and recurrent clot or embolism (eg, limb pain or edema, shortness of breath, hemoptysis, and syncope), and regarding how to notify a clinician if any of these events occur. Patients should be taught about the administration of LMWH, including the expectation of a small hematoma at the site of injection. The injection should be subcutaneous, not intramuscular, and the site of LMWH injection should be rotated using the antero-lateral and posterolateral abdominal wall. Patients should be taught about the storage of medications and equipment and the appropriate way to dispose of syringes and needles. Health care workers should arrange for the acquisition of LMWH, alcohol swabs, and a sharps container, and should schedule frequent INR testing [58], complete blood count monitoring [1], and follow-up visits.

Long-term therapy for venous thromboembolism with coumarins

To decrease the risk of recurrent VTE, patients require months of anticoagulation after the initial VTE and prolonged or indefinite therapy after a recurrent VTE [1] (see the article by Kearon elsewhere in this issue). Patients should generally be prescribed an oral coumarin during this period, because coumarins are more convenient and less expensive than parenteral therapy with UFHs or LMWHs. In North America, warfarin (Coumadin) or its generic equivalent is the only coumarin that is widely available; in other continents, acenocoumarol (Sinthrome) and phenprocoumon (Marcumar) are often prescribed. All coumarins have the same mechanism of action, that is, they inhibit the hepatic synthesis of vitamin K–dependent clotting factors (factors II [prothrombin], VII, IX, and X).

As is true for heparin, the dose of coumarin must be titrated carefully to provide an antithrombotic therapy effect without causing hemorrhage. The optimal INR that balances these risks is unclear but is thought to range from 2 to 3, and experts recommend a target INR value of 2.5 [1]. The dose of coumarin that achieves an INR of 2 to 3 is highly variable, and there is no way to predict the maintenance dose a priori. One effective strategy is to start patients on a typical dose (eg, 5 mg of warfarin [59]) and to check INRs frequently (eg, every other day initially). Patients who are elderly, petite, or taking certain medications (eg, amiodarone) have lower

Table 4
Checklist of information to review with patients when prescribing a coumarin

Your blood thinner (insert name here) can cause bleeding and bruising. If you develop excessive bruising or any bleeding (eg, pink urine or a black bowel movement), call your doctor.

The amount of vitamin K in your diet should be consistent. Bingeing on foods that are rich in vitamin K (eg, green leafy vegetables) counteracts the effect of your blood thinner.

Because alcohol interacts with your blood thinner and can cause stomach ulcers, you should consume alcohol only in moderation (ie, no more than two drinks per day).

Your blood thinner must be monitored every few weeks by a blood test called an INR.

If you miss one dose, take it as soon as possible. If you miss more than one dose, call your doctor for instructions.

Many drugs interact with blood thinner. When starting any new medication, including aspirin, check with your doctor or pharmacist to find out whether it is safe for you to take.

Women taking blood thinner pills must avoid pregnancy; if you intend to become pregnant, a blood thinner shot is safer for your baby.

Adapted from Gage BF, Fihn SD, White RH. Warfarin therapy for an octogenarian who has atrial fibrillation. Ann Intern Med 2001;134:466, with permission.

coumarin requirements and can be started on a lower initial dose. Patients beginning coumarin therapy should be educated about its use (Table 4). As the INR and coumarin dose stabilize, the frequency of INR monitoring should be decreased gradually, typically to every 3 or 4 weeks [58].

Asymptomatic patients with minimal INR elevations (eg, INR of 3.2) can be continued safely on the same dose. Patients with moderate INR elevations (eg, INR value around 3.5) can be treated with a modest (eg, 10%) reduction in the warfarin dose and a search for the underlying cause [60]. Greater INR elevations require temporary cessation of warfarin, and patients may benefit from administration of vitamin K_1. An oral dose of 1 mg of phytonadione is a safe and effective way to lower an INR ranging from 5 to 10 to near the therapeutic range [61].

Bleeding associated with anticoagulation requires aggressive therapy in addition to discontinuation of anticoagulation. For nonserious bleeding associated with coumarin therapy, vitamin K_1 (eg, 10 mg of intravenous phytonadione given slowly to avoid an anaphylactoid reaction) can lower the INR in 12 to 24 hours and typically should be repeated frequently because of the long half-life of coumarins [58]. Fresh-frozen plasma rapidly improves coagulation abnormalities in patients receiving LMWH, UFH, or a

coumarin. Clotting factor concentrates may be more effective than fresh-frozen plasma when complete and immediate correction of coumarin-associated coagulation defects is desired in patients with severe or life-threatening hemorrhage [62]. Protamine sulfate use should be considered in patients with severe or life-threatening bleeding associated with UFH. Protamine may be helpful in reversing the effect of LMWH but may not completely correct its inhibition of factor Xa [63]. Protamine does not reverse the action of coumarins.

Although many patients with a first-time VTE should be prescribed anticoagulants for 6 months, the duration of anticoagulation depends on patient preferences and the risk of adverse events. Factors that favor a shorter duration of treatment are a high risk of hemorrhage and a low risk of recurrence. Risk factors for hemorrhage can be identified by using the COUMARIN acronym (*see* Table 3). Patients in whom the initial VTE was caused by a transient risk factor (eg, surgery) are at lower risk for recurrence when compared with patients with VTE owing to a different etiology (eg, malignancy) [64]. Patients with a significant ongoing risk of recurrence may benefit from longer than 6 months of anticoagulant therapy.

Summary

Once- or twice-daily subcutaneous dosing of LMWHs without laboratory monitoring has facilitated outpatient VTE therapy. Clinical trials have demonstrated at least equivalent efficacy and safety and potential cost savings of outpatient therapy for uncomplicated proximal DVT with LMWH when compared with inpatient therapy. Explicit criteria exist for outpatient DVT therapy. Home therapy for PE requires further evaluation before it can be recommended outside of a trial or other supervised setting.

References

[1] Hyers T, Agnelli G, Hull R, Morris T, Samama M, Tapson V, et al. Antithrombotic therapy for venous thromboembolic disease. Chest 2001;119:176S–93S.

[2] Levine M, Gent M, Hirsh J, Leclerc J, Anderson D, Wietz J, et al. A comparison of low-molecular-weight heparin administered primarily at home with unfractionated heparin administered in the hospital for proximal deep-vein thrombosis. N Engl J Med 1996;334: 677–81.

[3] Koopman M, Prandoni P, Piovella F, Ockelford P, Brandjes D, Van Der Meer J, et al. Treatment of ve-

nous thrombosis with intravenous unfractionated heparin administered in the hospital as compared with subcutaneous low-molecular-weight heparin administered at home. N Engl J Med 1996;334:682–7.

[4] Columbus Investigators. Low-molecular-weight heparin in the treatment of patients with venous thromboembolism. N Engl J Med 1997;337:657–62.

[5] Belcaro G, Nicolaides A, Cesarone M, Laurora G, De Sanctis M, Incandela L, et al. Comparison of low-molecular-weight heparin, administered primarily at home, with unfractionated heparin, administered in hospital, and subcutaneous heparin, administered at home for deep-vein thrombosis. Angiology 1999;50: 781–7.

[6] Boccalon H, Elias A, Chale J, Cadene A, Gabriel S. Clinical outcome and cost of hospital vs home treatment of proximal deep vein thrombosis with a low-molecular-weight heparin. Arch Intern Med 2000; 160:1769–73.

[7] Wells P, Kovacs M, Bormanis J, Forgie M, Goudie D, Morrow B, et al. Expanding eligibility for outpatient treatment of deep venous thrombosis and pulmonary embolism with low-molecular-weight heparin. Arch Intern Med 1998;158:1809–12.

[8] Kovacs M, Anderson D, Morrow B, Gray L, Touchie D, Wells P. Outpatient treatment of pulmonary embolism with dalteparin. Thromb Haemost 2000;83: 209–11.

[9] Brandjes D, Heijboer H, Buller H, De Rijk M, Jagt H, Ten Cate J. Acenocoumarol and heparin compared with acenocoumarol alone in the initial treatment of proximal-vein thrombosis. N Engl J Med 1992;327: 1485–9.

[10] Hull RD, Raskob GE, Rosenbloom D, Panju A, Brill-Edwards P, Ginsberg J, et al. Heparin for 5 days as compared with 10 days in the initial treatment of proximal venous thrombosis. N Engl J Med 1990;322: 1260–4.

[11] White R, Zhou H, Romano P. Length of hospital stay for treatment of deep venous thrombosis and the incidence of recurrent thromboembolism. Arch Intern Med 1998;158:1005–10.

[12] Decousus H, Leizorovics A, Parent F, Page Y, Tardy B, Girard P, et al. A clinical trial of vena caval filters in the prevention of pulmonary embolism in patients with proximal deep-vein thrombosis. N Engl J Med 1998; 338:409–15.

[13] Bratt G, Tornebohm E, Granqvist S, Aberg W, Lockner D. A comparison between low molecular weight heparin (KABI2165) and standard heparin in the intravenous treatment of deep venous thrombosis. Thromb Haemost 1985;54:813–7.

[14] Holm H, Ly B, Handeland G, Abildgaard U, Arnesen K, Gottschalk P, et al. Subcutaneous treatment of deep venous thrombosis: a comparison of unfractionated heparin and low molecular weight heparin. Haemostasis 1986;16:30S–7S.

[15] Albada J, Niewwenhuis H, Sixma J. Treatment of acute venous thromboembolism with low molecular weight

heparin (fragmin): results of a double-blind randomized study. Circulation 1989;80:935–40.

[16] Duroux P, Beclere A. A randomized trial of subcutaneous low molecular weight heparin (CY 216) compared with intravenous unfractionated heparin in the treatment of deep vein thrombosis. Thromb Haemost 1991;65:251–6.

[17] Hull R, Raskob G, Pineo G, Green D, Trowbridge A, Elliot G, et al. Subcutaneous low molecular weight heparin compared with continuous intravenous heparin in the treatment of proximal vein thrombosis. N Engl J Med 1992;326:975–82.

[18] Prandoni P, Lensing A, Buller H, Carta M, Cogo A, Vigo M, et al. Comparison of subcutaneous low-molecular-weight heparin with intravenous standard heparin in proximal deep-vein thrombosis. Lancet 1992; 339:441–5.

[19] Holmström M, Berglund C, Granquist S, Bratt G, Tomebotim E, Lockner D. Fragmin once or twice daily subcutaneously in the treatment of deep venous thrombosis of the leg. Thromb Res 1992;67:49–55.

[20] Lopaciuk S, Meissner A, Filipecki S, Zawilska K, Sowier J, Ciesielski L, et al. Subcutaneous low molecular weight heparin versus subcutaneous unfractionated heparin in the treatment of deep vein thrombosis: a Polish multicenter trial. Thromb Haemost 1992;68:14–8.

[21] Simonneau G, Charbonnie B, Decousus H, Planchon B, Ninet J, Sie P, et al. Subcutaneous low-molecular-weight heparin compared with continuous intravenous unfractionated heparin in the treatment of proximal deep vein thrombosis. Arch Intern Med 1993;153: 1541–6.

[22] Lindmarker P, Holmström M, Granqvist S, Johnsson H, Lockner D. Comparison of once-daily subcutaneous fragmin with continuous intravenous unfractionated heparin in the treatment of deep vein thrombosis. Thromb Haemost 1994;72:186–90.

[23] Monreal M, Lafoz E, Olive A, del Rio L, Vedia C. Comparison of subcutaneous unfractionated heparin with a low molecular weight heparin (Fragmin) in patients with venous thromboembolism and contraindications to Coumarin. Thromb Haemost 1994;71:7–11.

[24] Alhenc-Gelas M, Jestin-Le Guernic C, Vitoux J, Kher A, Alach M, Fiessinger J. Adjusted versus fixed doses of the low-molecular-weight heparin Fragmin in the treatment of deep vein thrombosis. Thromb Haemost 1994;71:698–702.

[25] Fiessinger J, Lopez-Fernandez M, Gatterer E, Granqvist S, Kher A. Once-daily subcutaneous Dalteparin, a low molecular weight heparin, for the initial treatment of acute deep vein thrombosis. Thromb Haemost 1996; 76:195–9.

[26] Charbonnier B, Fiessinger J, Banga J, Wenzel E, d'Azemar P, Sagnard L. Comparison of a once daily with a twice daily subcutaneous low molecular weight heparin regimen in the treatment of deep vein thrombosis. Thromb Haemost 1998;79:897–901.

[27] Merli G, Spiro T, Olsson C, Abilgaard U, Davidson B,

Eldor A, et al. Subcutaneous enoxaparin once or twice daily compared with intravenous unfractionated heparin for treatment of venous thromboembolic disease. Ann Intern Med 2001;134:191–202.

[28] Simonneau G, Sors H, Charbonnier B, Page Y, Laaban J, Azarian R, et al. A comparison of low-molecular-weight heparin with unfractionated heparin for acute pulmonary embolism. N Engl J Med 1997;337:663–9.

[29] Gould M, Dembitzer A, Doyle R, Hastie T, Garber A. Low-molecular-weight heparins compared with unfractionated heparin for treatment of acute deep venous thrombosis: a meta-analysis of randomized, controlled trials. Ann Intern Med 1999;130:800–9.

[30] Dolovich L, Ginsberg J, Douketis J, Holbrook A, Cheah G. A meta-analysis comparing low-molecular-weight heparins with unfractionated heparin in the treatment of venous thromboembolism. Arch Intern Med 2000;160:181–8.

[31] Rocha E, Martinez-Gonzalez M, Montes R, Panizo C. Do the low molecular weight heparins improve efficacy and safety of the treatment of deep venous thrombosis? A meta-analysis. Haematologica 2000;85:935–42.

[32] Lindmarker P, Holmstrom M. Use of low molecular weight heparin (dalteparin), once daily, for the treatment of deep vein thrombosis: a feasibility and health economic study in an outpatient setting. J Intern Med 1996;240:395–401.

[33] Dedden P, Chang B, Nagel D. Pharmacy-managed program for home treatment of deep vein thrombosis with enoxaparin. Am J Health Syst Pharm 1997;54:1968–72.

[34] Harrison L, McGinnis J, Crowther M, Ginsberg J, Hirsh J. Assessment of outpatient treatment of deep-vein thrombosis with low-molecular-weight heparin. Arch Intern Med 1998;158:2001–3.

[35] Goldhaber S, Morrison R, Diran L, Creager M, Lee T. Abbreviated hospitalization for deep venous thrombosis with the use of ardeparin. Arch Intern Med 1998;158:2325–8.

[36] Ting S, Ziegenbein R, Gan T, Catalano J, Monagle P, Silvers J, et al. Dalteparin for deep venous thrombosis: a hospital-in-the-home program. Med J Australia 1998;168:272–6.

[37] Mattiasson I, Berntorp E, Bornhov S, Lagerstedt C, Lethagen S, Persson J, et al. Outpatient treatment of acute deep vein thrombosis. Int Angiol 1998;17:146–50.

[38] O'Shaughnessy D, Tovey C, Miller A, O'Neill V, Rana P, Akbar S, et al. Outpatient management of deep vein thrombosis. J Accid Emerg Med 1998;15:292–3.

[39] Pearson S, Blair R, Halper A, Eddy E, McKean S. An outpatient program to treat deep venous thrombosis with low-molecular-weight heparin. Effective Clinical Practice 1999;2:210–7.

[40] Blättler W, Kreis N, Blattler I. Practicability and quality of outpatient management of acute deep venous thrombosis. J Vasc Surg 2000;32:855–60.

[41] Dunn A, Schechter C, Gotlin A, Vomvolakis D, Jacobs E, Sacks H, et al. Outpatient treatment of deep venous thrombosis in diverse inner-city patients. Am J Med 2001;110:458–62.

[42] Grau E, Tenias J, Real E, Medrano J, Ferrer R, Pastor E, et al. Home treatment of deep venous thrombosis with low molecular weight heparin: long-term incidence of recurrent venous thromboembolism. Am J Hematol 2001;67:10–4.

[43] Vinson D, Berman D. Outpatient treatment of deep venous thrombosis: a clinical care pathway managed by the emergency department. Ann Emerg Med 2001;37:251–8.

[44] Douketis J, Foster G, Crowther M, Prins M, Ginsberg J. Clinical risk factors and timing of recurrent venous thromboembolism during the initial 3 months of anticoagulant therapy. Arch Intern Med 2000;160:3431–6.

[45] de Lissovoy G, Yusen R, Spiro T, Krupski W, Champion A, Sorensen S. Cost for inpatient care of venous thrombosis—a trial of enoxaparin vs standard heparin. Arch Intern Med 2000;160:3160–5.

[46] Gould M, Dembitzer A, Sanders G, Garber A. Low-molecular-weight heparins compared with unfractionated heparin for treatment of acute deep venous thrombosis: a cost-effectiveness analysis. Ann Intern Med 1999;130:789–99.

[47] Spyropoulos A, Hurley J, Ciesla G, de Lissovoy G. Management of acute proximal deep vein thrombosis: pharmacoeconomic evaluation of outpatient treatment with enoxaparin vs inpatient treatment with unfractionated heparin. Chest 2002;122:108–14.

[48] Hull R, Raskob G, Rosenbloom D, et al. Low-molecular-weight heparin was more cost-effective than intravenous heparin for treating proximal venous thrombosis. Arch Intern Med 1997;157:289–94.

[49] van den Belt A, Bossuyt P, Prins M, Gallus A, Buller H. Replacing inpatient care by outpatient care in the treatment of deep venous thrombosis—an economic evaluation. Thromb Haemost 1998;79:259–63.

[50] O'Brien B, Levine M, Willan A, Goeree R, Haley S, Blackhouse G, et al. Economic evaluation of outpatient treatment with low-molecular-weight heparin for proximal vein thrombosis. Arch Intern Med 1999;159:2298–304.

[51] Tillman D, Charland S, Witt D. Effectiveness and economic impact associated with a program for outpatient management of acute deep vein thrombosis in a group model health maintenance organization. Arch Intern Med 2000;160:2926–32.

[52] Huse D, Communis G, Taylor D, Russell M. Outpatient treatment of venous thromboembolism with low-molecular-weight heparin: an economic evaluation. Am J Manag Care 2002;8:S10–6.

[53] Rodger M, Bredeson C, Wells P, Beck J, Kearns B, Huebsch L. Cost-effectiveness of low-molecular-weight heparin and unfractionated heparin in treatment of deep vein thrombosis. CMAJ 1998;159:931–8.

[54] Bossuyt P, van den Belt A, Prins M. Out-of-hospital treatment of venous thrombosis: socioeconomic aspects and patients' quality of life. Haemostasis 1998; 28:100–7.

[55] Smith B, Weekley J, Pilotto L, Howe T, Beven R. Cost comparison of at-home treatment of deep vein thrombosis with low molecular weight heparin to inpatient treatment with unfractionated heparin. Int Med J 2002; 32:29–34.

[56] Douketis J, Kearon C, Bates S, Duku E, Ginsberg J. Risk of fatal pulmonary embolism in patients with treated venous thromboembolism. JAMA 1998;279: 458–62.

[57] Yusen R, Haraden B, Gage B, Woodward R, Rubin B, Botney M. Criteria for outpatient management of proximal lower extremity deep venous thrombosis. Chest 1999;115:972–9.

[58] Gage B, Fihn S, White R. Management and dosing of warfarin therapy. Am J Med 2000;109:481–8.

[59] Harrison L, Johnston M, Massicotte M, Crowther M, Moffat K, Hirsh J. Comparison of 5-mg and 10-mg loading doses in initiation of warfarin therapy. Ann Intern Med 1997;126:133–6.

[60] Banet G, Waterman A, Milligan P, Gatchel S, Gage B. Warfarin dose reduction versus watchful waiting for mild elevations in the international normalized ratio. Chest 2003;123:499–503.

[61] Crowther M, Douketis J, Schnurr T, Steidl L, Mera V, Ultori C, et al. Oral vitamin K lowers the international normalized ratio more rapidly than subcutaneous vitamin K in the treatment of warfarin-associated coagulopathy. Ann Intern Med 2002;137:251–4.

[62] Makris M, Greaves M, Phillips W, Kitchen S, Rosendaal F, Preston F. Emergency oral anticoagulation reversal: the relative efficacy of infusions of fresh frozen plasma and clotting factor concentrate on correction of the coagulopathy. Thromb Haemost 1997;77:477–80.

[63] Wolzt M, Weltermann A, Nieszpaur-Los M, Schneider B, Fassolt A, Lechner K, et al. Studies on the neutralizing effects of protamine on unfractionated and low molecular weight heparin (Fragmin) at the site of activation of the coagulation system in man. Thromb Haemost 1995;73:439–43.

[64] Hansson P, Sorbo J, Eriksson H. Recurrent venous thromboembolism after deep vein thrombosis. Arch Intern Med 2000;160:769–74.

Clin Chest Med 24 (2003) 63–72

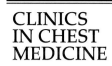

Duration of therapy for acute venous thromboembolism

Clive Kearon, MB, MRCPI, FRCPC, PhD

McMaster Clinic, Henderson General Hospital, Hamilton Health Sciences, 711 Concession Street, Hamilton, Ontario L8V 1C3, Canada

Following an episode of venous thromboembolism (VTE), treatment should be continued until the benefits of anticoagulation no longer outweigh the risks of therapy. The optimal duration of anticoagulation needs to be individualized. This assessment is dominated by the risk of recurrent VTE if anticoagulation is stopped and the risk of bleeding if treatment is continued. After considering these two competing risks, if the benefits of remaining on anticoagulant therapy are small or uncertain, patient preference and the cost of therapy also strongly influence this decision, particularly if indefinite anticoagulant therapy is being considered.

Risk factors for recurrent venous thromboembolism after stopping anticoagulant therapy

Reversibility of risk factors for venous thromboembolism

Probably the greatest advance in the assessment of the risk for recurrent VTE after anticoagulant therapy is stopped is the recent recognition that patients who have thrombosis provoked by a major reversible risk factor, such as surgery, have a low risk of recurrence (ie, approximately 3% per year), whereas patients with an unprovoked (idiopathic) episode of VTE or a persistent risk factor (eg, cancer) have a high risk (ie, approximately 10% per year) (Table 1) [1–7].

Dr. Kearon is a Research Scholar of the Heart and Stroke Foundation of Canada.
E-mail address: kearon@mcmaster.ca

Thrombophilia

Hereditary and acquired biochemical states that are associated with VTE (thrombophilia) are heterogeneous in terms of the frequency with which they occur in the normal population and the strength of their association with thrombosis [8–11] (Table 1). Although the presence of one of these abnormalities is often assumed an important risk factor for recurrent VTE and a strong indication for prolonged treatment, the evidence supporting this assumption is inconsistent.

Antiphospholipid antibodies

Antiphospholipid antibodies (anticardiolipin antibody [12,13] or lupus anticoagulant [13]) are associated with a twofold or greater risk of recurrent thrombosis after stopping anticoagulant therapy [12,13]. One study found that, owing to an excess of subsequent venous and arterial thrombosis following a first episode of VTE, the presence of an anticardiolipin antibody was associated with a higher mortality. Remaining on anticoagulant therapy seemed to reduce this risk [12].

Factor V Leiden and the G20210A prothrombin gene mutation

Factor V Leiden and the prothrombin gene mutation, singly in a heterozygous state, are of uncertain importance as risk factors for recurrent VTE. Two prospective studies found that factor V Leiden was associated with a twofold increase in the risk of recurrence [14,15], whereas three other studies found no such association [13,16,17]. Similarly, the prothrombin gene mutation was associated with an increase in the risk of recurrent VTE in two prospective studies [18,19], whereas it was not in two others [17,20]. Patients who are heterozygous for factor V

doi:10.1016/S0272-5231(02)00076-X

Table 1

Risk of recurrent venous thromboembolism after stopping anticoagulant therapy

Variable	Relative risk
Transient risk factor [1–5,7]	≤ 0.5
Persistent risk factor [1–5,7]	≥ 2
Unprovoked VTE [1–3,7,13]	≥ 2
Protein C, protein S, and antithrombin deficiencies [23]	1.4
Heterozygous for factor V Leiden [13–17]	1–2
Homozygous for factor V Leiden [17]	4.1
Heterozygous for G20210A mutation in the prothrombin gene [13,14,17–20]	1–2
Heterozygous for factor V Leiden and G20210A prothrombin gene [18,21,22]	2–5
Factor VIII level >200 IU/dL [25,26]	~6
Antiphospholipid antibodies [12,13]	2–4
Mild hyperhomo-cysteinemia [28]	2.7
Family history of VTE [3,17]	~1
Cancer [7,23,34]	~3
Chemotherapy [34]	~2
Discontinuation of estrogen [34,68,69]	<1
Proximal DVT versus PE [3,13]	~1
Distal DVT versus proximal DVT or PE [3,6]	0.5
Residual thrombosis [2,3,13,33,51]	1–2
Vena caval filter [38,53,54]	~1.8
Second versus first episode of VTE [38,52]	~1.4
Age [13,17,34,38]	~1
Gender [13,17,38]	~1
Asian [38]	~0.8

Abbreviations: DVT, deep vein thrombosis; PE, pulmonary embolism; VTE, venous thromboembolism.

Leiden and the prothrombin gene mutations [18, 21,22] or homozygous for factor V Leiden [17] seem to have a high risk for recurrent VTE (Table 1).

Deficiency of protein C, protein S, and antithrombin

Limited prospective data are available regarding the risk for recurrent VTE in patients with antithrombin, protein C, or protein S deficiency. One prospective study identified a hazard ratio of 1.4 for recurrent VTE in patients with one of these abnormalities or a lupus anticoagulant [23]. A retrospective family cohort study estimated that the presence of one of these abnormalities was associated with a 10% cumulative frequency of a recurrent VTE 1 year after diagnosis, rising to 23% after 5 years [24]. Nevertheless, because these three deficiency states are associated with a 20 to 50 fold increase in the risk for a first episode of VTE [8], they are thought to be clinically important risk factors for recurrent VTE.

Factor VIII

A markedly elevated level of factor VIII is a risk factor for recurrent thrombosis (Table 1) [25,26].

Hyperhomocysteinemia

Hyperhomocysteinemia, a condition that is related to hereditary and acquired risk factors [27], was associated with a 2.7-fold increased risk of recurrent VTE in one study of patients with unprovoked VTE [28]. Reversal of hyperhomocysteinemia with vitamin therapy may reduce the risk of recurrent VTE, a hypothesis that is currently being tested [29].

Cancer

Cancer is associated with a threefold increased risk of recurrent VTE during [30–33] and following [7,23,33,34] oral anticoagulant therapy (Table 1). Some evidence suggests that anticoagulant therapy may favorably alter the natural history of some cancers [35,36]. Schulman and colleagues [36] found that treatment of a first episode of VTE with oral anticoagulant therapy for 6 months versus 6 weeks was associated with a lower frequency of cancer (odds ratio, 0.6), especially urogenital, during 8 years of follow-up. This observation must be confirmed in other studies before it can be considered an argument in favor of more prolonged anticoagulant therapy for patients with VTE.

Pulmonary embolism versus deep vein thrombosis

Patients who present with pulmonary embolism (PE) have the same risk for a recurrent episode of

VTE as patients who present with proximal deep vein thrombosis (DVT) [3,34,37,38]. Nevertheless, patients with PE are about four times as likely to have a recurrence as PE when compared with patients who present initially with DVT [37–39], and this pattern of recurrence seems to persist long-term [38,39]. Approximately 10% of symptomatic PEs are thought to be rapidly fatal [40–42], and 5% or more of patients who have PE diagnosed and treated die of PE [38,39,43–46]. These observations suggest that, in patients who have completed 3 or more months of therapy for DVT or PE, recurrent VTE presenting as PE has a case–fatality rate of approximately 15%. The risk of dying of acute DVT because of subsequent PE or other complications (eg, bleeding, precipitation of myocardial infarction) seems to be 2% or less [23,38,39,44,47]. Based on these estimates for the proportion of recurrences that will be PE and DVT and the case–fatality rate associated with each presentation, the case–fatality rate associated with recurrent VTE that occurs 3 or months after a preceding PE is expected to be approximately 12% and the rate after a preceding DVT approximately 5%. Consistent with the latter estimate, an overview of randomized trials calculated a 5.1% case–fatality rate for recurrent VTE in patients with DVT who had completed 3 months of treatment [37]. Although the risk of a recurrence is the same after PE and proximal DVT, the consequence of a recurrence, including events that occur after the initial phase of treatment, seems to be much more severe after PE than after DVT.

Because they frequently have sustained recurrent episodes of PE and have a poor tolerance for further episodes of PE, patients with chronic thromboembolic pulmonary hypertension generally should be treated indefinitely [48].

Residual deep vein thrombosis

The resolution of DVT is often slow and incomplete. Approximately half of patients with proximal DVT have an abnormal compression ultrasound of the proximal veins 1 year after diagnosis and treatment [33,49,50]. The significance of residual DVT as a risk factor for recurrent VTE is unclear. After 3 months of treatment for unprovoked proximal DVT or PE in one study, residual DVT was not associated with subsequent recurrence (hazard ratio, 1.25; 95% confidence interval [CI], 0.5–3.3) [13]. Nevertheless, in a heterogeneous group of patients with proximal DVT, including those with asymptomatic thrombi or cancer, residual DVT after 3 months of treatment was associated with recurrence after stopping therapy (75% risk

in the ipsilateral leg) [33]. In that study, residual thrombosis was associated with initial large and symptomatic DVT and cancer [33].

In the duration of anticoagulation (DURAC) study that compared 6 weeks and 6 months of anticoagulant therapy for a first VTE, 59% of recurrent DVTs within 6 months of diagnosis involved the ipsilateral leg, whereas 31% of late recurrences were in the initially affected limb [51]. Most of the early recurrences were seen in patients who had stopped anticoagulants after 6 weeks of treatment. These observations suggest that early ipsilateral recurrences reflect inadequate initial treatment (ie, 6 weeks), whereas recurrences after adequate initial therapy (ie, 6 months) reflect a systemic predisposition to thrombosis. Patients with abnormal impedance plethysmography after 3 months of treatment for proximal DVT were not found to have a higher risk for recurrent VTE when compared with patients with normal plethysmography (relative risk, 1.3). This observation argues against residual DVT and local venous obstruction as a risk factor for recurrence [2].

Multiple previous episodes of venous thromboembolism

Intuitively, patients who have had more than one VTE, particularly if the interval between episodes is not long, are expected to have a higher risk of recurrence than patients with a first VTE. Contrary to this expectation, the DURAC investigators found a similar risk of recurrence during 2 years of follow-up after 6 months of treatment for a first and a second episode of VTE [3,52]. In contrast, in a large epidemiologic study of linked hospital discharge records, the risk of recurrence was approximately 50% higher during 2 years of follow-up after a second versus first DVT [53].

Vena caval filters

In a randomized trial that evaluated routine placement of vena caval filters as an adjunct to anticoagulant therapy in patients with proximal DVT, filters were shown to reduce the frequency of PE acutely (during the first 12 days) but almost doubled the long-term risk of recurrent DVT [54]. Despite increasing the risk of recurrent DVT, filters were not associated with more frequent PE. These findings are supported by another large epidemiologic study of linked hospital discharge records. In that study, a vena caval filter was an independent risk factor for recurrent DVT (odds ratio, 1.8) but not a risk factor for PE (odds ratio, 1.0) [38]. The filter-associated increase in DVT was largely confined to patients who presented initially with PE [53]. The findings of these two studies support the use of anticoagulant therapy in patients who have had a filter inserted when such therapy becomes safe (eg, bleeding risk resolves), and favor a more prolonged, but not necessarily indefinite, duration of such treatment (Table 1).

D-dimer and other factors

Laboratory evidence of increased activation of coagulation after withdrawal of anticoagulants may identify patients who are at a higher risk for recurrent VTE. A positive D-dimer level 1 or 3 months after stopping anticoagulant therapy was found to be associated with a two to threefold increase in recurrent VTE and seemed to be predictive of recurrence regardless of whether the initial VTE was unprovoked or provoked by a transient or persistent risk factor [7]. This approach to stratifying the risk for recurrent VTE requires confirmation and standardization before it can be recommended.

The influence of several other factors on the risk for recurrent VTE is noted in Table 1.

Risk factors for bleeding during anticoagulant therapy

Long-term anticoagulation targeted to an International Normalized Ratio (INR) of 2.0 to 3.0 is generally associated with an annual risk for major bleeding of approximately 3% [13,52,55,56]. Of these major bleeds, about one fifth are expected to be fatal (annual rate of fatal bleeding of approximately 0.6%) [55]. The risk of bleeding for individual patients may differ markedly from these estimates depending on the prevalence of risk factors for bleeding, such as the patient's age and gender (ie, female), the prevalence of certain comorbid conditions (eg, previous gastrointestinal bleeding or stroke, chronic renal disease, malignancy, alcohol-related disease, diabetes), and the use of concomitant antiplatelet therapy [55–60]. The risk of bleeding is highest shortly after starting anticoagulant therapy [55–57] and is higher if oral anticoagulation is difficult to control [56].

Recent randomized trials have demonstrated that better control of anticoagulant therapy can be achieved with computer-assisted dosing of warfarin versus traditional dosing by experienced medical staff alone [61] and by using a multicomponent intervention that promotes patient education and participation in anticoagulant management versus usual care [62].

The multicomponent intervention halved the frequency of major bleeding during the 6 months after anticoagulant therapy was started [62].

Two prospectively validated prediction rules have been published for assessing an individual's risk of major bleeding during the first 3 months of anticoagulant therapy [58,59] and thereafter [58]. Hereditary factors, such as polymorphisms that affect the cytochrome P-450 system of the liver, may increase sensitivity to warfarin and predispose the patient to anticoagulant-induced bleeding [63,64].

Relative importance of an episode of recurrent venous thromboembolism and an episode of major bleeding

When weighing the risks and benefits of anticoagulation in an individual patient, in addition to considering the absolute risk of thrombosis and major bleeding with and without anticoagulant therapy, the consequences associated with each of these outcomes need to be considered.

The consequences of recurrent VTE depend on whether the recurrence is a PE or DVT. Death is expected to result from 15% of PEs and 2% or less of DVTs. Initial presentation as a PE rather than DVT is the only factor other than previous insertion of a vena caval filter (risk factor for DVT only) that seems to influence markedly whether recurrent VTE is a PE versus DVT [38]. After the patient has completed 3 or more months of anticoagulant therapy, the case–fatality rate for recurrent VTE is expected to be 12% following PE and 5% following DVT.

The case–fatality rate associated with major bleeding during anticoagulant therapy is approximately 20% [55]. This rate is likely to be higher in patients with a history of ischemic stroke that is not caused by atrial fibrillation, because these patients are at a greater risk for intracerebral bleeding (case–fatality rate of approximately 50% [65]) than for other types of bleeding [65,66].

A comparison of associated case–fatality rates suggests that, on average, the consequence of a major bleed during long-term anticoagulation is about twice as severe as the consequence of a recurrent episode of VTE that occurs after a PE, and about four times as severe as the consequence of a recurrent episode of VTE that occurs after a DVT. The annual risk of recurrent VTE needs to exceed 6% after a PE and 12% after a DVT before one should consider long-term anticoagulation in patients with an average risk of bleeding (ie, approximately 3% per year [13,52,55,56]).

Direct comparisons of different durations of anticoagulant therapy

Short versus conventional durations of anticoagulant therapy

Four large trials have assessed the safety of shortening the duration of oral anticoagulant therapy from 3 or 6 months to 4 or 6 weeks [1–3,6]. The three studies that enrolled patients primarily with proximal DVT or PE found that shortening the duration of anticoagulation was associated with about double the frequency of recurrent VTE during follow-up [1–3]. Regardless of the duration of anticoagulation, major bleeding was uncommon in these three studies; therefore, it can be concluded that anticoagulant therapy should not be shortened to 4 or 6 weeks in patients with a first episode of VTE. Subgroup analyses of one study suggested that isolated calf vein thrombosis provoked by a major transient risk factor could be treated safely with only 6 weeks of therapy [3]. The fourth of these studies, which compared 6 versus 12 weeks of therapy in patients with isolated calf DVT (idiopathic or secondary), found that shortening therapy did not increase the risk of recurrence (relative risk, 0.58; 95% CI, 0.01–3.36) and was associated with a low frequency of recurrent VTE during follow-up (approximately 1.3% per year) [6].

Six or 12 months versus 3 months of anticoagulant therapy

Pinede and colleagues [6] compared 6 and 3 months of anticoagulant therapy in patients with a first episode of proximal DVT or PE (unprovoked or secondary). After 15 months of follow-up, the frequency of recurrent VTE did not differ between the two groups (relative risk, 0.93 in favor of 3 months; 95% CI, 0.53–1.65).

Agnelli and colleagues [67] compared stopping anticoagulant therapy at 3 months with continuing it for another 9 months after a first episode of unprovoked DVT. At the end of the first year, recurrent VTE was less frequent in the group that remained on anticoagulant therapy (3.0% versus 8.3%), but this benefit was lost 2 years after anticoagulant therapy was stopped (16% rate of recurrent VTE in both groups).

Prolonged versus conventional durations of anticoagulant therapy

Two trials have assessed long-term anticoagulation in different groups of patients believed to have

a high risk for recurrent VTE. Schulman and colleagues [52] compared 6 months versus 4 years of warfarin therapy in patients with a second episode of VTE. Recurrent VTE was markedly reduced by long-term oral anticoagulant therapy (0.65% versus 5.2% per year), but such therapy was associated with a higher frequency of major bleeding (2.2% versus 0.45% per year). Overall, there was no convincing benefit of long-term anticoagulation in this patient population.

Kearon and colleagues [13] compared an additional 2 years of anticoagulant therapy with placebo in patients with a first episode of idiopathic VTE who had completed 3 months of warfarin therapy. The trial was stopped after an average of 10 months of follow-up when an interim analysis revealed unexpectedly high recurrence rates (27% per year) in patients who discontinued warfarin after 3 months of treatment. Long-term warfarin therapy resulted in a 95% reduction in the risk of recurrent VTE but was associated with a 3.8% per year risk of major bleeding. It is not known whether the benefit accrued from the extended duration of therapy in this study could be achieved with less than 2 additional years of anticoagulation, or whether anticoagulants can be been stopped safely at the end of this period.

Recommended duration of anticoagulation in individual patients

Based on the previous analysis of risk factors for recurrent thrombosis and the findings of studies that have compared different durations of anticoagulation, an approach to selecting the optimal duration of anticoagulation for individual patients with VTE is outlined in Table 2. Because the presence or absence of a major reversible risk factor at the time of thrombosis seems to have the greatest prognostic influence on the risk for recurrence, this clinical categorization is the starting point. Factors that may modify the duration of anticoagulation within each category are then considered.

For patients who have VTE associated with a major transient risk factor, stopping anticoagulant therapy after 3 months of treatment is expected to be associated with a subsequent low risk of recurrent VTE of approximately 3% per year [1,2,5–7,23]. For patients who have unprovoked VTE, stopping anticoagulant therapy after 6 or more months of treatment is expected to be associated with a subsequent risk of recurrent VTE of approximately 10% per year [3,6,7,67]. The recurrence rate in such patients has tended to be lower than this estimate in European studies [6,7,67], and the rate seems to decrease over

Table 2
Recommended duration of anticoagulant therapy for venous thromboembolism

Recommended duration of therapy	Type of VTE and associated risk factors
VTE provoked by a major transient risk factor[a]	
3 months	Proximal DVT or PE
6 weeks	Isolated distal DVT
6 months	Protein C, protein S, antithrombin deficiencies; homozygous factor V Leiden or G20210A mutation in the prothrombin gene; antiphospholipid antibodies; combined thrombophilic abnormalities; concomitant cancer with a normal functional status; inferior vena cava filter; patient preference
VTE not provoked by a major transient risk factor	
6 months	Minor reversible risk factor (estrogen therapy, prolonged travel [4 hours], treated hyperhomocysteinemia); moderate risk of bleeding; patient preference
Long-term therapy[b]	More than one episode of idiopathic VTE; active cancer; protein C, protein S, antithrombin deficiencies; homozygous factor V Leiden or G20210A mutation in the prothrombin gene; antiphospholipid antibodies; combined thrombophilic abnormalities; severe immobilization; pulmonary embolism; pulmonary hypertension; severe postthrombotic syndrome; inferior vena cava filter; low risk of bleeding; patient preference
3 months	High risk for bleeding; isolated distal DVT; patient preference

Abbreviations: DVT, deep vein thrombosis; PE, pulmonary embolism; VTE, venous thromboembolism.

[a] Major transient risk factors include hospitalization, general anesthesia, 3 days of bedrest, leg fracture with or without plaster immobilization, all within 3 months.

[b] No upper limit to duration of anticoagulation. Decision to continue anticoagulant therapy may be changed if risk of bleeding increases or at patient's request.

time. For some patients, particularly those who have had a PE, this risk may be considered high enough to justify long-term therapy (Table 2). It is uncertain whether stopping anticoagulant therapy after 3 months rather than 6 months would be associated with a higher subsequent risk of recurrence in patients with unprovoked VTE. Although one study found a high risk of recurrence (approximately 27% per year) after 3 months of therapy in such patients [13], two others found much lower rates of recurrence after 3 months of treatment (approximately 7% per year), which were similar to the rates observed after 6 months [6] and 12 months [67] of treatment.

Summary

Prospective studies are providing a better understanding of the relative risk for recurrent thrombosis and anticoagulant-related bleeding in subgroups of patients with VTE, particularly during the extended phase of therapy. These findings in conjunction with the results of randomized trials evaluating specific anticoagulant and nonanticoagulant therapies are resulting in improvements in the management of VTE (Box 1). It is anticipated that ongoing studies will continue to identify clinical and biochemical risk factors for recurrent thrombosis and bleeding. Such research will determine whether lower intensities of oral anticoagulation (eg, INR < 2.0) are indicated for long-term secondary prophylaxis of VTE. The data obtained will clarify the role of extended-duration LMWH therapy in patients with and without cancer and may result in the development of novel antithrombotic agents that overcome the limitations of current therapies.

Box 1.

Key points

- Anticoagulant therapy should be stopped when its benefits (reduction of VTE) no longer clearly outweigh the risk of bleeding.
- Shortening the duration of anticoagulation from 3 [1,2] or 6 [3] months to 4 [1,2] or 6 [3] weeks results in a doubling of the frequency of recurrent VTE during 1 [1,2] to 2 [3] years of follow-up.

- Patients with VTE provoked by a transient risk factor have a lower (about one-third) risk of recurrence than do patients with an unprovoked VTE or a persistent risk factor [1–3, 5,7,23].
- Three months of anticoagulation is adequate treatment for VTE provoked by a transient risk factor; the subsequent risk of recurrence is 3% or less per patient-year [1,2,5–7,70].
- Three months of anticoagulation may not be adequate treatment for an unprovoked (idiopathic) episode of VTE; the subsequent early risk of recurrence has ranged from 5% to 25% per patient-year [3,6,7,13,67].
- After 6 months of anticoagulation, recurrent DVT is at least as likely to affect the contralateral leg; this observation suggests that systemic rather than local factors (including inadequate treatment) are responsible for recurrences after 6 months of treatment [51].
- There is a persistently elevated risk of recurrent VTE after a first episode; this risk is thought to be 5% to 12% per year after 6 or more months of treatment for an unprovoked episode [3,6,67].
- Oral anticoagulants targeted at an INR of approximately 2.5 are effective (risk reduction $\geq 90\%$) in preventing recurrent unprovoked VTE after the first 3 months of treatment [13,52].
- Indefinite anticoagulation is an option for patients with a first unprovoked VTE who have a low risk of bleeding.
- A second episode of VTE suggests a higher risk of recurrence but not necessarily high enough to justify indefinite anticoagulation [13,38].
- The risk of bleeding during anticoagulant therapy differs markedly among patients depending on the prevalence of risk factors (eg, advanced age, previous bleeding or stroke, renal failure, diabetes, anemia, antiplatelet therapy, malignancy, poor anticoagulant control) [57,58,60].

- The risk of PE is higher after an initial PE than after a DVT; this observation favors a longer duration of anticoagulation [38,39].
- The risk of recurrence is lower (about half) following an isolated calf (distal) DVT; this observation favors a shorter duration of treatment [3,6].
- The risk of recurrence is higher with antiphospholipid antibodies (anticardiolipin antibodies with or without lupus anticoagulants) [12,13], homozygous factor V Leiden [17], cancer [23], and, probably, antithrombin deficiency. These risk factors favor a longer duration of treatment.
- Heterozygous factor V Leiden and the G20210A prothrombin gene mutations do not seem to be clinically important risk factors for recurrence [17].
- Other abnormalities, such as elevated levels of clotting factors VIII, IX, and XI and homocysteine, and deficiencies of protein C and protein S, may be risk factors for recurrence; they have uncertain implications for the duration of treatment.
- For the purpose of influencing the duration of anticoagulant therapy, thrombophilia screening can be limited to situations in which the results of testing will change management, that is, (1) clinical assessment suggests an equivocal risk-to-benefit ratio for remaining on anticoagulants; and (2) test results have clear prognostic significance.

References

[1] Research Committee of the British Thoracic Society. Optimum duration of anticoagulation for deep-vein thrombosis and pulmonary embolism. Lancet 1992; 340:873–6.

[2] Levine MN, Hirsh J, Gent M, Turpie AG, Weitz J, Ginsberg J, et al. Optimal duration of oral anticoagulant therapy: a randomized trial comparing four weeks with three months of warfarin in patients with proximal deep vein thrombosis. Thromb Haemost 1995;74: 606–11.

[3] Schulman S, Rhedin A-S, Lindmarker P, Carlsson A,

Lärfars G, Nicol P, et al. A comparison of six weeks with six months of oral anticoagulant therapy after a first episode of venous thromboembolism. N Engl J Med 1995;332:1661–5.

[4] Prandoni P, Lensing AWA, Buller HR, Cogo A, Prins MH, Cattelan AM, et al. Deep-vein thrombosis and the incidence of subsequent symptomatic cancer. N Engl J Med 1992;327:1128–33.

[5] Pini M, Aiello S, Manotti C, Pattacini C, Quintavalla R, Poli T, et al. Low molecular weight heparin versus warfarin for the prevention of recurrence after deep vein thrombosis. Thromb Haemost 1994;72(2):191–7.

[6] Pinede L, Ninet J, Duhaut P, Chabaud S, Demolombe-Rague S, Durieu I, et al. Comparison of 3 and 6 months of oral anticoagulant therapy after a first episode of proximal deep vein thrombosis or pulmonary embolism and comparison of 6 and 12 weeks of therapy after isolated calf deep vein thrombosis. Circulation 2001;103:2453–60.

[7] Palareti G, Legnani C, Cosmi B, Guazzaloca G, Pancani C, Coccheri S. Risk of venous thromboembolism recurrence: high negative predictive value of D-dimer performed after oral anticoagulation is stopped. Thromb Haemost 2002;87:7–12.

[8] Kearon C, Crowther M, Hirsh J. Management of patients with hereditary hypercoagulable disorders. Annu Rev Med 2000;51:169–85.

[9] Lane DA, Mannucci PM, Bauer KA, Bertina RM, Bochkov NP, Boulyjenkov V, et al. Inherited thrombophilia. Part 1. Thromb Haemost 1996;76(5):651–62.

[10] Lane DA, Mannucci PM, Bauer KA, Bertina RM, Bochkov NP, Boulyjenkov V, et al. Inherited thrombophilia. Part 2. Thromb Haemost 1996;76(6):824–34.

[11] Rosendaal FR. Venous thrombosis: a multicausal disease. Lancet 1999;353:1167–73.

[12] Schulman S, Svenungsson E, Granqvist S. Anticardiolipin antibodies predict early recurrence of thromboembolism and death among patients with venous thromboembolism following anticoagulant therapy. Am J Med 1998;104:332–8.

[13] Kearon C, Gent M, Hirsh J, Weitz J, Kovacs MJ, Anderson DR, et al. A comparison of three months of anticoagulation with extended anticoagulation for a first episode of idiopathic venous thromboembolism. N Engl J Med 1999;340:901–7.

[14] Ridker PM, Miletich JP, Stampfer MJ, Goldhaber SZ, Lindpaintner K, Hennekens CH. Factor V Leiden and risks of recurrent idiopathic venous thromboembolism. Circulation 1995;92:2800–2.

[15] Simioni P, Prandoni P, Lensing AWA, Scudeller A, Sardella C, Prins MH, et al. The risk of recurrent venous thromboembolism in patients with an $Arg^{506} \rightarrow Gln$ mutation in the gene for factor V (factor V Leiden). N Engl J Med 1997;336:399–403.

[16] Eichinger S, Pabinger I, Stumpflen A, Hirschl M, Bialonczyk C, Schneider B, et al. The risk of recurrent venous thromboembolism in patients with and without factor V Leiden. Thromb Haemost 1997;77(4):624–8.

[17] Lindmarker P, Schulman S, Sten-Linder M, Wiman B, Egberg N, Johnsson H. The risk of recurrent venous thromboembolism in carriers and non-carriers of the G1691A allele in the coagulation factor V gene and the G20210A allele in the prothrombin gene. Thromb Haemost 1999;81:684–9.

[18] Miles JS, Miletich JP, Goldhaber SZ, Hennekens CH, Ridker PM. G20210A mutation in the prothrombin gene and the risk of recurrent venous thromboembolism. J Am Coll Cardiol 2001;37:215–8.

[19] Simioni P, Prandoni P, Lensing AW, Manfrin D, Tormene D, Gavasso S, et al. Risk for subsequent venous thromboembolic complications in carriers of the prothrombin or the factor V gene mutation with a first episode of deep-vein thrombosis. Blood 2000;96:3329–33.

[20] Eichinger S, Minar E, Hirschl M, Bialonczyk C, Stain M, Mannhalter C, et al. The risk of early recurrent venous thromboembolism after oral anticoagulant therapy in patients with the G20210A transition in the prothrombin gene. Thromb Haemost 1999;81:14–7.

[21] Margaglione M, Brancaccio V, Giuliani N, D'Andrea G, Cappucci G, Iannaccone L, et al. Increased risk for venous thrombosis in carriers of the prothrombin G–A 20210 gene variant [abstract]. Ann Intern Med 1998;129:89–93.

[22] DeStefano V, Martinelli I, Mannucci PM, Paciaroni K, Chiusolo P, Casorelli I, et al. The risk of recurrent deep venous thrombosis among heterozygous carriers of both factor V Leiden and the G20210A prothrombin mutation. N Engl J Med 1999;341:801–6.

[23] Prandoni P, Lensing AWA, Cogo A, Cuppini S, Villalta S, Carta M, et al. The long-term clinical course of acute deep venous thrombosis. Ann Intern Med 1996;125:1–7.

[24] Van den Belt AGM, Sanson BJ, Simioni P, Prandoni P, Buller HR, Girolami A, et al. Recurrence of venous thromboembolism in patients with familial thrombophilia. Arch Intern Med 1997;157:2227–32.

[25] Kryle P, Minar E, Hirschl M, Bialonczyk C, Stain M, Schneider B, et al. High plasma levels of factor VIII and the risk of recurrent venous thromboembolism. N Engl J Med 2000;343:457–62.

[26] Kraaijenhagen RA, in't Anker PS, Koopman MM, Reitsma PH, Prins MH, van den EA, et al. High plasma concentration of factor VIIIc is a major risk factor for venous thromboembolism. Thromb Haemost 2000;83:5–9.

[27] Cattaneo M. Hyperhomocysteinemia, atherosclerosis and thrombosis. Thromb Haemost 1999;81:165–76.

[28] Eichinger S, Stumpflen A, Hirschl M, Bialonczyk C, Herkner K, Stain M, et al. Hyperhomocysteinemia is a risk factor of recurrent venous thromboembolism. Thromb Haemost 1998;80:566–9.

[29] Willems HP, Den Heijer M, Bos GM. Homocysteine and venous thrombosis: outline of a vitamin intervention trial. Semin Thromb Hemost 2000;26:297–304.

[30] Hutten BA, Prins M, Gent M, Ginsberg J, Tijssen J, Buller H. Incidence of recurrent thromboembolic and bleeding complications among patients with venous

thromboembolism in relation to both malignancy and achieved international normalized ratio: a retrospective analysis. J Clin Oncol 2000;18:3078–83.

[31] Merli G, Spiro TE, Olsson CG, Abildgaard U, Davidson BL, Eldor A, et al. Subcutaneous enoxaparin once or twice daily compared with intravenous unfractionated heparin for treatment of venous thromboembolic disease. Ann Intern Med 2001;134:191–202.

[32] Palareti G, Legnani C, Lee A, Manotti C, Hirsh J, D'Angelo A, et al. A comparison of the safety and efficacy of oral anticoagulation for the treatment of venous thromboembolic disease in patients with or without malignancy. Thromb Haemost 2000;84:805–10.

[33] Piovella F, Crippa L, Barone M, Vigano DS, Serafini S, Galli L, et al. Normalization rates of compression ultrasonography in patients with a first episode of deep vein thrombosis of the lower limbs: association with recurrence and new thrombosis. Haematologica 2002; 87:515–22.

[34] Heit JA, Mohr DN, Silverstein MD, Petterson TM, O'Fallon WM, Melton III LJ. Predictors of recurrence after deep vein thrombosis and pulmonary embolism: a population-based cohort study. Arch Intern Med 2000;160:761–8.

[35] Zacharski LR, Ornstein DL. Heparin and cancer. Thromb Haemost 1998;80:10–23.

[36] Schulman S, Lindmarker P, for the Duration of Anticoagulation Trial. Incidence of cancer after prophylaxis with warfarin against recurrent venous thromboembolism. N Engl J Med 2000;342:1953–8.

[37] Douketis JD, Kearon C, Bates S, Duku EK, Ginsberg JS. Risk of fatal pulmonary embolism in patients with treated venous thromboembolism. JAMA 1998;279: 458–62.

[38] Murin S, Romano PS, White RH. Comparison of outcomes after hospitalization for deep vein thrombosis or pulmonary embolism. Thromb Haemost 2002;88: 407–14.

[39] Kniffin Jr WD, Baron JA, Barrett J, Birkmeyer JD, Anderson FA. The epidemiology of diagnosed pulmonary embolism and deep venous thrombosis in the elderly. Arch Intern Med 1994;154:861–6.

[40] Bell WR, Simon TL. Current status of pulmonary embolic disease: pathophysiology, diagnosis, prevention, and treatment. Am Heart J 1982;103:239–61.

[41] Stein PD, Henry JW. Prevalence of acute pulmonary embolism among patients in a general hospital and at autopsy. Chest 1995;108:978–81.

[42] Kearon C. Natural history of venous thromboembolism. Seminars in Vascular Medicine 2001;1:27–37.

[43] Goldhaber SZ, Visni L, De Rosa M. Acute pulmonary embolism: clinical outcomes in the International Cooperative Pulmonary Embolism Registry (ICOPER). Lancet 1999;353:1386–9.

[44] Heit JA, Silverstein MD, Mohr DN, Petterson TM, O'Fallon WM, Melton III LJ. Predictors of survival after deep vein thrombosis and pulmonary embolism: a population-based, cohort study. Arch Intern Med 1999;159:445–53.

[45] Ribeiro A, Lindmarker P, Juhlin-Dannfelt A, Johnsson H, Jorfeldt L. Echocardiography Doppler in pulmonary embolism: right ventricular dysfunction as a predictor of mortality rate. Am Heart J 1997;134:479–87.

[46] Bell CM, Redelmeier DA. Mortality among patients admitted to hospitals on weekends as compared with weekdays. N Engl J Med 2002;345:663–8.

[47] Beyth RJ, Cohen AM, Landefeld CS. Long-term outcomes of deep-vein thrombosis. Arch Intern Med 1995;155:1031–7.

[48] Fedullo PF, Auger WR, Kerr KM, Rubin LJ. Chronic thromboembolic pulmonary hypertension. N Engl J Med 2001;345:1465–72.

[49] Heijboer H, Jongbloets LMM, Buller HR, Lensing AWA, ten Cate JW. Clinical utility of real-time compression ultrasonography for diagnostic management of patients with recurrent venous thrombosis. Acta Radiol 1992;33:297–300.

[50] Prandoni P, Cogo A, Bernardi E, Villalta S, Polistena P, Simioni P, et al. A simple ultrasound approach for detection of recurrent proximal vein thrombosis. Circulation 1993;88:1730–5.

[51] Lindmarker P, Schulman S. The risk of ipsilateral versus contralateral recurrent deep vein thrombosis in the leg: the DURAC Trial Study Group. J Intern Med 2000;247:601–6.

[52] Schulman S, Granqvist S, Holmstrom M, Carlsson A, Lindmarker P, Nicol P, et al. The duration of oral anticoagulant therapy after a second episode of venous thromboembolism. N Engl J Med 1997;336:393–8.

[53] White RH, Zhou H, Kim J, Romano PS. A population-based study of the effectiveness of inferior vena cava filter use among patients with venous thromboembolism. Arch Intern Med 2000;160:2033–41.

[54] Decousus H, Leizorovicz A, Parent F, Page Y, Tardy B, Girard P, et al. A clinical trial of vena caval filters in the prevention of pulmonary embolism in patients with proximal deep-vein thrombosis. N Engl J Med 1998; 338:409–15.

[55] Landefeld CS, Beyth RJ. Anticoagulant-related bleeding: clinical epidemiology, prediction, and prevention. Am J Med 1993;95:315–28.

[56] Palareti G, Leali N, Coccheri S, Poggi M, Manotti C, D'Angelo A, et al. Bleeding complications of oral anticoagulant treatment: an inception-cohort, prospective collaborative study (ISCOAT). Lancet 1996;348: 423–8.

[57] White RH, Beyth RJ, Zhou H, Romano PS. Major bleeding after hospitalization for deep-venous thrombosis. Am J Med 1999;107:414–24.

[58] Beyth RJ, Quinn LM, Landefeld S. Prospective evaluation of an index for predicting the risk of major bleeding in outpatients treated with warfarin. Am J Med 1998;105:91–9.

[59] Kuijer PMM, Hutten BA, Prins MH, Buller HR. Prediction of the risk of bleeding during anticoagulant treatment for venous thromboembolism. Arch Intern Med 1999;159:457–60.

[60] Pengo V, Legnani C, Noventa F, Palareti G. Oral anti-

coagulant therapy in patients with nonrheumatic atrial fibrillation and risk of bleeding: a multicenter inception cohort study. Thromb Haemost 2001;85:418–22.

[61] Poller L, Shiach CR, MacCallum PK, Johansen AM, Munster AM, Magalhaes A, et al. Multicentre randomised study of computerised anticoagulant dosage: European Concerted Action on Anticoagulation. Lancet 1998;352:1505–9.

[62] Beyth RJ, Quinn L, Landefeld CS. A multicomponent intervention to prevent major bleeding complications in older patients receiving warfarin: a randomized controlled trial. Ann Intern Med 2000;133:687–95.

[63] Margaglione M, Colaizzo D, D'Andrea G, Brancaccio V, Ciampa A, Grandone E, et al. Genetic modulation of oral anticoagulation with warfarin. Thromb Haemost 2000;84:775–8.

[64] Aithal GP, Day CP, Kesteven PJ, Daly AK. Association of polymorphisms in the cytochrome P450 CYP2C9 with warfarin dose requirement and risk of bleeding complications. Lancet 1999;353:717–9.

[65] Hylek EM, Singer DE. Risk factors for intracranial hemorrhage in outpatients taking warfarin. Ann Intern Med 1994;120:897–902.

[66] The Stroke Prevention In Reversible Ischemia Trial (SPIRIT) Study Group. A randomized trial of anticoagulants versus aspirin after cerebral ischemia of presumed arterial origin. Ann Neurol 1997;42: 857–65.

[67] Agnelli G, Prandoni P, Santamaria MG, Bagatella P, Iorio A, Bazzan M, et al. Three months versus one year of oral anticoagulant therapy for idiopathic deep vein thrombosis. N Engl J Med 2001;345:165–9.

[68] Grady D, Wenger NK, Herrington D, Khan S, Furberg C, Hunninghake D, et al. Postmenopausal hormone therapy increases risk for venous thromboembolic disease: the Heart and Estrogen/progestin Replacement Study. Ann Intern Med 2000;132:689–96.

[69] Hoibraaten E, Qvigstad E, Arnesen H, Larsen S, Wickstrom E, Sandset PM. Increased risk of recurrent venous thromboembolism during hormone replacement therapy – results of the randomized, double-blind, placebo- controlled estrogen in venous thromboembolism trial (EVTET). Thromb Haemost 2000;84:961–7.

[70] Pinede L, Duhaut P, Cucherat M, Ninet J, Pasquier J, Boissel JP. Comparison of long versus short duration of anticoagulant therapy after a first episode of venous thromboembolism: a meta-analysis of randomized, controlled trials. J Intern Med 2000;247:553–62.

Clin Chest Med 24 (2003) 73–91

CLINICS
IN CHEST
MEDICINE

Local and systemic thrombolytic therapy for acute venous thromboembolism

Selim M. Arcasoy, MD, FCCP, FACP[a,b,*], Anil Vachani, MD[c]

[a]Pulmonary, Allergy, and Critical Care Division, Columbia University College of Physicians and Surgeons,
622 West 168th Street, New York, NY 10032, USA
[b]Lung Transplantation Program, New York Presbyterian Hospital of Columbia and Cornell University,
622 West 168th Street, New York, NY 10032, USA
[c]Pulmonary, Allergy, and Critical Care Division, University of Pennsylvania School of Medicine, 3400 Spruce Street,
Philadelphia, PA 19104, USA

Pulmonary embolism (PE) and deep venous thrombosis (DVT), collectively referred to as venous thromboembolism (VTE), are common disorders associated with substantial morbidity and mortality. PE is estimated to occur in approximately 600,000 patients annually in the United States, causing or contributing to 50,000 to 200,000 deaths [1–3]. Autopsy series have shown that PE is responsible for, or at least accompanies, as many as 15% of all in-hospital deaths, further highlighting the significance of this problem [2,4,5]. Moreover, a disturbingly small fraction of patients with this common and lethal disorder is recognized antemortem, with the majority of deaths occurring in the first few hours of presentation [6–9].

The importance of DVT stems from its short- and long-term local complications in the affected extremity, as well as its frequent association with PE, which is seen in as many as 40% to 50% of patients with symptomatic proximal DVT [10–12]. Acutely, DVT results in considerable symptoms. In a small number of cases, extensive venous obstruction may lead to limb-threatening ischemia, known as phlegmasia cerulea dolens. Long-term, the two major consequences of DVT are recurrent VTE and the development of postthrombotic syndrome (PTS) [13–17].

Currently, anticoagulation remains the standard of care for VTE. Anticoagulation prevents clot propagation and allows endogenous fibrinolytic activity to dissolve existing thrombi, a process that typically occurs over several weeks or months. Nonetheless, incomplete resolution is not uncommon after several months and may result in organization of thromboemboli and obliteration of the pulmonary or deep venous vascular system [18–24].

Thrombolytic therapy, by actively dissolving thromboemboli, offers several potential advantages over anticoagulation in the treatment of patients with VTE (Fig. 1) [25]. By virtue of its ability to produce more rapid clot lysis, thrombolysis may result in earlier improvement in pulmonary perfusion, hemodynamic alterations, gas exchange, and right ventricular function in patients with PE. Thrombolysis also may eliminate venous thrombi, the source of PE, thereby reducing the risk of recurrence. Furthermore, rapid and more complete clot resolution may prevent the development of chronic vascular obstruction and thromboembolic pulmonary hypertension. Through all of these mechanisms, thrombolytic therapy offers the potential to reduce morbidity and mortality from PE. Likewise, thrombolysis offers similar benefits in the treatment of DVT by rapidly improving short-term venous patency, which, in turn, may result in a

* Corresponding author. Pulmonary, Allergy, and Critical Care Division, Columbia University College of Physicians and Surgeons, 622 West 168th Street, New York, NY 10032.
E-mail address: sa2059@columbia.edu (S.M. Arcasoy).

0272-5231/03/$ – see front matter © 2003, Elsevier Inc. All rights reserved.
doi:10.1016/S0272-5231(02)00051-5

Venous Thromboembolism

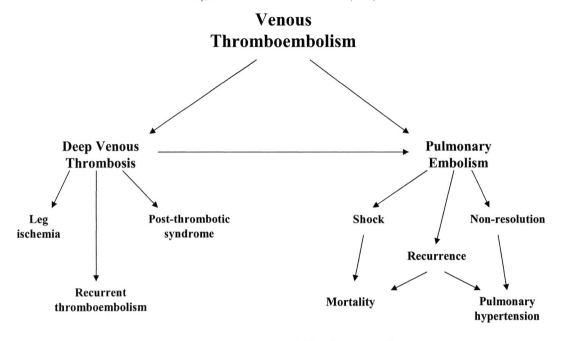

Fig. 1. Adverse outcomes of VTE with potential benefit from thrombolytic therapy.

decrease in the risk of embolization and the development of PTS.

Despite its potential advantages, the widespread interest in its use, and more than 3 decades of investigation, the role of thrombolytic therapy in VTE remains unsettled. A recent report from the Sixth American College of Chest Physicians (ACCP) Consensus Conference on Antithrombotic Therapy suggested a highly individualized approach to the use of thrombolytic agents in the treatment of VTE, recommending thrombolysis in patients at low risk for bleeding with hemodynamically unstable PE or massive iliofemoral thrombosis [26].

This article provides a comprehensive review of the literature evaluating the efficacy and safety of thrombolytic therapy in patients with VTE, with a focus on PE. Using data drawn primarily from randomized controlled trials and large registries, the following topics in PE thrombolysis are discussed and recommendations for the use of thrombolytic therapy are provided:

- Efficacy of thrombolytic therapy
- Comparison of thrombolytic agents
- Methods of delivery
- Timing of PE thrombolysis
- Hemorrhagic complications
- Practical aspects of PE thrombolysis
- Special circumstances

Thrombolytic therapy for DVT is discussed briefly, with an emphasis on its short- and long-term efficacy and complications.

Pulmonary embolism

Efficacy of thrombolytic therapy

Data from randomized trials

The National Institutes of Health–sponsored Urokinase Pulmonary Embolism Trial (UPET) was the first study to evaluate PE thrombolysis in a controlled fashion [18]. In this large prospective trial, 160 patients with angiographically documented PE were randomized to receive either a 12-hour infusion of urokinase followed by heparin or heparin alone. At 24 hours, the degree of improvement in hemodynamic measurements and pulmonary blood flow as assessed by angiography and perfusion scan was significantly greater in patients who had received urokinase. Nevertheless, serial perfusion scans performed over 12 months revealed that the quantitative difference in resolution between the two groups decreased progressively after 24 hours such that no difference was found beyond 5 days. Furthermore, no difference in mortality or the rate of PE recurrence was detected between the two groups.

A small subset of 40 patients who were enrolled in either the UPET or the subsequent Urokinase–Streptokinase Embolism Trial (USET) underwent measurements of diffusing capacity and pulmonary capillary blood volume as surrogate markers of small vessel patency 2 weeks and 1 year after therapy with heparin or thrombolytic agents [27]. Although no difference in the degree of perfusion scan resolution had been evident, both of these measurements were initially low in the heparin arm and remained unchanged at 1 year, whereas both values were within the normal range at 2 weeks and improved further by 1 year in the thrombolytic therapy arm. These results are suggestive of more complete resolution of emboli by thrombolysis in small peripheral vessels that are beyond the resolution of perfusion scanning or angiography.

Long-term effects of thrombolytic therapy were assessed by clinical follow-up and hemodynamic studies in the same group of 40 patients more than 7 years after their initial PE [28]. At the end of the follow-up period, more patients in the heparin group had recurrent VTE and dyspnea on exertion when compared with the patients treated with thrombolysis. Twenty-three patients underwent right-sided heart catheterization and measurement of resting and exercise hemodynamics. The group that had received heparin alone had elevated resting pulmonary artery pressure and pulmonary vascular resistance, both of which increased significantly with exercise. The group treated with thrombolytic agents demonstrated normal resting values and normal response to exercise. The observations from this small study suggest that thrombolytic therapy prevents the development of pulmonary hypertension by achieving more complete resolution of emboli and decreasing the risk of subsequent PE recurrence.

Since the UPET trial, eight smaller randomized studies have prospectively compared the efficacy and safety of various thrombolytic agents with heparin in patients with PE [29–36]. In general, these studies, which are summarized in Table 1, were not designed to assess survival as a primary endpoint but focused on various surrogate markers of the degree and rate of clot resolution. The total numbers of patients treated with thrombolysis and heparin were 241 and 220, respectively. The vast majority of the studies revealed that, in the first 24 hours, thrombolytic therapy resulted in more rapid clot resolution than treatment with heparin alone as assessed by angiography, perfusion scan, and hemodynamic measurements [25]. Within 5 to 7 days, both treatments produced similar improvements in pulmonary perfusion as assessed by perfusion scan. Although most of the studies demonstrated no significant differences in

mortality or PE recurrence rates, this finding may be related to inadequate power to detect a difference. Two of the PE thrombolysis studies deserve more detailed discussion.

In 1993, Goldhaber et al reported the results of a randomized trial of 101 normotensive patients treated with either alteplase (rt-PA) or heparin [35]. Baseline right ventricular function was assessed by echocardiography, which was repeated 3 and 24 hours after the start of therapy. In addition, perfusion scans were obtained before and 24 hours after the initiation of treatment. Patients receiving rt-PA had a greater improvement in right ventricular function and pulmonary perfusion than patients receiving heparin alone. Moreover, in the group receiving heparin, there were two fatal and three nonfatal clinically suspected PE recurrences during the first 14 days. None of the patients treated with rt-PA experienced a recurrence, and this difference approached, but did not reach, statistical significance ($P = 0.06$). It is important to note that all of the recurrences occurred in patients with right ventricular dysfunction on baseline echocardiography.

Two years later, Jerjes-Sanchez et al reported the results of a small study in which eight patients with shock owing to massive PE were randomized to receive bolus streptokinase or heparin [36]. No deaths occurred in the streptokinase group, whereas all of the patients receiving heparin alone died, resulting in a statistically significant difference between treatment groups and premature termination of the study. This study was the first and only randomized trial to demonstrate a survival advantage with thrombolytic therapy. Nevertheless, the results are difficult to interpret, because patients receiving heparin presented initially with hemodynamic stability but then experienced severe respiratory failure and shock owing to massive PE recurrence. Therefore, there was a much longer interval between the onset of symptoms and randomization in the heparin group when compared with the patients receiving streptokinase. Additionally, patients receiving streptokinase did not have a PE recurrence before enrollment in the study.

Risk stratification and right ventricular dysfunction

Conflicting data and the lack of a clear advantage of thrombolytic therapy over anticoagulation in reducing clinically important adverse outcomes suggest the possibility that only a subset of patients with PE may benefit from aggressive therapy with thrombolysis. Clearly, the risk–benefit ratio of thrombolytic therapy is expected to be most favorable in patients who are at highest risk for mortality from PE. Hemodynamic instability, defined as hypotension

Table 1
Randomized trials comparing thrombolytic and heparin therapy for pulmonary embolism

Author (year)	Number of patients	Treatment regimens[a,b]	Mortality, n (%)	Recurrent PE[c], n (%)	Major hemorrhage[d], n (%)
UPET (1970) [18]	78	Heparin	7 (8.9)	15 (19)	21 (27)
	82	UK, 2000 U/lb bolus, 2000 U/lb/h for 12 h	6 (7.3)	12 (15)	37 (45)
Tibbutt et al (1974) [29]	17	Intrapulmonary heparin	1 (5.8)	1 (5.8)	1 (5.8)
	13	Intrapulmonary SK, 600,000 U bolus, 100,000 U/h for 72 h	0	0	1 (8)
Ly et al (1978) [30]	11	Heparin	2 (18.2)	ND	2 (18.2)
	14	SK, 250,000 U bolus, 100,000 U/h for 72 h	1 (7.1)	ND	4 (29)
Marini et al (1988) [31]	10	Heparin	0	0	0
	10	UK, 800,000 U/d infused over 12 h for 3 d	0	0	0
	10	UK, 3,300,000 U infused over 12 h	0	0	0
PIOPED (1990) [32]	4	Heparin	0	ND	0
	9	rt-PA, 40–80 mg over 40–90 min and concomitant heparin	1 (11.1)	ND	1 (11.1)
Levine et al (1990) [33]	25	Heparin	0	0	0
	33	rt-PA, 0.6 mg/kg over 2 min	1 (3)	0	0
PAIMS 2: Dalla-Volta et al (1992) [34]	16	Heparin	1 (6.3)	3 (18.8)	2 (12.5)
	20	rt-PA, 100 mg over 2 h	2 (10)	1 (5)	3 (15)
Goldhaber et al (1993) [35]	55	Heparin	2 (3.6)	5 (9.1)	1 (1.8)
	46	rt-PA, 100 mg over 2 h	0	0	2 (4.3)
Jerjes-Sanchez et al (1995) [36]	4	Heparin	4 (100)	ND	0
	4	SK, 1,500,000 U over 1 h	0[e]	ND	0

Abbreviations: ND, no data; PE, pulmonary embolism; rt-PA, alteplase; SK, streptokinase; UK, urokinase.

[a] Unless specified, treatment was administered intravenously.

[b] In all studies, heparin was adjusted to maintain a therapeutic partial thromboplastin time. In most of the studies, thrombolytic therapy was followed by heparin infusion.

[c] Recurrent PE rate includes clinically suspected but unconfirmed cases as well as those episodes confirmed by objective tests.

[d] The definition of major hemorrhage varied between trials but usually included intracranial hemorrhage, bleeding that required surgery, transfusion, or resulted in death, or a decrease in hematocrit of more than 10 or 15 percentage points.

[e] $P < 0.05$. All other comparisons did not reach statistical significance.

Adapted from Arcasoy SM, Kreit JW. Thrombolytic therapy of pulmonary embolism: a comprehensive review of current evidence. Chest 1999;115:1695–707; with permission.

with or without shock, is present in 5% to 10% of patients with PE and has been identified repeatedly as a strong predictor of death, with mortality rates exceeding 50% in hemodynamically unstable patients [18,37–40]. Although thrombolysis has proven beneficial in the setting of hemodynamic instability, these patients represent only a small subset of patients with PE, because the vast majority of deaths occur before the recognition of PE [36]. This fact has led to the investigation of other markers of adverse outcomes in the remaining majority of patients who are hemodynamically stable. Although several patient and clinical characteristics, including older age, underlying cardiopulmonary disease, certain electrocardiographic findings, elevated cardiac troponins, and the identification of a patent foramen ovale, have been identified as prognostic markers, the echocardiographic finding of right ventricular dysfunction has gained increasing popularity as a component of risk assessment and treatment decisions [40–47]. Recent studies suggest that right ventricular dysfunction is a frequent finding in acute PE, detected in 30% to 50% of patients who undergo echocardiography [40,47–49]. Most of these studies have identified the presence of right ventricular dysfunction in hemodynamically stable patients as a marker of poor prognosis.

Wolfe et al investigated the relationship between right ventricular hypokinesis and the extent of perfusion defects on the initial lung scan in 90 hemodynamically stable patients [48]. Thirty-eight patients (42%) had right ventricular hypokinesis, which was typically identified when the perfusion defect exceeded 30%. All five patients with recurrent symptomatic PE were in the group with right ventricular hypokinesis.

In a study of 126 consecutive patients with PE, echocardiography on the day of diagnosis revealed moderate-to-severe right ventricular dysfunction in 70 (56%) [49]. The overall in-hospital mortality rate was 7.9%, with deaths occurring exclusively in patients with significant right ventricular dysfunction. On multivariate analysis, right ventricular dysfunction was associated with in-hospital and 1-year mortality; however, because systemic blood pressure was not reported, this study does not provide adequate information to determine the independent impact of right ventricular dysfunction on prognosis in patients with PE.

In 1999, the results of the International Cooperative Pulmonary Embolism Registry (ICOPER), investigating the prognostic impact of baseline clinical factors on 3-month mortality were published. In this registry of 2454 consecutive patients with PE, 40% of the patients who underwent baseline echocardiography had right ventricular hypokinesis [40]. The presence of right ventricular hypokinesis was an independent predictor of mortality, doubling the risk of death during the follow-up period.

Recently, Grifoni et al investigated 209 consecutive patients with PE and identified right ventricular dysfunction in 31% of patients with normal systemic blood pressure [47]. In that group, shock owing to PE developed in 10%, resulting in death in half of these patients. In contrast, none of the normotensive patients with normal right ventricular function had a PE-related death.

The initial evidence of the efficacy of thrombolytic therapy in the setting of PE and isolated right

ventricular dysfunction came from the study of Goldhaber et al, as discussed in the previous section. Further support for this concept emerged from the analysis of the Management Strategy and Prognosis of Pulmonary Embolism Registry (MAPPET), which included 1001 patients [50]. The clinical course of 719 patients presenting with right ventricular dysfunction with or without pulmonary hypertension, excluding those with shock, was reported in 1997. In this nonrandomized study, 169 patients initially received thrombolytic therapy, whereas 550 were treated with heparin alone. There were important baseline differences between treatment groups, including older age and a higher frequency of underlying cardiopulmonary disease in the heparin arm. Moreover, the treatment decision was left to the discretion of the attending physician, with a potential for selection bias. In the group undergoing thrombolysis, mortality at 30 days and the rate of recurrent PE were significantly lower than in the heparin-treated group, but the bleeding rate was much higher. Despite its shortcomings, this study was the first to demonstrate a survival advantage with thrombolytic therapy in patients without shock and supports the trend noted previously by Goldhaber and colleagues for thrombolysis to reduce the risk of recurrent PE.

The findings of Goldhaber et al and the MAPPET have provided justification for thrombolytic therapy in normotensive patients with PE and right ventricular dysfunction [46,51]. The proponents of this approach believe that patients with right ventricular dysfunction have "impending hemodynamic instability" with a larger clot burden and a lower likelihood of tolerating recurrent PE. They argue that rapid improvement in pulmonary blood flow, reversal of right ventricular dysfunction, and elimination of the source of recurrent emboli by thrombolytic therapy will improve the outcomes in this setting. However, although rapid reversal of right ventricular dysfunction can be achieved by thrombolytic therapy, it has never been demonstrated conclusively that the PE recurrence rate can be reduced by thrombolysis [35,52,53]. More importantly, right ventricular dysfunction has a low positive predictive value for mortality; the majority of hemodynamically stable patients with right ventricular dysfunction have a good prognosis and survive when treated with anticoagulation alone [47,54]. The extension of thrombolytic therapy to this large subset of patients with a good prognosis would lead to a significantly increased incidence of bleeding, outweighing any potential benefits of thrombolysis.

Furthermore, a recent report from a single-center registry of 128 patients with massive PE and right ventricular dysfunction sharply contradicts the results of the MAPPET [55]. In this study, patients treated with thrombolytic therapy had significantly worse outcomes when compared with patients treated with anticoagulation. Although the PE recurrence rate was the same in both groups, significantly higher rates of in-hospital mortality and intracranial and other severe hemorrhage were observed in the thrombolysis arm.

Recommended indications for thrombolytic therapy

Based on the ability of thrombolytic therapy to reduce clot burden rapidly and improve hemodynamic abnormalities and on the survival advantage demonstrated by Jerjes-Sanchez and colleagues, patients with PE and circulatory shock should be treated with thrombolytic therapy unless an overwhelming contraindication exists [25]. Thrombolysis has never been proven to reduce mortality or the risk of recurrent PE in hemodynamically stable patients. Given the increased risk of major hemorrhage that accompanies thrombolytic therapy, patients in this category should generally be treated with heparin alone. As discussed previously, PE thrombolysis based solely on the presence of right ventricular dysfunction in hemodynamically stable patients is controversial, because insufficient data are available

Table 2
Randomized trials comparing the efficacy and safety of thrombolytic agents

Author (year)	Number of patients	Treatment regimens[a]	Mortality, n (%)	Recurrent PE[b], n (%)	Major hemorrhage[c], n (%)
USET Phase 2 (1974) [37]	59	UK, 2000 U/lb bolus, 2,000 U/lb/h for 12 h	4 (7)	1 (1)	8 (14)
	54	UK, 2000 U/lb bolus, 2,000 U/lb/h for 24 h	5 (9)	4 (7)	10 (19)
	54	SK, 250,000 U bolus, 100,000 U/h for 24 h	5 (9)	2 (4)	6 (11)
Goldhaber et al (1988) [56]	23	UK, 2000 U/lb bolus, 2000 U/lb/h for 24 h	2 (8.7)	1 (4)	11 (48)
	22	rt-PA, 100 mg over 2 h	2 (8.7)	0	4 (18)
Meyer et al (1992) [57]	29	UK, 4400 U/kg bolus, 4400 U/kg/h for 12 h	1 (3.4)	2 (6.9)	8 (28)
	34	rt-PA, 80–100 mg over 2 h	3 (8.8)	2 (5.9)	7 (21)
Goldhaber et al (1992) [58]	46	UK, 1,000,000 U over 10 min, 2,000,000 U over 110 min	1 (?)	3 (6 5)	6 (13)
	44	rt-PA, 100 mg over 2 h	2 (4.5)	0	9 (20)
Meneveau et al (1997) [59]	25	SK, 250,000 U bolus, 100,000 U/h for 12 h	1 (4)	2 (8)	3 (12)
	25	rt-PA, 100 mg over 2 h	1 (4)	0	4 (16)
Meneveau et al (1998) [60]	43	SK, 1,500,000 U over 2 h	0	1 (2.3)	3 (7.0)
	23	rt-PA, 100 mg over 2 h	0	2 (8.7)	5 (21.7)
Tebbe et al (1999) [61]	23	Reteplase, 10 U, two injections 30 min apart	1 (4)	0	4 (17.4)
	13	rt-PA, 100 mg over 2 h	2 (15)	1 (7.7)	1 (7.7)

Abbreviations: PE, pulmonary embolism; rt-PA, alteplase; SK, streptokinase; UK, urokinase.

[a] In all studies, heparin was adjusted to maintain a therapeutic partial thromboplastin time. In most of the studies, thrombolytic therapy was followed by heparin infusion.

[b] Recurrent PE rate includes clinically suspected but unconfirmed cases as well as those episodes confirmed by objective tests.

[c] The definition of major hemorrhage varied between trials but usually included intracranial hemorrhage, bleeding that required surgery, transfusion, or resulted in death, or a decrease in hematocrit of more than 10 or 15 percentage points.

Adapted from Arcasoy SM, Kreit JW. Thrombolytic therapy of pulmonary embolism: a comprehensive review of current evidence. Chest 1999;115:1695–707; with permission.

to support this practice. Clearly, a large prospective randomized trial is needed to settle this issue and to identify precisely the subset of patients with right ventricular dysfunction and a higher risk of mortality who would benefit most from thrombolysis. The authors believe that, until such data are available, right ventricular dysfunction alone is not an indication for thrombolytic therapy. Lastly, many experts would consider severe respiratory failure with refractory hypoxemia as another potential indication for thrombolytic therapy, although this view has never been investigated formally.

Comparison of thrombolytic agents

Randomized controlled trials comparing streptokinase, urokinase, rt-PA, and reteplase are summarized in Table 2 [37,56–61]. The earliest and largest of these trials was the USET, which included 167 patients with angiographically demonstrated PE [37]. Patients were randomized to treatment with 12 hours of urokinase, 24 hours of urokinase, or 24 hours of streptokinase. Similar improvements in angiographic severity scores, hemodynamic variables, and perfusion scans were found in all groups at 24 hours, although no difference in the resolution of lung scan defects between groups was detected at 3 or 6 months. The rates of mortality, recurrent PE, and major hemorrhage were not significantly different.

Six subsequent trials have compared 2-hour infusions of rt-PA with 24-, 12-, and 2-hour regimens of urokinase, 12- and 2-hour infusions of streptokinase, and, most recently, two bolus injections of reteplase [56–61]. These trials revealed that a 2-hour infusion of rt-PA resulted in more rapid clot lysis when compared with the 12- or 24-hour regimens of urokinase and streptokinase; however, these agents have comparable efficacy and safety when equivalent doses are delivered at the same rate within the same time period. Similarly, the efficacy and safety of rt-PA and reteplase do not seem to be significantly different. The thrombolytic regimens available for the treatment of VTE are listed in Table 3. Three thrombolytic agents with specific regimens are approved by the United States Food and Drug Administration (FDA) for the treatment of PE.

Methods of delivery

Thrombolytic agents can be administered systemically or locally into the pulmonary artery. Interest in the local delivery of thrombolytic agents is based on several potential advantages over systemic administration [62–66]. Delivery of the drug directly into the

Table 3
Thrombolytic regimens used for treatment of venous thromboembolism

Drug	Regimen[a]
Streptokinase	250,000 U over 30 min followed by 100,000 U/h for 24 h[b,c] 250,000 U over 30 min followed by 100,000 U/h for 12 h 1,500,000 U over 1 to 2 h
Urokinase	4400 U/kg over 10 min followed by 4400 U/kg/h for 24 h[b] 4400 U/kg over 10 min followed by 4400 U/kg/h for 12 h[b] 1,000,000 U over 10 min followed by 2,000,000 U over 110 min
rt-PA	100 mg over 2 h[b]
Reteplase	Two injections of 10 U 30 min apart

Abbreviations: rt-PA, alteplase.
[a] All agents are administered as a continuous peripheral intravenous infusion.
[b] Approved by the US Food and Drug Administration for pulmonary embolism thrombolysis.
[c] A 72-hour infusion using the same dose is approved for the treatment of deep venous thrombosis.

pulmonary artery might be accompanied by more rapid or more complete clot lysis and, because of high local drug concentrations, low doses might be able to achieve the same degree of thrombolysis as higher systemic doses. Furthermore, local therapy might reduce the risk of bleeding, especially if lower doses are used. The major disadvantage of local therapy is the requirement for pulmonary artery catheterization, which is associated with an increased risk of bleeding from the vascular access site.

Only one controlled study has compared intrapulmonary and systemic thrombolysis. Verstraete et al randomized patients with angiographically proven massive PE to receive 50 mg of either intrapulmonary or intravenous rt-PA over 2 hours [67]. Angiography was then repeated, and a second dose of 50 mg was infused over 5 hours if sufficient improvement had not occurred. The rate and degree of improvement in pulmonary hemodynamics and perfusion and the incidence of major hemorrhage were not influenced by the route of drug administration.

A potentially more effective role of local thrombolysis is the combined use of a low-dose thrombolytic agent and mechanical adjuncts to assist in clot disruption, especially in patients with a higher bleeding risk. Local pharmacomechanical thrombolysis using low doses of urokinase or rt-PA and either intraembolic infusion or mechanical clot disruption has been used in several case series [62–64,66]. In one report, six patients with contraindications to systemic thrombolysis received low-dose intraembolic thrombolytic therapy using specialized catheters, which resulted in an impressive degree of angiographic improvement in all patients and no bleeding [64]. In a more recent larger series of 59 patients with massive PE, mechanical fragmentation and intrapulmonary thrombolysis led to clinical improvement in 56 patients [66].

Bolus thrombolysis is another approach that has been suggested to improve clot lysis and decrease the risk of bleeding by achieving a higher drug concentration over a shorter period of time. Two prospective randomized trials comparing bolus dose rt-PA with the traditional 2-hour regimen revealed no significant intergroup differences in the rate of angiographic, lung scan, and hemodynamic improvement, and bleeding rates [68–70].

In summary, the limited available controlled data do not support the use of bolus therapy or the use of intrapulmonary versus systemic thrombolytic therapy. Further research is needed to determine the precise role of local pharmacomechanical thrombolysis employing low doses of thrombolytic agents, especially in the treatment of patients with PE who are at high risk for bleeding complications.

Timing of pulmonary embolism thrombolysis

Contemporary studies of PE thrombolysis have included patients with symptoms up to 14 days before the diagnosis. Daniels et al combined data from 308 patients who participated in five multicenter trials to study the relationship between the duration of symptoms and the efficacy of thrombolytic therapy [71]. Based on perfusion lung scan improvement, this analysis documented a progressive decrease in the efficacy of thrombolytic therapy with increasing symptom duration; therefore, once the diagnosis is established, thrombolytic therapy should be carried out as early as possible. However, it is important to note that the benefit of thrombolysis extends up to 14 days after symptom onset.

Hemorrhagic complications

Hemorrhage following thrombolytic therapy most commonly occurs at vascular puncture sites, although spontaneous hemorrhage, especially gastrointestinal, retroperitoneal, and intracranial, may also occur. Older age, a higher body mass index, and the performance of pulmonary angiography have been identified as sig-

nificant predictors of bleeding [72]. As shown in Tables 1 and 2, the reported rate of major hemorrhage with thrombolytic and heparin therapy has ranged from 0% to 48% and 0% and 27%, respectively [25]. This wide range can be explained by more aggressive diagnostic and follow-up protocols in earlier studies and by variable definitions of "major hemorrhage." When major hemorrhage is defined arbitrarily as fatal hemorrhage, intracranial hemorrhage, or bleeding that requires surgery or transfusion, a review of controlled studies comparing thrombolysis and heparin yields an average incidence of 6.3% and 1.8%, respectively (see Table 1) [25]. When data from randomized studies comparing different thrombolytic agents are also considered, the overall incidence of major hemorrhage with PE thrombolysis increases to approximately 12%, with no significant differences in risk between the three agents (Table 2) [25].

The most dreaded bleeding complication is intracranial hemorrhage. An intracranial neoplasm or aneurysm, a recent cerebrovascular accident, and recent central nervous system trauma or surgery clearly increase the risk of intracranial hemorrhage. In addition, an overview of five previously published studies identified elevated diastolic blood pressure at the time of presentation as an additional risk factor for intracranial hemorrhage [73]. Pooled data from 19 randomized studies in which 932 patients received thrombolytic therapy revealed that the overall incidence of intracranial hemorrhage was 1.2%, with death occurring in about half of these patients. It is important to point out that in the ICOPER, the rate of intracranial hemorrhage was much higher at 3% in 304 patients treated with thrombolysis [40]. This higher rate of intracranial hemorrhage based on registry data may be more reflective of the real risk in routine clinical practice, because randomized controlled trials are equipped with multiple mechanisms to ensure safety and prevent complications [45].

Practical aspects of pulmonary embolism thrombolysis

Diagnosis of pulmonary embolism before thrombolytic therapy

A detailed discussion of the diagnostic evaluation of PE is beyond the scope of this article. The comments herein are limited to diagnostic techniques performed in the context of massive PE when thrombolytic therapy is considered. Because thrombolysis is accompanied by a significant risk of major hemorrhage, it is essential to confirm the presence of PE before the initiation of treatment, preferably with noninvasive imaging techniques. For instance, in the presence of a high pretest clinical suspicion, a high-probability ventilation–perfusion scan is sufficient to establish the diagnosis of PE; however, definitive diagnostic combinations of clinical and ventilation–perfusion scan probabilities are not observed in most patients. Spiral computed tomography of the chest, either as an initial study or in patients with a non-diagnostic ventilation–perfusion scan, is an attractive alternative modality for the detection of emboli in central (segmental or larger) pulmonary arteries. For the diagnosis of central PE, studies comparing spiral CT with angiography have demonstrated positive and negative predictive values exceeding 90% [74–77]. Despite an increased risk of bleeding, pulmonary angiography remains the diagnostic gold standard and should be considered when PE cannot be reliably diagnosed or excluded using noninvasive testing.

In hemodynamically unstable patients who cannot leave the intensive care unit for ventilation–perfusion scanning, spiral CT, or pulmonary angiography, diagnosis must be based on clinical evaluation supplemented by indirect evidence of PE. In this regard, bedside duplex ultrasound of extremities and echocardiography are potential options. Transthoracic or transesophageal echocardiography is extremely useful because of its ability to demonstrate signs of right ventricular pressure overload, including right ventricular hypokinesis or dilatation, interventricular septal flattening and paradoxical motion, and an elevated transtricuspid gradient, and to rule out other causes of shock, such as pericardial tamponade, left ventricular failure, aortic dissection, and valvular insufficiency [78]. Other more specific echocardiographic signs of PE are an altered pattern of right ventricular systolic flow velocity and regional hypokinesis of the right ventricular mid free wall [78–80]. Although it is rare for central emboli to be visualized directly by transthoracic echocardiography, transesophageal echocardiography can identify proximal thromboemboli with sensitivity and specificity figures exceeding 80% in cases of massive PE associated with right ventricular dilatation [81,82]. Finally, right-sided cardiac catheterization may also strengthen the suspicion of massive PE while excluding other causes of shock by demonstrating elevated pulmonary artery and right ventricular pressures, a normal or low pulmonary artery occlusion pressure, and a low cardiac index.

Guidelines for the administration of thrombolytic agents

The drug regimens available for PE thrombolysis are shown in Table 3. Based on studies demonstrating more rapid clot lysis, the authors believe that, among the FDA-approved regimens, rt-PA is the thrombolytic

agent of choice. Other effective alternatives are bolus infusion of streptokinase and the newer agent reteplase. Before therapy is initiated, patients must undergo a thorough evaluation to elicit factors that increase the risk of major hemorrhage (Table 4) [25]. This evaluation includes a detailed history and physical examination to detect signs of intracranial, gastrointestinal, or other organ system disorders that may predispose the patient to a higher risk of bleeding. Initial laboratory tests should include measurement of hemoglobin, hematocrit, platelet count, prothrombin time, and partial thromboplastin time (PTT). A blood sample should be obtained for blood typing in anticipation of the need for transfusion. The decision to use thrombolytic therapy must be based on a careful evaluation of its potential benefits and risks. No contraindication is absolute in the setting of massive PE and shock, and the decision to use thrombolytic therapy must be individualized. As an example, successful thrombolysis has been reported in pregnant and postoperative patients, including postneurosurgical patients [83–85].

Unlike in thrombolytic therapy for myocardial infarction, heparin is generally not infused during PE thrombolysis. Because all regimens employ fixed or weight-based dosages, there is no need to monitor coagulation parameters during the infusion. Following the completion of thrombolytic therapy, the PTT should be measured. Heparin should be started when

Table 4
Relative contraindications to thrombolytic therapy for venous thromboembolism

Recent (within 2 months) cerebrovascular accident, or intracranial or intraspinal trauma or surgery
Active intracranial disease (aneurysm, vascular malformation, neoplasm)
Major internal bleeding within the past 6 months
Uncontrolled hypertension (systolic blood pressure ≥ 200 or diastolic blood pressure ≥ 110 mm Hg)
Bleeding diathesis, including that associated with severe renal or hepatic disease
Recent (<10 days) major surgery, puncture of a noncompressible vessel, organ biopsy, or obstetric delivery
Recent major and minor trauma, including cardiopulmonary resuscitation
Infective endocarditis
Pregnancy
Hemorrhagic retinopathy
Pericarditis
Aneurysm

From Arcasoy SM, Kreit JW. Thrombolytic therapy of pulmonary embolism: a comprehensive review of current evidence. Chest 1999;115:1695–707; with permission.

Table 5
Randomized trials comparing systemic thrombolytic and heparin therapy for deep venous thrombosis

| Author (year) | Number of patients | | Treatment[a] | Venographic results[b] | | | Mortality, n (%) | PE[c], n (%) | Major hemorrhage[d], n (%) |
	Total	Evaluable[e]		Complete, n (%)	Partial, n (%)	None, n (%)			
Robertson et al (1968) [105]	16	8	Heparin[f]	0	3 (37)	5 (63)	1 (13)	ND	1 (13)
		8	SK	0	7 (87)	1 (13)	0	ND	3 (38)
Kakkar et al (1969) [106]	20	9	Heparin	2 (22)	2 (22)	5 (56)	2 (20)	1 (10)	2 (20)
		9	SK	6 (67)[g]	1 (11)	2 (22)	0	0	2 (20)
Robertson (1970) [107][h]	16	7	Heparin[f]	2 (29)		5 (71)	0	0	1 (14)
		9	SK	6 (67)		3 (33)	1 (11)	4 (44)	ND
Tsapogas (1973) [108][h]	34	15	Heparin	1 (7)		14 (93)	0	1 (7)	ND
		19	SK	10 (53)		9 (47)	0	0	ND
Porter et al (1975) [109]	50	26	Heparin	1 (4)	20 (77)	5 (19)	0	0	1 (4)
		23	SK	6 (26)	15 (65)	2 (9)	1 (4)	0	4 (17)
Arnesen et al (1978) [110][h]	42	21	Heparin	5 (24)		16 (76)	0	0	3 (14)
		21	SK	15 (71)		6 (29)	0	1 (5)	3 (14)
Elliot et al (1979) [111]	51	25	Heparin	0	ND	ND	2 (8)	2 (8)	0
		23	SK	9 (39)	12 (52)	2 (9)	0	1 (4)	2 (8)
Schulman et al (1986) [112]	38	19	Heparin	2 (11)	ND	ND	0	0	1 (5)
		17	SK	7 (41)	ND	ND	0	0	3 (18)

Study	N	Treatment	n						
Turpie I (1990) [113][h]	24	Heparin	12		2 (17)[i]	10 (83)	0	ND	1 (8)
		rt-PA	12		9 (75)	3 (25)	0	ND	4 (33)
Turpie II (1990) [113][h]	59	Heparin	30		7 (23)	23 (77)	0	ND	1 (3)
		rt-PA + heparin	28		13 (46)	15 (54)	0	ND	1 (3)
Goldhaber et al (1990) [114]	65	Heparin	11	0[j]	2 (18)	9 (82)	0	ND	0
		rt-PA	32	2 (6)	18 (56)	12 (38)	0	ND	1 (3)
		rt-PA + heparin	17	1 (6)	8 (47)	8 (47)	0	ND	0
Schweizer et al (2000) [115]	150	Heparin	50	1 (2)	9 (18)	40 (80)	0	0	0
		UK + heparin	50	17 (34)	23 (46)	10 (20)	0	4 (8)	4 (8)
		SK + heparin	50	20 (40)	20 (40)	10 (20)	0	5 (10)	5 (10)

Abbreviations: ND, no data; PE, pulmonary embolism; rt-PA, alteplase; SK, streptokinase; UK, urokinase.

[a] In most of the studies, thrombolytic therapy was followed by heparin infusion.

[b] Venographic patency was defined as follows: complete (100% resolution), partial (1%–99% resolution), none (no resolution or worse).

[c] PE rates include clinically suspected but unconfirmed cases as well as those episodes confirmed by objective tests. PE rates are based on the total number of patients randomized.

[d] The definition of major hemorrhage varied between trials but usually included intracranial hemorrhage, retroperitoneal hemorrhage, bleeding that required transfusion, surgery, or resulted in death, or a decrease in the hemoglobin of 2 g or greater. Hemorrhage rates are based on the total number of patients randomized.

[e] Evaluable patients include those patients who finished therapy and underwent follow-up venography.

[f] Heparin was not adjusted to maintain a therapeutic partial thromboplastin time.

[g] P = 0.05.

[h] Results for venographic patency did not distinguish between complete or partial response.

[i] When venographic results are reported as > 50% resolution (0 patients in the heparin group versus 7 patients in the rt-PA group), there is a statistically significant difference between groups, P = 0.002.

[j] P = 0.04.

the PTT is less than 2.5 times the control value and adjusted to maintain the PTT in the range of 1.5 to 2.5 times control. If the initial PTT exceeds this upper limit, it should be remeasured every 2 to 4 hours until it returns to the therapeutic range, at which time heparin may safely be started [25,86,87]. When PTT measurements are not readily available, the authors recommend that heparin infusion be started immediately after the completion of thrombolytic therapy and adjusted based on PTT results.

During thrombolytic therapy, the avoidance of unnecessary invasive procedures minimizes the risk of hemorrhage. Management of hemorrhage depends on its location, severity, and cause. Bleeding from vascular access sites can usually be controlled with manual pressure or compression dressings. In clinically important major hemorrhage, the thrombolytic agent should be discontinued. Cryoprecipitate, fresh frozen plasma, or both may need to be administered to reverse any associated coagulopathy. If an altered mental status or focal neurologic findings develop during or after thrombolysis, the diagnosis of intracranial hemorrhage should be considered, and an emergent noncontrast CT scan of the brain should be obtained. In addition to measures to stop the bleeding, a neurosurgical consultation must be requested.

Special circumstances

Right-sided heart thromboemboli

With the increased use of echocardiography in patients with PE, right-sided heart thromboemboli (RHTE), also referred to as "emboli in transit," have been identified more frequently, with a reported incidence of 3% to 23%. The majority are found in the right atrium [88–92]. Most, but not all, reports of RHTE suggest a higher mortality rate in patients with this condition and recommend the use of aggressive therapeutic measures, such as surgery or thrombolytic therapy [88,93–96]. Nevertheless, it is unclear whether the presence of RHTE independently increases the risk of mortality or is simply a marker of severe accompanying PE, which is present in the vast majority of patients who have RHTE. A recent systematic review identified 177 patients with RHTE and reported an overall mortality rate of 27.1% [88]. The mortality rates in patients treated with anticoagulation, surgery, or thrombolytic therapy were 28.6%, 23.8%, and 11.3%, respectively. On multivariate analysis, thrombolytic therapy resulted in an odds ratio for mortality of 0.33 (95% confidence interval, 0.11–0.98) when anticoagulation was used as a reference. Previous studies have reported conflicting findings, with better or similar outcomes after

surgery or anticoagulation when compared with thrombolysis [96–98]; therefore, the optimal management strategy for RHTE remains unclear.

Cardiac arrest

Acute PE and myocardial infarction collectively account for 50% to 70% of out-of-hospital cardiac arrests not related to trauma [99]. Several case reports and series have revealed successful stabilization and long-term survival in patients with cardiac arrest owing to PE after thrombolytic therapy [100–102]. In a recent retrospective study, PE was identified as the cause of 4.8% of all cardiac arrests [103]. The initial rhythm was pulseless electrical activity or asystole in the majority of patients with PE, and clinical diagnosis was made antemortem in 42 patients (70% of those with PE). One half of these patients were treated with 100 mg of rt-PA. Although the rate of return of spontaneous circulation was significantly higher in the thrombolysis group (81% versus 43%, $P = 0.03$), only 2 of 21 patients survived to hospital discharge. More recent studies of thrombolysis in cardiac arrest victims have not differentiated patients with PE from those with other disorders and have yielded contrasting and less optimistic results [99,104].

Clearly, thrombolytic therapy for PE leads to much faster improvement in patients with pulmonary vascular obstruction and hemodynamic abnormalities than does treatment with anticoagulation alone. Nevertheless, it has not been established conclusively that this benefit results in a reduction in morbidity or mortality in all patients with PE. In the subset of patients with shock owing to massive PE, the potential benefits of thrombolysis almost certainly prevail over the risk of significant hemorrhage. In patients with small emboli that produce no hemodynamic impact, the risk of thrombolytic therapy is clearly not warranted. Additional information is required to determine the most appropriate therapy for patients who fall between these two extremes, focusing on the role of thrombolytic therapy in patients with right ventricular dysfunction who have no clinical signs of systemic hypoperfusion.

Deep venous thrombosis

Efficacy of thrombolytic therapy

Short-term results

The results of randomized controlled trials assessing the short-term efficacy of streptokinase and rt-PA compared with heparin are summarized in Table 5 [105–115]. Most of these trials demonstrate that systemic thrombolytic therapy leads to complete or partial resolution more often than does heparin therapy. Overall, some degree of lysis was achieved in approximately 70% of patients treated with thrombolysis compared with 24% of heparin-treated patients. Complete lysis occurred in 28% and 4% of patients, respectively. Data suggest that newer and nonocclusive thrombi are more likely to undergo successful lysis when compared with older and occlusive thrombi [108,109,111]. Although no differences in the rates of PE and mortality have been reported, studies have not been designed to assess these outcomes adequately.

Long-term results on the development of postthrombotic syndrome

Randomized controlled trials comparing the effects of thrombolytic therapy and heparin on the

Table 6
Long-term results of thrombolytic therapy: postthrombotic syndrome

| | Number of patients | | | | Results | | |
| | | | | | Venograms | | |
Author (year)	Initial	Long-term follow-up	Mean duration of follow-up (range)	Treatment	Normal, n (%)	Venographic, PTS, n (%)	Clinical PTS, n (%)
Kakkar et al	20	8	6–12 Months	Heparin	1 (13)	7 (87)	ND
(1969) [116]		7		SK	4 (57)	3 (43)	ND
Bieger et al	10	5	3–4 Months	Heparin	1 (20)	4 (80)	2 (40)
(1976) [117]		5		SK	4 (80)	1 (20)	0
Common et al	50	12	7 Months	Heparin	1 (8)	11 (92)	6 (50)
(1976) [118]		15	(4–18)	SK	6 (40)	9 (60)	5 (33)
Johansson et al	57	3	10 Years	Heparin	2 (66)	1 (33)	2 (66)
(1979) [119]		5[a]	(9–12)	SK	0	3 (100)	4 (80)
Elliot et al	51	20	19 Months	Heparin	ND	ND	18 (90)
(1979) [111]		23[b]		SK	10 (50)	10 (50)	8 (35)
Arnesen et al	42	18	6.5 Years	Heparin	0[e]	18 (100)	12 (67)
(1982) [120]		17[c]		SK	7 (44)	9 (56)	4 (24)
Schulman et al	38	18[d]	60 Months	Heparin	4 (36)	7 (64)	11 (61)
(1986) [112]		17	(2–108)	SK	1 (14)	6 (86)	11 (65)
Schweizer et al	69	22	12 Months	Heparin	ND	ND	18 (82)
(1998) [121]		22		UK + heparin	ND	ND	12 (54)
		22		rt-PA + heparin	ND	ND	16 (73)
Schweizer et al	250	46	12 Months	Heparin	5 (11)[f]	41 (89)	41 (89)
(2000) [115]		46		SK (systemic) + heparin	23 (50)	23 (50)	23 (50)
		46		UK (systemic) + heparin	14 (30)	32 (70)	32 (70)
		50		UK (locoregional) + heparin	13 (26)	37 (74)	37 (74)
		50		rt-PA + heparin	11 (22)	39 (78)	39 (78)

Abbreviations: ND, no data; PTS, posthrombotic syndrome; rt-PA, alteplase; SK, streptokinase; UK, urokinase.

[a] Venographic data available for three patients.

[b] Venographic data available for 20 patients.

[c] Venographic data available for 16 patients.

[d] Venographic results at 1 month. Venographic data available for 11 patients in the heparin arm and 7 patients in the SK arm.

[e] $P = 0.004$.

[f] $P < 0.001$ for systemic thrombolytic therapy (SK or UK) versus controls (heparin).

development of PTS are summarized in Table 6 [111,112,115–121]. In most of the studies, thrombolytic therapy reduced the rate of venographic PTS, which frequently translated into an improvement in the rate of clinical PTS [116–118,120]. The data also suggest that the long-term benefit of thrombolytic therapy on the development of PTS is observed primarily in patients with an early response to treatment. Nevertheless, these data suffer from several important limitations, including small study populations, variable patient follow-up, and nonstandardized clinical assessment at the time of follow-up.

Methods of delivery

Local delivery of thrombolytic agents for the treatment of DVT has been investigated for reasons similar to those discussed in the section on PE. The two main strategies for local therapy that have been employed are regional administration of thrombolytic agents via a peripheral vein in the affected limb and catheter-directed thrombolysis. Limited data from controlled studies do not demonstrate any clear advantages of the use of regional versus systemic therapy [115,122]. Recently, catheter-directed thrombolysis has shown promising results in nonrandomized patient series. In a large registry of 473 patients, catheter-directed urokinase resulted in a "marked" (defined as more than 50%) lysis rate in 83% of patients and complete lysis in 31%. The primary patency rate was 60% at 1 year [123]. The technique and indications for catheter-directed thrombolysis merit further research.

Dosage

The three controlled studies directly comparing different dosages of thrombolytic agents, two using streptokinase and one using rt-PA, demonstrated no evidence of superior efficacy or decreased bleeding rate with the use of lower dosages [124–126]. Currently, streptokinase should be administered in dosages approved by the FDA, that is, a 250,000 U bolus followed by an infusion of 100,000 U/hour for 72 hours (see Table 3). The recommended dosage of rt-PA is 0.5 mg/kg over 8 hours, which can be repeated once 24 hours later if necessary.

Hemorrhagic complications

The rates of major hemorrhage with thrombolytic therapy are listed in Table 5. Pooled data from randomized trials of DVT thrombolysis demonstrate rates of major hemorrhage similar to those reported in the PE thrombolysis literature, that is, an average incidence of 10% (range, 0% to 38%) with thrombolytic therapy and 5% (range, 0% to 22%) with heparin. The overall incidence of intracranial hemorrhage is 0.5% with thrombolytic therapy and 1.2% with heparin. The incidence of intracranial hemorrhage with DVT thrombolysis seems to be somewhat lower than the incidence reported in controlled clinical trials of PE, most likely reflecting differences in patient populations and treatment regimens [25].

When compared with anticoagulation, thrombolytic therapy for DVT leads to superior short-term venous patency and a higher risk of major hemorrhage but no difference in the rates of PE and mortality. The data also suggest a lower incidence of PTS following thrombolysis, although it is unclear whether the potential benefit of improved early patency and lower incidence of PTS outweighs the risk of increased bleeding and cost associated with thrombolytic therapy. Limited data do not show any advantage of locoregional versus systemic thrombolytic therapy, although catheter-directed techniques warrant further investigation.

Summary

Thrombolytic therapy unquestionably leads to more rapid and complete clot lysis with a significantly higher risk of bleeding when compared with anticoagulation. The most definite indication for thrombolytic therapy in patients with VTE is massive PE associated with hemodynamic instability. Other potential indications, although not widely accepted or proven, include PE-related respiratory failure with severe hypoxemia and massive iliofemoral thrombosis with the risk of phlegmasia cerulea dolens. Routine use of thrombolytic therapy in all other cases of PE and DVT cannot be justified. Future research using randomized controlled studies should focus on the following key questions:

- Do hemodynamically stable patients with PE and right ventricular dysfunction benefit from thrombolysis, and, if so, is there a subset of patients within this group who are most likely to benefit?
- Does thrombolytic therapy improve long-term outcomes of DVT with a favorable risk-to-benefit ratio, and, if so, which patients are most likely to benefit long-term?

- What is the precise role of catheter-directed thrombolysis in the treatment of VTE, particularly the use of a low-dose thrombolytic agent in conjunction with mechanical clot disruption to minimize bleeding in patients at high risk?

Until these questions are answered, clinicians must approach decision-making regarding the use of thrombolytic therapy in PE and DVT with careful consideration of the potential risks and benefits for the patient within the framework of currently available data.

References

[1] Coon WW, Willis PW. Deep venous thrombosis and pulmonary embolism: prediction, prevention and treatment. Am J Cardiol 1959;4:611–21.

[2] Dalen JE, Alpert JS. Natural history of pulmonary embolism. Prog Cardiovasc Dis 1975;17:259–70.

[3] Lilienfield DE, Chan E, Ehland J, Godbold JH, Landrigan PJ, Marsh G. Mortality from pulmonary embolism in the United States: 1962 to 1984. Chest 1990; 98:1067–72.

[4] Morrell MT, Dunnill MS. The post-mortem incidence of pulmonary embolism in a hospital population. Br J Surg 1968;55:347–52.

[5] Uhland H, Goldberg LM. Pulmonary embolism: a commonly missed clinical entity. Dis Chest 1964;45: 533–6.

[6] Stein PD, Henry JW. Prevalence of acute pulmonary embolism among patients in a general hospital and at autopsy. Chest 1995;108:978–81.

[7] Pineda LA, Hathwar VS, Grant BJ. Clinical suspicion of fatal pulmonary embolism. Chest 2001;120:791–5.

[8] Wood KE. Major pulmonary embolism: review of a pathophysiologic approach to the golden hour of hemodynamically significant pulmonary embolism. Chest 2002;121:877–905.

[9] Goldhaber SZ, Hennekens CH, Evans DA, Newton EC, Godleski JJ. Factors associated with correct antemortem diagnosis of major pulmonary embolism. Am J Med 1982;73:822–6.

[10] Huisman MV, Buller HR, ten Cate JW, van Royen EA, Vreeken J, Kersten MJ, et al. Unexpected high prevalence of silent pulmonary embolism in patients with deep venous thrombosis. Chest 1989;95:498–502.

[11] Moser KM, Fedullo PF, LitteJohn JK, Crawford R. Frequent asymptomatic pulmonary embolism in patients with deep venous thrombosis. JAMA 1994;271: 223–5.

[12] Decousus H, Leizorovicz A, Parent F, Page Y, Tardy B, Girard P, et al. A clinical trial of vena caval filters in the prevention of pulmonary embolism in patients with proximal deep-vein thrombosis: Prevention du Risque d'Embolie Pulmonaire par Interruption Cave Study Group. N Engl J Med 1998;338:409–15.

[13] Douketis JD, Kearon C, Bates S, Duku EK, Ginsberg JS. Risk of fatal pulmonary embolism in patients with treated venous thromboembolism. JAMA 1998;279: 458–62.

[14] Prandoni P, Lensing AW, Cogo A, Cuppini S, Villalta S, Carta M, et al. The long-term clinical course of acute deep venous thrombosis. Ann Intern Med 1996;125: 1–7.

[15] Ginsberg JS, Hirsh J, Julian J, Vander LaandeVries M, Magier D, MacKinnon B, et al. Prevention and treatment of postphlebitic syndrome: results of a 3-part study. Arch Intern Med 2001;161:2105–9.

[16] Brandjes DP, Buller HR, Heijboer H, Huisman MV, de Rijk M, Jagt H, et al. Randomised trial of effect of compression stockings in patients with symptomatic proximal-vein thrombosis. Lancet 1997;349:759–62.

[17] Bernardi E, Prandoni P. The post-thrombotic syndrome. Curr Opin Pulm Med 2000;6:335–42.

[18] Urokinase Pulmonary Embolism Trial. Phase 1 results: a cooperative study. JAMA 1970;214:2163–72.

[19] Paraskos JA, Adelstein SJ, Smith RE, Rickman FD, Grossman W, Dexter L, et al. Late prognosis of acute pulmonary embolism. N Engl J Med 1973;289:55–8.

[20] Dalen JE, Banas JS, Brooks HL, Evans GL, Paraskos JA, Dexter L. Resolution rate of acute pulmonary embolism in man. N Engl J Med 1969;280:1194–9.

[21] Fred HL, Axelrad MA, Lewis JM, Alexander JK. Rapid resolution of pulmonary thromboemboli in man: angiographic study. JAMA 1966;196:1137–9.

[22] Tow DE, Wagner NHJ. Recovery of pulmonary arterial blood flow in patients with pulmonary embolism. N Engl J Med 1967;276:1053–9.

[23] Prandoni P, Cogo A, Bernardi E, Villalta S, Polistena P, Simioni P, et al. A simple ultrasound approach for detection of recurrent proximal-vein thrombosis. Circulation 1993;88:1730–5.

[24] Heijboer H, Jongbloets LM, Buller HR, Lensing AW, ten Cate JW. Clinical utility of real-time compression ultrasonography for diagnostic management of patients with recurrent venous thrombosis. Acta Radiol 1992;33:297–300.

[25] Arcasoy SM, Kreit JW. Thrombolytic therapy of pulmonary embolism: a comprehensive review of current evidence. Chest 1999;115:1695–707.

[26] Hyers TM, Agnelli G, Hull RD, Morris TA, Samama M, Tapson V, et al. Antithrombotic therapy for venous thromboembolic disease. Chest 2001;119:176S–93S.

[27] Sharma GVRK, Burleson VA, Sasahara AA. Effect of thrombolytic therapy on pulmonary-capillary blood volume in patients with pulmonary embolism. N Engl J Med 1980;303:842–5.

[28] Sharma GV, Folland ED, McIntyre KM, Sasahara AA. Long-term benefit of thrombolytic therapy in patients with pulmonary embolism. Vasc Med 2000;5:91–5.

[29] Tibbutt DA, Davies JA, Anderson JA, Fletcher EWL, Hamill J, Holt JM, et al. Comparison by controlled clinical trial of streptokinase and heparin in treatment of life-threatening pulmonary embolism. BMJ 1974; 1:343–7.

[30] Ly B, Arnesen H, Erie H, Hol R. A controlled trial of streptokinase and heparin in the treatment of major pulmonary embolism. Acta Med Scand 1978;203: 465–70.

[31] Marini C, Di Ricco G, Rossi G, Rindi M, Palla R, Giuntini C. Fibrinolytic effects of urokinase and heparin in acute pulmonary embolism: a randomized clinical trial. Respiration 1988;54:162–73.

[32] A collaborative study by the PIOPED investigators: Tissue plasminogen activator for the treatment of acute pulmonary embolism. Chest 1990;97:528–33.

[33] Levine M, Hirsh J, Weitz J, Cruickshank M, Neemeh J, Turpie AG, et al. A randomized trial of a single bolus dosage regimen of recombinant tissue plasminogen activator in patients with acute pulmonary embolism. Chest 1990;98:1473–9.

[34] Dalla-Volta S, Palla A, Santolicandro A, Giuntini C, Pengo V, Visioli O, et al. PAIMS 2: alteplase combined with heparin versus heparin in the treatment of acute pulmonary embolism. Plasminogen Activator Italian Multicenter Study 2. J Am Coll Cardiol 1992; 20:520–6.

[35] Goldhaber SZ, Haire WD, Feldstein ML, Miller M, Toltzis R, Smith JL, et al. Alteplase versus heparin in acute pulmonary embolism: randomised trial assessing right-ventricular function and pulmonary perfusion. Lancet 1993;341:507–11.

[36] Jerjes-Sanchez C, Ramirez-Rivera A, Garcia MDL, Arriaga-Nava R, Valencia S, Rosado-Buzzo A, et al. Streptokinase and heparin versus heparin alone in massive pulmonary embolism: a randomized controlled trial. J Thromb Thrombolysis 1995;2:227–9.

[37] Urokinase-Streptokinase Embolism Trial. Phase 2 results: a cooperative study. JAMA 1974;229:1606–13.

[38] The PIOPED Investigators. Value of the ventilation/ perfusion scan in acute pulmonary embolism: results of the Prospective Investigation of Pulmonary Embolism Diagnosis (PIOPED). JAMA 1990;263:2753–9.

[39] Alpert JS, Smith R, Carlson J, Ockene IS, Dexter L, Dalen JE. Mortality in patients treated for pulmonary embolism. JAMA 1976;236:1477–80.

[40] Goldhaber SZ, Visani L, De Rosa M. Acute pulmonary embolism: clinical outcomes in the International Cooperative Pulmonary Embolism Registry (ICOPER). Lancet 1999;353:1386–9.

[41] Ferrari E, Imbert A, Chevalier T, Mihoubi A, Morand P, Baudouy M. The ECG in pulmonary embolism: predictive value of negative T waves in precordial leads–80 case reports. Chest 1997;111:537–43.

[42] Meyer T, Binder L, Hruska N, Luthe H, Buchwald AB. Cardiac troponin I elevation in acute pulmonary embolism is associated with right ventricular dysfunction. J Am Coll Cardiol 2000;36:1632–6.

[43] Giannitsis E, Muller-Bardorff M, Kurowski V, Weidtmann B, Wiegand U, Kampmann M, et al. Independent prognostic value of cardiac troponin T in patients with confirmed pulmonary embolism. Circulation 2000;102:211–7.

[44] Konstantinides S, Geibel A, Kasper W, Olschewski M, Blumel L, Just H. Patent foramen ovale is an important predictor of adverse outcome in patients with major pulmonary embolism. Circulation 1998; 97:1946–51.

[45] Goldhaber SZ. Unsolved issues in the treatment of pulmonary embolism. Thromb Res 2001;103:V245–55.

[46] Cannon CP, Goldhaber SZ. Cardiovascular risk stratification of pulmonary embolism. Am J Cardiol 1996; 78:1149–51.

[47] Grifoni S, Olivotto I, Cecchini P, Pieralli F, Camaiti A, Santoro G, et al. Short-term clinical outcome of patients with acute pulmonary embolism, normal blood pressure, and echocardiographic right ventricular dysfunction. Circulation 2000;101:2817–22.

[48] Wolfe MW, Lee RT, Feldstein ML, Parker JA, Come PC, Goldhaber SZ. Prognostic significance of right ventricular hypokinesis and perfusion lung scan defects in pulmonary embolism. Am Heart J 1994;127: 1371–5.

[49] Ribeiro A, Lindmarker P, Juhlin-Dannfelt A, Johnsson H, Jorfeldt L. Echocardiography Doppler in pulmonary embolism: right ventricular dysfunction as a predictor of mortality rate. Am Heart J 1997;134: 479–87.

[50] Konstantinides S, Geibel A, Olschewski M, Heinrich F, Grosser K, Rauber K, et al. Association between thrombolytic treatment and the prognosis of hemodynamically stable patients with major pulmonary embolism: results of a multicenter registry. Circulation 1997;96:882–8.

[51] Goldhaber SZ. Pulmonary embolism thrombolysis: broadening the paradigm for its administration. Circulation 1997;96:716–8.

[52] Come PC, Kim D, Parker JA, Goldhaber SZ, Braunwald E, Markis JE. Early reversal of right ventricular dysfunction in patients with acute pulmonary embolism after treatment with intravenous tissue plasminogen activator. J Am Coll Cardiol 1987;10:971–8.

[53] Konstantinides S, Tiede N, Geibel A, Olschewski M, Just H, Kasper W. Comparison of alteplase versus heparin for resolution of major pulmonary embolism. Am J Cardiol 1998;82:966–70.

[54] Simonneau G, Sors H, Charbonnier B, Page Y, Laaban JP, Azarian R, et al. A comparison of low-molecular-weight heparin with unfractionated heparin for acute pulmonary embolism. The THESEE Study Group. Tinzaparine ou Heparine Standard: Evaluations dans l'Embolie Pulmonaire. N Engl J Med 1997;337:663–9.

[55] Hamel E, Pacouret G, Vincentelli D, Forissier JF, Peycher P, Pottier JM, et al. Thrombolysis or heparin therapy in massive pulmonary embolism with right ventricular dilation: results from a 128-patient monocenter registry. Chest 2001;120:120–5.

[56] Goldhaber SZ, Kessler CM, Heit J, Markis J, Sharma GVRK, Dawley D, et al. Randomised controlled trial of recombinant tissue plasminogen activator versus urokinase in the treatment of acute pulmonary embolism. Lancet 1988;2:293–8.

[57] Meyer G, Sors H, Charbonnier B, Kasper W, Bassand J-P, Kerr IH, et al. Effects of intravenous urokinase versus alteplase on total pulmonary resistance in acute massive pulmonary embolism: a European multicenter double-blind trial. J Am Coll Cardiol 1992;19: 239–45.

[58] Goldhaber SZ, Kessler CM, Heit JA, Elliot CG, Friedenberg WR, Heiselman DE, et al. Recombinant tissue-type plasminogen activator versus a novel dosing regimen of urokinase in acute pulmonary embolism: a randomized controlled multicenter trial. J Am Coll Cardiol 1992;20:24–30.

[59] Meneveau N, Schiele F, Vuillemenot A, Valette B, Grollier G, Bernard Y, et al. Streptokinase vs alteplase in massive pulmonary embolism: a randomized trial assessing right heart haemodynamics and pulmonary vascular obstruction. Eur Heart J 1997;18:1141–8.

[60] Meneveau N, Schiele F, Metz D, Valette B, Attali P, Vuillemenot A, et al. Comparative efficacy of a two-hour regimen of streptokinase versus alteplase in acute massive pulmonary embolism: immediate clinical and hemodynamic outcome and one-year follow-up. J Am Coll Cardiol 1998;31:1057–63.

[61] Tebbe U, Graf A, Kamke W, Zahn R, Forycki F, Kratzsch G, et al. Hemodynamic effects of double bolus reteplase versus alteplase infusion in massive pulmonary embolism. Am Heart J 1999;138:39–44.

[62] Fava M, Loyola S, Flores P, Huete I. Mechanical fragmentation and pharmacologic thrombolysis in massive pulmonary embolism. J Vasc Interv Radiol 1997;8:261–6.

[63] Stock KW, Jacob AL, Schnabel KJ, Bongartz G, Steinbrich W. Massive pulmonary embolism treatment with thrombus fragmentation and local fibrinolysis with recombinant human-tissue plasminogen activator. Cardiovasc Interv Radiol 1997;20:364–8.

[64] Tapson VF, Davidson CJ, Bauman R, Newman GE, O'Connor CM, Stack RS. Rapid thrombolysis of massive pulmonary emboli without systemic fibrinogenolysis: intraembolic infusion of thrombolytic therapy. Am Rev Respir Dis 1992;145:A719.

[65] Sze DY, Carey MB, Razavi MK. Treatment of massive pulmonary embolus with catheter-directed tenecteplase. J Vasc Interv Radiol 2001;12:1456–7.

[66] De Gregorio MA, Gimeno MJ, Mainar A, Herrera M, Tobio R, Alfonso R, et al. Mechanical and enzymatic thrombolysis for massive pulmonary embolism. J Vasc Interv Radiol 2002;13:163–9.

[67] Verstraete M, Miller GAH, Bounameaux H, Charbonnier B, Colle JP, Lecorf G, et al. Intravenous and intrapulmonary recombinant tissue-type plasminogen activator in the treatment of acute massive pulmonary embolism. Circulation 1988;77:353–60.

[68] Goldhaber SZ, Feldstein ML, Sors H. Two trials of reduced bolus alteplase in the treatment of pulmonary embolism: an overview. Chest 1994;106:725–6.

[69] Goldhaber SZ, Agnelli G, Levine MN. Reduced dose bolus alteplase vs conventional alteplase infusion for pulmonary embolism thrombolysis: an international multicenter randomized trial. Chest 1994; 106:718–24.

[70] Sors H, Pacouret G, Azarian R, Meyer G, Charbonnier B, Simonneau G. Hemodynamic effects of bolus vs 2-h infusion of alteplase in acute massive pulmonary embolism: a randomized controlled multicenter trial. Chest 1994;106:712–7.

[71] Daniels LB, Parker JA, Patel SR, Grodstein F, Goldhaber SZ. Relation of duration of symptoms with response to thrombolytic therapy in pulmonary embolism. Am J Cardiol 1997;80:184–8.

[72] Mikkola KM, Patel SR, Parker JA, Grodstein F, Goldhaber SZ. Increasing age is a major risk factor for hemorrhagic complications after pulmonary embolism thrombolysis. Am Heart J 1997;134:69–72.

[73] Kanter DS, Mikkola KM, Patel SR, Parker JA, Goldhaber SZ. Thrombolytic therapy for pulmonary embolism: frequency of intracranial hemorrhage and associated risk factors. Chest 1997;111:1241–5.

[74] Goodman LR, Curtin JJ, Mewissen MW, Foley WD, Lipchik RJ, Crain MR, et al. Detection of pulmonary embolism in patients with unresolved clinical and scintigraphic diagnosis: helical CT versus angiography. AJR Am J Roentgenol 1995;164:1369–74.

[75] Blum AG, Delfau F, Grignon B, Beurrier D, Chabot F, Claudon M, et al. Spiral-computed tomography versus pulmonary angiography in the diagnosis of acute massive pulmonary embolism. Am J Cardiol 1994;74:96–8.

[76] Remy-Jardin M, Remy J, Deschildre F, Artaud D, Beregi JP, Hossein-Foucher C, et al. Diagnosis of pulmonary embolism with spiral CT: comparison with pulmonary angiography and scintigraphy. Radiology 1996;200:699–706.

[77] Stein PD, Hull RD, Pineo GF. The role of newer diagnostic techniques in the diagnosis of pulmonary embolism. Curr Opin Pulm Med 1999;5:212–5.

[78] Goldhaber SZ. Echocardiography in the management of pulmonary embolism. Ann Intern Med 2002;136: 691–700.

[79] Torbicki A, Kurzyna M, Ciurzynski M, Pruszczyk P, Pacho R, Kuch-Wocial A, et al. Proximal pulmonary emboli modify right ventricular ejection pattern. Eur Respir J 1999;13:616–21.

[80] McConnell MV, Solomon SD, Rayan ME, Come PC, Goldhaber SZ, Lee RT. Regional right ventricular dysfunction detected by echocardiography in acute pulmonary embolism. Am J Cardiol 1996;78:469–73.

[81] Pruszczyk P, Torbicki A, Pacho R, Chlebus M, Kuch-Wocial A, Pruszynski B, et al. Noninvasive diagnosis of suspected severe pulmonary embolism: transesophageal echocardiography vs spiral CT. Chest 1997;112:722–8.

[82] Steiner P, Lund GK, Debatin JF, Steiner D, Nienaber C, Nicolas V, et al. Acute pulmonary embolism: value of transthoracic and transesophageal echocardiography in comparison with helical CT. AJR Am J Roentgenol 1996;167:931–6.

[83] Molina JE, Hunter DW, Yedlicka JW, Cerra FB.

Thrombolytic therapy for postoperative pulmonary embolism. Am J Surg 1992;163:375–80.

[84] Severi P, Lo Pinto G, Poggio R, Andrioli G. Urokinase thrombolytic therapy of pulmonary embolism in neurosurgically treated patients. Surg Neurol 1994; 42:469–70.

[85] Ahearn GS, Hadjiliadis D, Govert JA, Tapson VF. Massive pulmonary embolism during pregnancy successfully treated with recombinant tissue plasminogen activator: a case report and review of treatment options. Arch Intern Med 2002;162:1221–7.

[86] Goldhaber SZ. Contemporary pulmonary embolism thrombolysis. Chest 1995;107:45S–51S.

[87] Goldhaber SZ. Thrombolytic therapy in venous thromboembolism: clinical trials and current indications. Clin Chest Med 1995;16:307–20.

[88] Rose PS, Punjabi NM, Pearse DB. Treatment of right heart thromboemboli. Chest 2002;121:806–14.

[89] Greco F, Bisignani G, Serafini O, Guzzo D, Stingone A, Plastina F. Successful treatment of right heart thromboemboli with IV recombinant tissue-type plasminogen activator during continuous echocardiographic monitoring: a case series report. Chest 1999; 116:78–82.

[90] Chakko S, Richards 3rd F. Right-sided cardiac thrombi and pulmonary embolism. Am J Cardiol 1987;59: 195–6.

[91] Diebold J, Lohrs U. Venous thrombosis and pulmonary embolism: a study of 5039 autopsies. Pathol Res Pract 1991;187:260–6.

[92] Lindblad B, Sternby NH, Bergqvist D. Incidence of venous thromboembolism verified by necropsy over 30 years. BMJ 1991;302:709–11.

[93] Casazza F, Bongarzoni A, Centonze F, Morpurgo M. Prevalence and prognostic significance of right-sided cardiac mobile thrombi in acute massive pulmonary embolism. Am J Cardiol 1997;79:1433–5.

[94] Pandey AS, Rakowski H, Mickleborough LL, Butany JW, Omran A, Parker TG. Right heart pulmonary embolism in transit: a review of therapeutic considerations. Can J Cardiol 1997;13:397–402.

[95] Chartier L, Bera J, Delomez M, Asseman P, Beregi JP, Bauchart JJ, et al. Free-floating thrombi in the right heart: diagnosis, management, and prognostic indexes in 38 consecutive patients. Circulation 1999;99: 2779–83.

[96] Kinney EL, Wright RJ. Efficacy of treatment of patients with echocardiographically detected right-sided heart thrombi: a meta-analysis. Am Heart J 1989;118: 569–73.

[97] Farfel Z, Shechter M, Vered Z, Rath S, Goor D, Gafni J. Review of echocardiographically diagnosed right heart entrapment of pulmonary emboli-in-transit with emphasis on management. Am Heart J 1987;113:171–8.

[98] Chapoutot L, Nazeyrollas P, Metz D, Maes D, Maillier B, Jennesseaux C, et al. Floating right heart thrombi and pulmonary embolism: diagnosis, outcome and therapeutic management. Cardiology 1996;87: 169–74.

[99] Bottiger BW, Bode C, Kern S, Gries A, Gust R, Glatzer R, et al. Efficacy and safety of thrombolytic therapy after initially unsuccessful cardiopulmonary resuscitation: a prospective clinical trial. Lancet 2001;357:1583–5.

[100] Bottiger BW, Reim SM, Diezel G, Bohrer H, Martin E. High-dose bolus injection of urokinase: use during cardiopulmonary resuscitation for massive pulmonary embolism. Chest 1994;106:1281–3.

[101] Bottiger BW, Bohrer H, Bach A, Motsch J, Martin E. Bolus injection of thrombolytic agents during cardiopulmonary resuscitation for massive pulmonary embolism. Resuscitation 1994;28:45–54.

[102] Langdon RW, Swicegood WR, Schwartz DA. Thrombolytic therapy of massive pulmonary embolism during prolonged cardiac arrest using recombinant tissue-type plasminogen activator. Ann Emerg Med 1989;18:678–80.

[103] Kurkciyan I, Meron G, Sterz F, Janata K, Domanovits H, Holzer M, et al. Pulmonary embolism as a cause of cardiac arrest: presentation and outcome. Arch Intern Med 2000;160:1529–35.

[104] Abu-Laban RB, Christenson JM, Innes GD, van Beek CA, Wanger KP, McKnight RD, et al. Tissue plasminogen activator in cardiac arrest with pulseless electrical activity. N Engl J Med 2002;346:1522–8.

[105] Robertson BR, Nilsson IM, Nylander G. Value of streptokinase and heparin in treatment of acute deep venous thrombosis: a coded investigation. Acta Chir Scand 1968;134:203–8.

[106] Kakkar VV, Flanc C, Howe CT, O'Shea M, Flute PT. Treatment of deep vein thrombosis: a trial of heparin, streptokinase, and arvin. BMJ 1969;1:806–10.

[107] Robertson BR, Nilsson IM, Nylander G. Thrombolytic effect of streptokinase as evaluated by phlebography of deep venous thrombi of the leg. Acta Chir Scand 1970;136:173–80.

[108] Tsapogas MJ, Peabody RA, Wu KT, Karmody AM, Devaraj KT, Eckert C. Controlled study of thrombolytic therapy in deep vein thrombosis. Surgery 1973; 74:973–84.

[109] Porter JM, Seaman AJ, Common HH, Rosch J, Eidemiller LR, Calhoun AD. Comparison of heparin and streptokinase in the treatment of venous thrombosis. Am Surg 1975;41:511–9.

[110] Arnesen H, Heilo A, Jakobsen E, Ly B, Skaga E. A prospective study of streptokinase and heparin in the treatment of deep vein thrombosis. Acta Med Scand 1978;203:457–63.

[111] Elliot MS, Immelman EJ, Jeffery P, Benatar SR, Funston MR, Smith JA, et al. A comparative randomized trial of heparin versus streptokinase in the treatment of acute proximal venous thrombosis: an interim report of a prospective trial. Br J Surg 1979;66:838–43.

[112] Schulman S, Granqvist S, Juhlin-Dannfelt A, Lockner D. Long-term sequelae of calf vein thrombosis treated with heparin or low-dose streptokinase. Acta Med Scand 1986;219:349–57.

[113] Turpie AG, Levine MN, Hirsh J, Ginsberg JS, Cruick-shank M, Jay R, et al. Tissue plasminogen activator (rt-PA) vs heparin in deep vein thrombosis: results of a randomized trial. Chest 1990;97:172S–5S.

[114] Goldhaber SZ, Meyerovitz MF, Green D, Vogelzang RL, Citrin P, Heit J, et al. Randomized controlled trial of tissue plasminogen activator in proximal deep venous thrombosis. Am J Med 1990;88:235–40.

[115] Schweizer J, Kirch W, Koch R, Elix H, Hellner G, Forkmann L, et al. Short- and long-term results after thrombolytic treatment of deep venous thrombosis. J Am Coll Cardiol 2000;36:1336–43.

[116] Kakkar VV, Howe CT, Laws JW, Flanc C. Late results of treatment of deep vein thrombosis. BMJ 1969;1: 810–1.

[117] Bieger R, Boekhout-Mussert RJ, Hohmann F, Loe-liger EA. Is streptokinase useful in the treatment of deep vein thrombosis? Acta Med Scand 1976;199: 81–8.

[118] Common HH, Seaman AJ, Rosch J, Porter JM, Dotter CT. Deep vein thrombosis treated with streptokinase or heparin: follow-up of a randomized study. Angiology 1976;27:645–54.

[119] Johansson L, Nylander G, Hedner U, Nilsson IM. Comparison of streptokinase with heparin: late results in the treatment of deep venous thrombosis. Acta Med Scand 1979;206:93–8.

[120] Arnesen H, Hoiseth A, Ly B. Streptokinase or heparin in the treatment of deep vein thrombosis: follow-up results of a prospective study. Acta Med Scand 1982; 211:65–8.

[121] Schweizer J, Elix H, Altmann E, Hellner G, Fork-mann L. Comparative results of thrombolysis treatment with rt-PA and urokinase: a pilot study. Vasa 1998;27:167–71.

[122] Schwieder G, Grimm W, Siemens HJ, Flor B, Hilden A, Gmelin E, et al. Intermittent regional therapy with rt-PA is not superior to systemic thrombolysis in deep vein thrombosis (DVT)–a German multicenter trial. Thromb Haemost 1995;74:1240–3.

[123] Mewissen MW, Seabrook GR, Meissner MH, Cynamon J, Labropoulos N, Haughton SH. Catheter-directed thrombolysis for lower extremity deep venous thrombosis: report of a national multicenter registry. Radiology 1999;211:39–49.

[124] Schulman S, Lockner D, Granqvist S, Bratt G, Paul C, Nyman D. A comparative randomized trial of low-dose versus high-dose streptokinase in deep vein thrombosis of the thigh. Thromb Haemost 1984;51: 261–5.

[125] Heinrich F, Heinrich U. North Baden venous lysis trial (NBVL): multicentre prospective randomized phlebographically controlled trial on the effect of ultra-high versus conventional doses of streptokinase in fresh leg-pelvis venous thromboses. Vasc Med 1998; 3:87–94.

[126] Bounameaux H, Banga JD, Bluhmki E, Coccheri S, Fiessinger JN, Haarmann W, et al. Double-blind, randomized comparison of systemic continuous infusion of 0.25 versus 0.50 mg/kg/24 h of alteplase over 3 to 7 days for treatment of deep venous thrombosis in heparinized patients: results of the European Thrombolysis with rt-PA in Venous Thrombosis (ETTT) trial. Thromb Haemost 1992;67:306–9.

CLINICS
IN CHEST
MEDICINE

Clin Chest Med 24 (2003) 93–101

Venous thromboembolism prophylaxis in the medically ill patient

Franklin A. Michota, MD

Department of General Internal Medicine, The Cleveland Clinic Foundation, 9500 Euclid Avenue, Cleveland, OH 44195, USA

Venous thromboembolism (VTE), which includes the entities of deep vein thrombosis (DVT) and pulmonary embolism (PE), is a common disease that affects more than 2 million people each year and may be responsible for up to 200,000 deaths annually [1]. Almost all PEs originate from existing clots in the deep venous system of the legs, of which more than half are clinically silent [2]. In fact, the first manifestation of the disease may be fatal PE. Identifying patients at risk and applying preventive measures is the only way to decrease VTE-related morbidity and mortality.

Scope of the problem

Venous thromboembolism accounts for 10% of all in-hospital mortality, with a long-term case fatality rate of 19% at 1 year [3]. In elderly patients, PE is associated with a 1-year mortality rate of 39%. Approximately three of four fatal PEs occur in medical patients, and autopsy series demonstrate that, over the past 2 decades, the incidence of fatal PE has remained constant for nonsurgical patients [4]. VTE survivors are at increased risk for VTE recurrence and for chronic postthrombotic syndrome (PTS). PTS is characterized by chronic pain, edema, skin induration, and ulceration of the lower extremities and is estimated to occur in one-third of VTE survivors within 10 years [5]. In economic terms, the cost of a primary DVT is similar to that of an acute myocardial infarction or stroke [6]. The additional long-term health care cost of PTS is approximately 75% of the cost of a primary DVT.

The need for prophylaxis

Prevention of VTE has become widely accepted as an effective and worthwhile strategy. Nevertheless, most protocols for VTE prophylaxis have primarily addressed surgical patients, because the assessment of the prevention of VTE is less developed in medical populations. Nearly 100,000 surgical patients have been included in trials concerning the prevention of VTE, whereas only 15,000 patients receiving medical care have been included in such trials [7]. Medically ill patients accounted for fewer than 10% of patients identified as prophylaxis candidates in the 2001 American College of Chest Physicians (ACCP) recommendations for anticoagulation [8]. Unfortunately, even when guidelines exist, the use of preventive measures remains highly variable. A recent survey found that 28% of medical inpatients with risk factors for VTE were receiving prophylaxis [9]. General medical patients represent a heterogeneous group and are thought to have a lower incidence of VTE than surgical patients; however, evidence is mounting that all hospitalized patients, medical as well as surgical, should be protected from VTE. In another recent study, factors associated with institutionalization independently accounted for more than half of all cases of VTE in the community [10]. Hospitalization for surgery accounted for no more than 24% of cases, and 74% of patients had risk factors other than hospitalization or surgery.

Clinical risk factors

Knowledge of the clinical risk factors for VTE forms the basis for the appropriate use of prophylaxis.

E-mail address: michotf@ccf.org

0272-5231/03/$ – see front matter © 2003, Elsevier Inc. All rights reserved.
doi:10.1016/S0272-5231(02)00078-3

As early as 1856, Virchow described the well-known triad of factors that predisposes patients to VTE—venous stasis, endothelial injury, and hypercoagulability. Numerous other independent risk factors have been identified [8] and are summarized in Box 1.

Cancer is a common comorbidity in the medically ill population. Patients with cancer, patients receiving chemotherapy, and patients with a history of cancer in remission are at increased risk for VTE. Hemostatic abnormalities are often associated with malignancy. In addition to the hypercoagulability seen in cancer, the presence of indwelling central venous catheters increases the risk for VTE.

Many aspects of cardiovascular disease represent independent risk factors for VTE. Acute myocardial infarction, ischemic and nonischemic cardiomyopathy, congestive heart failure secondary to valvular disease, and chronic idiopathic dilated cardiomyopathy increase the risk for VTE. The risk for VTE is especially high in patients with stages III to IV New York Heart Association heart failure.

Acute respiratory failure also increases the risk for VTE. Several conditions can produce, or are associated with, respiratory failure, including acute exacerbations of chronic obstructive pulmonary disease, adult respiratory distress syndrome, community acquired or nosocomial pneumonia, lung cancer, interstitial lung disease, and pulmonary hypertension [11].

Most hospitalized patients are aged more than 40 years, and this factor represents an independent risk for VTE. Patients aged 60 years and older are at the highest risk. Hospitalized elderly patients are often frail, immobile, or have restricted mobility. Advancing age also predisposes patients to venous stasis and the presence of venous varicosities. As the population ages, the number of cases of VTE can be expected to increase.

Restricted mobility can range from limited ambulation to bed rest and represents one of the most important risk factors for VTE. In a study of primarily medical patients, patients confined to bed rest for fewer than 5 days had a 21% occurrence rate of VTE compared with a 36% occurrence rate for patients restricted to bed rest for more than 10 days [12]. Patients with a lower limb paralysis associated with ischemic stroke have a DVT incidence of more than 50% in the paralyzed limb [8]. Patients with spinal cord injuries are similarly at high risk owing to immobility. Nevertheless, complete bed rest or paralysis is not needed to increase greatly the risk of VTE owing to restricted mobility. Medical patients who simply have restricted mobility seem to be at risk.

Most serious systemic infections increase the risk for VTE, including pneumonia and urinary tract, skin,

---

Box 1. Risk factors for venous thromboembolism

Venous stasis
　Advanced age (>40 years)
　Immobilization/reduced mobility
　Varicose veins
　Acute myocardial infarction
　Congestive heart failure
　Stroke
　Paralysis
　Spinal cord injury
　Hyperviscosity syndromes
　Polycythemia
　Anesthesia
　Severe chronic obstructive
　　pulmonary disease
Endothelial injury
　Surgery
　Previous VTE
　Trauma
　Central venous catheters
Hypercoagulability
　Cancer
　Obesity
　Estrogens (contraceptives, hormone
　　replacement therapy)
　Pregnancy/postpartum
　Family history
　Inflammatory bowel disease
　Systemic infections
　Nephrotic syndrome
　Thrombophilia
　　Activated protein C resistance
　　Prothrombin gene
　　　20210A mutation
　　Antithrombin deficiency
　　Protein C and S deficiency
　　Heparin-induced
　　　thrombocytopenia
　　Antiphospholipid syndrome
　　Homocysteinemia
　　Lupus anticoagulant

---

and abdominal infections [11]. Seriously ill medical patients admitted to the intensive care unit (ICU) are at increased risk; this setting is also an independent risk factor for VTE.

Disorders of coagulation regulation predispose patients to VTE. These disorders can be inherited or acquired and include deficiencies in protein C and S, antithrombin, and plasminogen. Purely inherited disorders, such as the presence of factor V Leiden or resistance to activated protein C, also increase VTE risk. The prevalence of the Leiden genetic mutation is 5% in the general population, making it the most common inherited disorder associated with VTE [13]. The risk for recurrent VTE is approximately 40% in heterozygotes compared with 18% in persons without the mutation. Another inherited risk factor recently described is the prothrombin gene mutation, which leads to elevated prothrombin levels and an increased risk for VTE in heterozygous carriers. This gene mutation occurs in 2% to 4% of the general population, with a southern European ethnic predominance [14]. An abnormality in the metabolism of homocysteine resulting in increased serum and urine levels of this product is another recognized clinical risk factor for VTE [15].

In the current hospital environment, virtually all medical patients are acutely ill and compromised by restricted mobility. Most patients have multiple risk factors, and the risks are cumulative [16]. A history of previous VTE confers risk for a future event, because approximately 20% of patients with confirmed VTE have had prior DVT or PE [17]. Anderson et al [18] demonstrated that one of five hospitalized patients had at least three VTE risk factors a decade ago. Currently, medical inpatients are older, sicker, and more complex, and as many as 90% or more of medical patients may be eligible for prophylaxis [19].

Nonpharmacologic prevention strategies

The use of nonpharmacologic VTE prevention strategies, such as elastic stockings (ES) or intermittent pneumatic compression (IPC) devices, has not been studied in heterogeneous medical populations and is not recommended for routine prophylaxis. Nevertheless, disease-specific trials have used ES or IPC alone or in combination with pharmacologic approaches. In a study by Kierkegaard and Norgren [20], 80 patients with acute myocardial infarction wore ES on one leg, with the contralateral extremity serving as a control. Eight of the control legs had an abnormal fibrinogen uptake scan, whereas there were no abnormalities in the legs on which ES were worn ($P = 0.003$). In a nonrandomized prospective study of 681 ischemic stroke patients, the combination of low-dose unfractionated heparin (LDUH), ES, and IPC was associated with fewer symptomatic VTEs when compared with LDUH plus ES [21]. Nevertheless, Hirsch et al [22] demonstrated in the medical ICU that IPC was no better than no prophylaxis at all. Upper- or lower-limb DVT was diagnosed in 32% of patients receiving no prophylaxis versus

33% of patients using IPC devices. Marik et al [23] also found IPC to be ineffective in the ICU setting. Lower-limb DVT was diagnosed by Doppler ultrasonography in 25% of patients receiving no prophylaxis versus 19% of patients using IPC ($P = 0.42$). Extrapolating further from the data obtained in trials in surgical patients, ES and IPC will most likely modulate the risk for VTE and carry no risk for hemorrhage [8]. Nevertheless, ES alone are unlikely to be helpful, because they yield only modest risk reductions in low-risk surgical populations. IPC has produced satisfactory risk reduction in high-risk surgical groups, but these devices have several significant limitations in the medically ill population. First, the mechanical devices must be worn continuously to maintain a protective effect, and this requirement increases VTE risk from immobility. Second, the devices may be uncomfortable to wear, thereby destroying sleep hygiene. Poor sleep hygiene has been associated with episodes of delirium in hospitalized elderly patients [24]. Third, the devices have not been studied adequately to recommend their use in place of pharmacologic strategies that have established efficacy. The use of ES or IPC strategies for the prevention of VTE in the medically ill population should be limited to situations in which the risk for bleeding is believed to exceed the risk for thrombosis.

Pharmacologic strategies

The most comprehensively studied patients with medical conditions have sustained myocardial infarction or ischemic stroke. Nevertheless, in myocardial infarction, the current use of fibrinolytics, systemic anticoagulation with heparins, antiplatelet agents, or combinations of these drugs has made the prevention of VTE a secondary goal. In general medical patients with risk factors for VTE, the ACCP recommends either LDUH twice or three times per day or low molecular weight heparin (LMWH) [8]. The following sections review the major trial evidence that supports this recommendation.

Low-dose unfractionated heparin versus placebo

Most data comparing LDUH with placebo are decades old. In ischemic stroke patients, two separate trials demonstrated a 71% risk reduction in DVT relative to control patients [25,26]. Belch et al [27] compared LDUH given every 8 hours with placebo in 100 patients with heart failure and respiratory disease and found a significant reduction in DVT by fibrinogen uptake scanning (4% versus 26%, P = 0.01). There was no increase in major bleeding. Cade [28] compared LDUH given every 12 hours with placebo in 250 medical and ICU patients and demonstrated a significant reduction in DVT by fibrinogen uptake scanning (13% versus 29%, P < 0.05). Safety endpoints were not evaluated. Ibarra-Perez and Sandset [29] compared given LDUH every 12 hours with placebo in 85 ICU patients and showed a significant reduction in DVT by venography (26% versus 3%, P < 0.002) with no increase in major hemorrhage. More recent work has been less clear in the medical ICU setting. Hirsh and colleagues [22] found LDUH given twice daily to be no better than no prophylaxis by Doppler ultrasonography (40% versus 32%). Marik et al [23] found that LDUH given twice daily significantly reduced the risk for VTE by Doppler ultrasonography (7% versus 25%, P < 0.05). No safety endpoints were evaluated in either of the previous studies. Kupfer et al [30] compared LDUH given every 8 hours with placebo and demonstrated a significant reduction in VTE in the LDUH group by serial duplex scanning (11% versus 31%, P = 0.001).

Two randomized trials assessed the effect of LDUH on mortality. Halkin et al [31] gave 1358 consecutive general medical patients LDUH twice daily versus no prophylaxis for the duration of hospitalization or until the patients were fully mobile. The primary outcome was all-cause mortality without reporting of thromboembolic events. The mortality rates were significantly lower in the LDUH group (7.8% versus 10.9%, P < 0.05). Garlund and colleagues [32] randomized 11,693 patients with acute infections who were admitted to six Swedish hospitals to treatment with LDUH twice daily or no prophylaxis until discharge. In the intention-to-treat analysis, mortality rates were similar in the LDUH and placebo groups (5.3% versus 5.6%, P = 0.4); however, there were fewer nonfatal VTE events in the LDUH group (70 versus 116, P = 0.001).

Low molecular weight heparin versus placebo

Two early studies performed on ischemic stroke patients compared dalteparin with placebo [33,34]. One study demonstrated significant efficacy for dalteparin, whereas the other did not. The pooled DVT rates in these two trials were 40% for placebo patients and 26% for the dalteparin group. More recently, two randomized and blinded trials have compared enoxaparin with placebo in the medically ill population. Dahan et al [35] compared 60 mg of enoxaparin daily with placebo in 270 medically ill patients and found a significant reduction in DVT by fibrinogen scanning

(10% versus 3%, P = 0.04) with no increase in major bleeding. The mortality rate was 4.4% in the enoxaparin and placebo groups. Samama and colleagues [36] compared two different doses of enoxaparin (20 or 40 mg) daily with placebo in the Comparison of Enoxaparin with Placebo for the Prevention of Venous Thromboembolism in Acutely Ill Medical Patients (MEDENOX) trial. The trial evaluated thromboprophylaxis in 1102 acutely ill medical patients who were at risk for thromboembolic complications owing to severely restricted mobility. The trial included general medical patients with acute disorders (average of 2.3 clinical risk factors) who were believed to have a moderate risk for DVT and who were older than age 40 years, had a projected hospital stay of less than 6 days, and had been immobilized previously for fewer than 3 days. Patients were randomized to placebo; enoxaparin, 20 mg daily; or enoxaparin, 40 mg daily for 6 to14 days. The overall incidence of venographically detectable VTE was 14.9% in the placebo group (5% proximal DVT) versus 5.5% in the enoxaparin group (P < 0.001). In this patient population, the 40-mg dose reduced the risk of VTE by 63%. No significant differences were found in the enoxaparin 20-mg dose and placebo groups with regard to efficacy. There was no increase in major bleeding or thrombocytopenia with either dose of enoxaparin when compared with placebo. Mortality was not significantly different in any of the treatment groups; however, there was a 2.5% absolute risk reduction in the overall risk of death at 3 months in the group assigned to 40 mg of enoxaparin (Fig. 1).

Low-dose unfractionated heparin versus low molecular weight heparin

Several randomized trials have been performed comparing LDUH with dalteparin or enoxaparin. Harenburg et al [37] compared 2500 U of dalteparin daily with LDUH given every 8 hours in 166 medical patients and found no significant difference in DVT by serial plethysmography and Doppler ultrasound scanning (4.8% versus 3.4%; P, not significant). Nevertheless, LDUH was associated with significantly more episodes of major bleeding.

Bergmann and Neuhart [38] compared enoxaparin, 20 mg daily, with LDUH given every 12 hours in 442 hospitalized elderly patients and demonstrated no significant difference in VTE by fibrinogen scanning (4.8% versus 4.6%; P, not significant) with a similar safety profile. This result is intriguing, because Samama found the 20-mg enoxaparin dose to be no better than placebo.

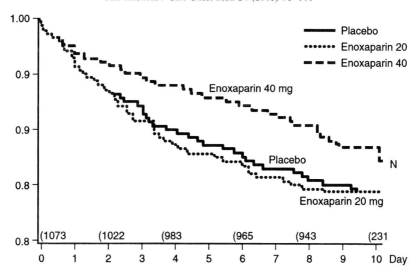

Fig. 1. Kaplan-Meier estimate of the probability of survival in the MEDENOX trial (log-rank test; $P = 0.31$; hazard ratio, 0.90; confidence interval, 0.7 to 1.1). The risk of death was lower in the group assigned to 40 mg of enoxaparin than in the group assigned to placebo. (*Adapted from* Samama MM, Cohen AT, Darmon J-Y, et al. A comparison of enoxaparin with placebo for the prevention of VTE in acutely ill medical patients. N Engl J Med 1999;341:793–800; with permission.)

Lechler et al [39] compared 40 mg of enoxaparin daily with LDUH given every 8 hours in the Prophylaxis in Internal Medicine with Enoxaparin (PRIME) study. This multicenter, randomized, double-blind controlled trial was performed on 959 patients who were immobilized for 7 days in addition to having another risk factor for VTE (ie, congestive heart failure, malignancy, obesity, or age over 60 years). There was no significant difference in the two strategies on duplex ultrasonography (0.2% versus 1.4%; *P*, not significant); however, there was more bleeding in the LDUH group.

Kleber et al [40] compared 40 mg of enoxaparin once daily with LDUH given every 8 hours in 665 patients with severe respiratory disease or congestive heart failure. Patients with elevated levels of D-dimer or soluble fibrin underwent venography. Thromboembolic events were detected in 8.4% of patients receiving enoxaparin and 10.4% of those treated with LDUH ($P = 0.6$). Substudy analysis found the enoxaparin strategy to be significantly more effective in reducing VTE in the setting of congestive heart failure when compared with LDUH (9.7% versus 16.1%, $P = 0.01$). In addition, overall bleeding occurred significantly more in the LDUH group when compared with the enoxaparin group (3.6% versus 1.5%, $P < 0.05$).

Using venographic endpoints, Harenburg et al [41] compared 40 mg of enoxaparin daily with LDUH given every 8 hours in 877 medically ill patients and found a significant reduction in a com-

posite endpoint of VTE and death with enoxaparin (15% versus 22%, $P = 0.04$). Also using venographic endpoints, Hillbom et al [42] compared 40 mg of enoxaparin daily with LDUH given every 8 hours in 212 ischemic stroke patients and found a significant reduction in DVT with enoxaparin without an increase in bleeding.

Mismetti et al [7] recently performed a meta-analysis of nine trials comparing LMWH with unfractionated heparin (n = 4669) and demonstrated no significant difference in DVT, clinical PE, or mortality. Nevertheless, LMWH was associated with significantly less bleeding (0.4% versus 1.2%, $P = 0.049$), representing a 52% risk reduction.

Evidence-based recommendations

The intensity of the prophylaxis should match the VTE risk in the general medical patient. Patients with medical conditions are thought to be at moderate risk for VTE based on epidemiologic data revealing DVT in 10% to 26% of general medical patients [8]. The MEDENOX trial found a 5% rate of proximal DVT in a heterogeneous cohort of general medical patients with an average of more than two clinical risk factors. Extrapolating from epidemiologic data obtained in surgical populations, the average medical patient would be at high risk for VTE. Autopsy-proven fatal PE was found in 2.5% of medical patients observed prospectively without prophylaxis [43]. Using epidemiologic data obtained in surgical populations, the general medical patient would be in the very high-risk category for VTE. Understanding the true level of VTE risk in the medical patient is critical in attempts to apply the appropriate pharmacologic prevention strategy. LDUH given twice daily is not efficacious enough in high-risk surgical populations; LDUH every 8 hours is recommended [8]. In very high-risk surgical populations, LDUH is not recommended at all owing to the lack of efficacy data.

Using surgical evidence as a guide, LDUH given every 12 hours does not seem to be efficacious enough to prevent VTE in general medical patients who are at high to very high risk for VTE. Most of the studies suggesting the efficacy of LDUH given twice daily when compared with placebo were completed 20 years ago [27,28]. Given the increased acuity seen in hospitals today, it is unclear whether the earlier data remain applicable. The Bergmann data raised further questions by demonstrating that LDUH given twice daily was equivalent to a placebo

dose of LMWH [38]. All other direct comparisons between LDUH and LMWH used a regimen of LDUH three times daily. In each comparison, LMWH was at least as efficacious and was safer to administer. Harenberg [41], Hillbom [42], and Kleber [40] and their colleagues all found the LMWH strategy to be superior to LDUH three times daily in the specific medical conditions of ischemic stroke and heart failure. Indirect data also question the efficacy of LDUH. Goldhaber et al [12] demonstrated in a recent case series (n = 384) of secondary DVT at Brigham and Women's Hospital that 52% of the study population had received some form of prophylaxis. Almost two thirds of the group receiving prophylaxis was given unfractionated heparin with or without mechanical devices.

A proposed algorithm presents a rational approach to the use of prophylactic anticoagulation in medical patients (Fig. 2). Patients should be assessed for VTE risk. If two or more clinical risk factors are present, the patient is probably at high to very high risk for

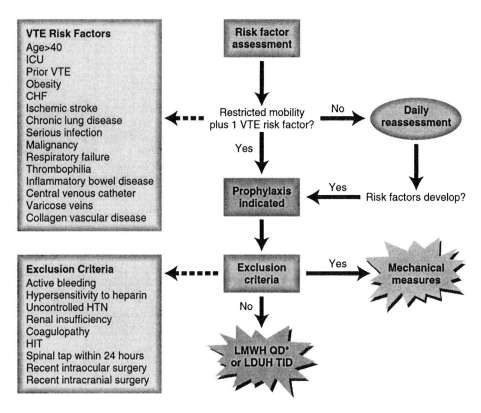

Fig. 2. Venous thromboembolism prophylaxis in the hospitalized medical patient. All patients should be screened and considered for VTE prophylaxis. LMWH is the preferred strategy owing to superior efficacy and safety. CHF, congestive heart failure; HIT, heparin-induced thrombocytopenia; HTN, hypertension; ICU, intensive care unit; LDUH, low-density unfractionated heparin; LMWH, low molecular weight heparin; VTE, venous thromboembolism. (*Adapted from* American Health Consultants and DVT-Free Clinical Consensus Panel, Victor Tapson, MD, Panel Chairman; with permission.)

VTE. In this setting, for the purpose of efficacy and safety, LMWH is the preferred pharmacologic preventive approach. Of the LMWH preparations, only enoxaparin is currently approved by the United States Food and Drug Administration for VTE prevention in the medically ill population with restricted mobility.

Low molecular weight heparin has not been studied adequately in clinical trials in several important patient populations. These special groups include patients with morbid obesity (>150 kg) and those with severe renal insufficiency (creatinine clearance <30 mL/minute). Morbidly obese patients are at increased risk for VTE [8]. Fixed doses of LMWH administered once daily may not be sufficient in morbidly obese patients. In addition, patients with severe renal insufficiency may be at increased risk for bleeding with pharmacologic prophylaxis when compared with non–renally impaired patients. LMWH is cleared by the kidneys, and patients with renal impairment experience a prolonged elimination of the drug that can lead to unintended high heparin levels over time, increasing the risk for hemorrhage. Ultimately, in all patient assessments, the risk for bleeding must be weighed against the risk for thrombosis. Patients with a high to very high risk for hemorrhage should probably not receive pharmacologic VTE prevention strategies; nonpharmacologic approaches would be preferred.

In most VTE prevention trials, study patients have received prophylaxis for at least 7 to 10 days [8]; however, shorter or longer durations of prophylaxis may be appropriate depending on clinical factors or the length of hospitalization. Many patients are still at risk for VTE at the time of hospital discharge. The convalescent phase of medical illness is often accompanied by limited mobility. Extending VTE prophylaxis out of the hospital following recent acute illness is being investigated in the Extended VTE Prophylaxis in Acutely Ill Medical Patients with Prolonged Immobilization trial. This double-blind, placebo-controlled, parallel multicenter study is being performed on acutely ill medical patients with prolonged immobilization.

Pharmacoeconomic data

Pharmacoeconomic data suggest that the increased initial cost of LMWH is more than offset by the benefits of lower morbidity and reduced hospitalization costs owing to a reduction in VTE complications, recurrence, or adverse events related to prophylaxis [43,44]. A recently proposed cost-analytic model indicates that thromboprophylaxis with 40 mg of enoxaparin daily is cost-effective in acutely ill medical patients when compared with no prophylaxis [44]. The effectiveness analysis in this model is consistent with the large body of clinical evidence demonstrating a better risk-to-benefit ratio when using LMWH versus unfractionated heparin for VTE prevention. Moreover, when compared with thromboprophylaxis using unfractionated heparin, enoxaparin prophylaxis was found to be cost neutral.

Summary

All general medical patients should be assessed for clinical risk factors for VTE. The ACCP has recommended that general medical patients with clinical risk factors receive either LDUH twice or three times daily or once-daily LMWH. Current evidence suggests that twice-daily LDUH may not be efficacious enough in the acutely ill medical inpatient. LDUH three times daily may be efficacious in most medical patients; however, it is associated with an increased risk for bleeding. The preferred strategy for prevention in the medically ill population at high to very high risk for VTE is LMWH. For patients who have a high to very high risk for bleeding, nonpharmacologic strategies such as ES or IPC devices are recommended.

References

[1] Hirsh J, Hoak J. Management of deep vein thrombosis and pulmonary embolism: a statement for healthcare professionals. Council on Thrombosis, American Heart Association. Circulation 1996;93:2212–45.

[2] Hull RD, Pineio GF. Clinical features of deep venous thrombosis. In: Hull RD, Raskob GE, Pineo GF, editors. VTE: an evidence-based atlas. Armonk (NY): Futura Publishing; 1996. p. 87–91.

[3] Anderson Jr FA, Wheeler HB, Goldberg RJ, et al. A population-based perspective of the hospital incidence and case-fatality rates of deep vein thrombosis and pulmonary embolism: the Worcester DVT Study. Arch Intern Med 1991;151:933–8.

[4] Sandler DA, Martin JF. Autopsy proven pulmonary embolism in hospital patients: are we detecting enough deep vein thrombosis? J R Soc Med 1989;82:203–5.

[5] Prandoni P, Lensing AWA, Cogo A, et al. The long-term clinical course of acute deep venous thrombosis. Ann Intern Med 1996;82:1251–7.

[6] Bergqvist D, Jendteg S, Johansen L, et al. Cost of long-term complications of deep venous thrombosis of the lower extremities: an analysis of a defined pa-

tient population in Sweden. Ann Intern Med 1997; 126:454–7.

[7] Mismetti P, Laporte-Simitsidis S, Tardy B, et al. Prevention of venous thromboembolism in internal medicine with unfractionated or low-molecular weight heparins: a meta-analysis of randomised clinical trials. Thromb Haemost 2000;83:14–9.

[8] Geerts WH, Heit JA, Clagett GP, et al. Prevention of venous thromboembolism. Chest 2001;119: 132S–75S.

[9] Tapson V, Elliot G, Turpe AGG, et al. Suspicions and subtleties in venous thromboembolism: are clinical models and strategies effective? Medical Crossfire 2000;2:35–45.

[10] Heit JA, O'Fallon M, Petterson T, et al. Relative impact of risk factors for deep vein thrombosis and pulmonary embolism. Arch Intern Med 2002;162: 1245–8.

[11] Bosker G. Thrombosis prophylaxis in seriously ill medical patients: evidence-based management, patient risk stratification, and outcome optimizing pharmacologic management. Internal Medicine Consensus Reports 2001:1–8.

[12] Goldhaber SZ, Dunn K, MacDougall RC. New onset of venous thromboembolism among hospitalized patients at Brigham and Women's Hospital is caused more often by prophylaxis failure than by withholding treatment. Chest 2000;118:1680–4.

[13] Middledorp S, Meinardi JR, Koopman MM, et al. A prospective study of asymptomatic carriers of the factor V Leiden mutation to determine the incidence of venous thromboembolism. Ann Intern Med 2001;135: 322–7.

[14] Martinelli I. Risk factors in venous thromboembolism. Thromb Haemost 2001;86:395–403.

[15] Bertina RM. The prothrombin 20210 G to A variation and thrombosis. Curr Opin Hematol 1998;5:339–42.

[16] Salzman EW, Hirsh J. The epidemiology, pathogenesis, and natural history of venous thrombosis. In: Colman RW, Hirsh J, Marder VJ, et al, editors. Hemostasis and thrombosis, basic principles and clinical practice, 3rd edition. Philadelphia: Lippincott; 1994. p. 1275–96.

[17] Kim V, Spandorfer J. Epidemiology of venous thromboembolic disease. Emerg Med Clin North Am 2001; 19:839–59.

[18] Anderson Jr FA, Wheeler HB, Goldberg RJ, et al. Prevalence of venous thromboembolism risk in a typical hospital population. Arch Intern Med 1992;152: 1660–4.

[19] The mandate to prevent venous thromboembolism: nursing-based risk stratification and prevention of deep vein thrombosis and pulmonary embolism in the hospitalized medical patient. Nursing Clinical Consensus Report. June 2002. American Health Consultants.

[20] Kierkegaard A, Norgren L. Graduated compression stocking in the prevention of deep vein thrombosis in patients with acute myocardial infarction. Eur Heart J 1993;14:1365–8.

[21] Kamran SI, Downey D, Ruff RL. Pneumatic sequential compression reduces the risk of deep vein thrombosis in stroke patients. Neurology 1998;50:1683–8.

[22] Hirsch DR, Ingenito EP, Goldhaber SZ. Prevalence of deep venous thrombosis among patients in medical intensive care. JAMA 1995;274:335–7.

[23] Marik PE, Andrews L, Maini B. The incidence of deep venous thrombosis in ICU patients. Chest 1997;111: 661–4.

[24] Inouye SK, Schlesinger M, Lydon T. Delirium: a symptom of how hospital care is failing older persons and a window to improve quality of hospital care. Am J Med 1999;106:565–73.

[25] McCarthy ST, Turner JJ, Robertson D, et al. Low-dose heparin as a prophylaxis against deep-vein thrombosis after acute stroke. Lancet 1977;2:800–1.

[26] McCarthy ST, Turner JJ. Low-dose subcutaneous heparin in the prevention of deep vein thrombosis and pulmonary emboli following acute stroke. Age Ageing 1986;15:84–8.

[27] Belch JJ, Lowe GDO, Ward AG, et al. Prevention of deep vein thrombosis in medical patients by low dose heparin. Scott Med J 1981;26:115–7.

[28] Cade JF. High-risk of the critically ill for VTE. Crit Care Med 1982;10:448–50.

[29] Ibarra-Perez K, Sandset PM. A double-blind and randomized placebo-controlled trial of low dose heparin in the intensive care unit. Semin Thromb Haemost 1988;11:25–33.

[30] Kupfer Y, Anwar J, Senenviratne C, et al. Prophylaxis with subcutaneous heparin significantly reduces the incidence of deep venous thrombophlebitis in the critically ill [abstract]. Am J Respir Crit Care Med 1999; 159(suppl):A519.

[31] Halkin H, Goldberg J, Mordan M, et al. Reduction of mortality in general medical inpatients by low-dose heparin prophylaxis. Ann Intern Med 1982;96:561–5.

[32] Garlund B for the Heparin Prophylaxis Study Group. Randomised, controlled trial of low-dose heparin for prevention of fatal pulmonary embolism in patients with infectious diseases. Lancet 1996;347:1357–61.

[33] Prins MH, Gelsema R, Sing AK, et al. Prophylaxis of deep venous thrombosis with a low-molecular weight heparin in stroke patients. Haemostasis 1989;19: 245–50.

[34] Sandset PM, Dahl T, Stiris M, et al. A double-blind and randomized placebo-controlled trial of low molecular weight heparin once daily to prevent deep-vein thrombosis in acute ischemic stroke. Semin Thromb Haemost 1990;16(suppl):25–33.

[35] Dahan R, Houlbert D, Caulin C, et al. Prevention of deep vein thrombosis in elderly medical patients by a low molecular weight heparin: a randomized double-blind trial. Haemostasis 1986;16:159–64.

[36] Samama MM, Cohen AT, Darmon J-Y, et al. A comparison of enoxaparin with placebo for the prevention of VTE in acutely ill medical patients. N Engl J Med 1999;341:793–800.

[37] Harenberg J, Kallenbach B, Martin U, et al. Randomized controlled study of heparin and low molecular

weight heparin for prevention of deep-vein thrombosis in medical patients. Thromb Res 1990;59:639–50.

[38] Bergmann J-F, Neuhart E. A multicenter randomized double-blind study of enoxaparin compared with unfractionated heparin in the prevention of venous thromboembolic disease in elderly inpatients bedridden for an acute medical illness. Thromb Haemost 1996;76: 529–34.

[39] Lechler E, Schramm W, Flosbach CW, et al. The venous thrombotic risk in non-surgical patients: epidemiological data and efficacy/safety profile of a low-molecular weight heparin. Haemostasis 1996;26(suppl 2):49–56.

[40] Kleber FX, Witt C, Flosbach CW, et al. Study to compare the efficacy and safety of the LMWH enoxaparin and standard heparin in the prevention of thromboembolic events in medical patients with cardiopulmonary diseases [abstract]. Ann Hematol 1998; 76(suppl 1):A93.

[41] Harenberg J, Schomaker U, Flosbach CW, et al. Enoxaparin is superior to unfractionated heparin in the prevention of thromboembolic events in medical patients at increased thromboembolic risk [abstract]. Blood 1999;94(suppl 1):399a.

[42] Hillbom M, Erila T, Sotaniemi CW, et al. Comparison of the efficacy and safety of the low-molecular-weight heparin enoxaparin with unfractionated heparin in the prevention of deep venous thrombosis in patients with acute ischemic stroke [abstract]. Blood 1999; 94(suppl 1):183a.

[43] Lamy A, Wang X, Kent R, et al. Economic evaluation of the MEDENOX trial: a Canadian perspective. Can Respir J 2002;9:169–77.

[44] Lloyd AC, Anderson PM, Quinlan DJ, et al. Economic evaluation of the use of enoxaparin for thromboprophylaxis in acutely ill medical patients. J Med Econ 2001;4:99–112.

Clin Chest Med 24 (2003) 103–122

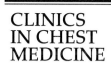

CLINICS
IN CHEST
MEDICINE

Venous thromboembolism in intensive care patients

Ana T. Rocha, MD*, Victor F. Tapson, MD

Division of Pulmonary and Critical Care Medicine, Duke University Medical Center, Box 3221, Durham, NC 27710, USA

Venous thromboembolism (VTE) represents a spectrum of disease that encompasses deep venous thrombosis (DVT), pulmonary embolism (PE), and, in critically ill patients, often includes central venous catheter (CVC)–associated thrombosis. PE is the most serious manifestation of VTE and remains one of the leading causes of unexpected deaths in hospitalized patients [1,2]. Although critically ill medical patients are thought to be at a higher risk for VTE, this population is heterogeneous and underinvestigated [3].

This article reviews particular aspects of the epidemiology, risk factors, prophylaxis, diagnosis, and treatment of VTE in critically ill patients.

Epidemiology

Venous thromboembolic events are considerably more common in hospitalized and severely ill patients than in the outpatient setting [4]. The reported rate of DVT ranges from 22% to almost 80% depending on patients' underlying clinical characteristics. In general medical wards, DVT is reported in 9% to 27.5% of patients without prevention [5,6]. Likewise, without prophylaxis, postoperative DVT can be detected in 6% to 22% of general surgical patients and in as many as 50% of patients with multisystem or major trauma [7,8]. The estimated prevalence of DVT is 22% to 35% in neurosurgical patients and exceeds 50% to 80% in acute spinal cord injury patients [9].

Most patients in the intensive care unit (ICU) have multiple risk factors for VTE, but only a few studies have focused on this complex population

(Table 1). When routine screening for DVT with either fibrinogen leg scanning or serial Doppler ultrasonography is performed in medical–surgical ICU patients, DVT is detected in 26% to 32% of patients receiving no prophylaxis [10–15]. Ten percent to 30% of medical–surgical ICU patients experience DVT within the first week of admission, and approximately 60% of trauma patients have DVT within the first 2 weeks, most of which are silent episodes [9]. Hirsch et al [14] assessed the risk for VTE in 100 consecutive medical ICU patients who received VTE prophylaxis (61%). Seventy percent of DVTs could be detected with a single screening ultrasound within the initial 5 days of hospitalization, resulting in therapeutic interventions in two thirds of events. The incidence of VTE in patients treated with intermittent pneumatic compression (IPC) devices or any heparin regimen did not differ from the incidence in patients receiving no prophylaxis (34% and 32%, respectively). Nevertheless, the lack of randomization and the small sample size in this study limit any conclusions about the efficacy of individual methods of prophylaxis.

Although the risk for VTE found in previous studies has been unexpectedly high, the incidence of DVT may still be underestimated. The screening techniques that have been used have limited sensitivity for isolated calf and pelvic thrombi, leading to a high percentage of false-negative results. Nevertheless, fewer DVT can be detected by clinical assessment alone. In an observational study of medical–surgical ICU patients in whom no imaging screening was performed, the incidence of clinically relevant DVT or PE was much lower than the incidence in the previous studies (5.4%) [16]. This finding could be anticipated, because the clinical signs and symptoms of DVT and PE are frequently underinvestigated.

---

* Corresponding author.
E-mail address: rocha002@mc.duke.edu (A.T. Rocha).

doi:10.1016/S0272-5231(02)00056-4

Table 1
Studies of the incidence of deep venous thrombosis in intensive care patients

Study (year)	Population	DVT screening test	Design	Number/total (%) with DVT		
				No prophylaxis	LDUH[a] or LMWH[b]	SCD
Moser et al (1981)	34 respiratory ICU patients, 76% were intubated	Fib I daily for 3–6 days	Prospective cohort	3/34 (9)	NA	NA
Cade (1982)	119 coronary and medical ICU patients	Fib I daily for 8 days (range, 4–10)	Blind RCT	NR/NR (29)	NR/NR (13)[a]	NA
Ibarra-Perez et al (1988)	192 high-risk pulmonary patients	Fib I, Doppler US, SGP daily until ambulatory	Prospective cohort	12/46 (26)	1/39 (2.6)[a]	0/39 (0)
Hirsch et al (1995)	100 medical ICU patients, 80% were intubated	Doppler US twice weekly	Prospective cohort	10/31 (32)	17/43 (40)[a]	6/18(33)
Marik et al (1997)	102 medical–surgical ICU patients, 68% were intubated	Single Doppler US at day 4–7	Prospective cohort	2/8 (25)	5/68 (7)[a]	5/26 (19)
Fraisse et al (2000)	223 medical ICU patients with COPD, 100% were intubated	Doppler US weekly until completion of the study	Multicenter, double-blind RCT	24/85 (28.2)	13/84 (15.5)[b]	NA

Abbreviations: COPD, chronic obstructive pulmonary disease; DVT, deep venous thrombosis; Fib I, fibrinogen I 125 scan of the legs; ICU, intensive care unit; LDUH, low-dose unfractionated heparin; LMWH, low molecular weight heparin; NA, not applicable; NR, not reported; RCT, randomized controlled trial; SCD, sequential compression devices; IPG, impedance plethysmography; US, ultrasonography.

[a] LDUH, 5000 U subcutaneously, twice daily.

[b] LMWH, nadroparin, 3800 anti-Xa IU or 5700 anti-Xa IU according to body weight, subcutaneously, once daily.

Mortality

Postmortem studies show that most fatal emboli arise from the deep venous system in the lower limbs, but only a minority of these patients have symptoms of DVT, and even a smaller percentage undergo an investigation for these symptoms before death [2]. Approximately 48% to 60% of DVT found in ICU patients are located above the knee and carry greater risk for embolization [12,14]. Even though the rate of symptomatic PE in high-risk trauma patients is low (0.7% to 2%), PE can be found in a much larger percentage of patients at autopsy [8,9]. In one study, PE was identified in 17 of 66 ICU patients (27%) undergoing autopsy, and only half of these events were diagnosed before death [17].

Several experts suggest that not all PE are clinically relevant. Nonetheless, in the study by Hirsch and colleagues [14] in which 100 medical ICU patients had ultrasound screening until discharge from the ICU, the inhospital mortality rate among patients with DVT was 50% higher than the rate for patients without DVT. Confirmation of this trend toward an increased mortality among patients with symptomatic and silent VTE needs to be confirmed in larger cohorts of ICU patients.

Morbidity

In many clinical settings, undetected and clinically evident VTE can impact on the morbidity of severely ill patients [18,19]. Significant additional morbidity from DVT relates to local complications such as stasis ulcers or recurrent thrombosis, which are sequelae of the postphlebitic syndrome, CVC-related thrombosis with associated line malfunctioning, and potential CVC-related infection [20]. Furthermore, recovery from the original critical illness (eg, weaning from mechanical ventilation) can be affected adversely by these complications [3].

Risk factors

Most critically ill patients have one or more recognizable risk factors for VTE. In one cohort of 225 patients admitted to a medical–surgical ICU, the average number of risk factors was four [21]. Surgical ICU patients, multiple trauma victims, and patients with severe head or injury are at extremely high risk for VTE [22]; however, less than 30% of patients hospitalized because of VTE are surgical.

Some nonsurgical situations, such as ischemic strokes and acute myocardial infarction, have been clearly identified as associated with an increased risk for VTE [23]. Acute and chronic illness, immobility, advanced age, respiratory failure, and procedural and pharmacologic interventions may also predispose ICU patients to VTE. The at-risk situations in nonsurgical patients are less well defined, and traditionally recognized DVT risk factors have failed to identify patients in whom VTE developed in some series. In a prospective ultrasound series of 100 medical ICU patients, there was no difference in age, gender, body mass index, diagnosis of cancer, recent surgery, duration of hospitalization before DVT, and use of DVT prophylaxis in patients with DVT and those without [14]. In another series of 119 medical–surgical ICU patients, DVT was found mainly in men and was associated with circulatory impairment, respiratory failure, and recent vascular and cancer surgery [11]. Cook and co-workers [16] demonstrated that, among 93 mixed medical–surgical ICU patients, acquired VTE risk factors were mechanical ventilation, immobility, a femoral venous catheter, sedatives, and paralytic drugs. In contrast, heparin prophylaxis, aspirin, and thromboembolic disease stockings conferred a lower risk, but only warfarin and intravenous heparin were associated with a statistically lower risk of VTE (odds ratio [OR], 0.07 and 0.04, respectively).

The assessment of VTE risk in surgical and medical patients requires a consideration of individual risk factors and their interactions to assist in developing adequate recommendations for prophylaxis and treatment [24]. Table 2 lists several of the general risk factors for the development of VTE in adult patients. Special factors that are unique to the ICU patient, including CVC-related thrombosis, infections complicating CVC-related thrombosis,

Table 2
Risk factors for venous thromboembolism

Previous venous thromboembolism	Inherited hypercoagulable states
Increased age (> 40 years)	Protein C deficiency
Obesity	Protein S deficiency
Malignancy	Antithrombin III deficiency
Pregnancy	Dysfibrinogenemia
Congestive heart failure	Factor V Leiden mutation
Immobilization	Prothrombin gene mutation
Recent surgery	Hyperhomocysteinemia
Trauma	Acquired hypercoagulable states
Mechanical ventilation	Lupus anticoagulant
Central venous catheterization	Anticardiolipin antibody

and upper extremity DVT, are discussed in the following sections.

Central venous catheter–related venous thromboembolism

Central venous catheter–related DVT is an important complication of intensive care, because venous catheters are commonly placed in the ICU patient, and thrombosis follows 35% to 67% of long-term catheterizations [25,26]. CVC-related thrombosis may develop as soon as 1 day after canulation and is initially asymptomatic [27,28]. Despite inconsistency from study to study, some investigators have identified factors that increase the risk for thrombotic complications related to CVC use. These conditions can be described as technical factors and host factors (Table 3).

Animal studies have linked some older catheter materials, such as Teflon, polyethylene, and polyvinyl, with higher rates of thrombosis than seen with silicone and Silastic [29]. Most contemporary catheters are made of polyurethane coated with hydromer, which is highly biocompatible and generates the least amount of thrombin formation [30,31].

According to recent studies, the rate of CVC-related thrombosis seems to vary slightly with the site of insertion. Femoral catheters have been associated with a higher incidence of thrombosis, with rates as high as 25% and abnormal Doppler ultrasound findings in as many as 48% of screened patients [32]. Nevertheless, in a study of mixed medical–surgical ICU patients undergoing an intensive ultrasound screening protocol, the incidence of femoral CVC-related DVT was much lower (9.6%) [28]. In that study, the risk of thrombosis was unrelated to the number of insertion attempts, arterial puncture or hematoma, the duration of catheterization, coagulation status, or the type of infused medications. Martin and colleagues [33] reported that the incidence of CVC-related axillary vein thrombosis was 11.6%, and that the risk increased when catheter-

ization exceeded 6 days. Thrombosis rates ranging from 4% to 28% have been reported after subclavian vein canulation [34–37] and rates from 4% to 33% after internal jugular vein catheterization [37,38].

Although catheterization of the femoral vein is convenient and has potential advantages, this practice seems to be associated with a greater risk of thrombotic events than catheterization of the upper body venous system. Nevertheless, questions regarding the frequency of clinically meaningful complications secondary to CVC-related femoral thrombosis, such as PE, remain unanswered.

Infections complicating central venous catheter–related thrombosis

Nosocomial blood stream infections are noteworthy causes of morbidity and mortality among ICU patients and frequently complicate the use of CVCs. In a prospective study of ICU adult patients with a CVC, the total days of hospitalization and the total number of intermittent infusions through the CVC were the best predictors of nosocomial infections [39]. CVC thrombosis also has been associated with an increased incidence of blood stream infection in an autopsy series of cancer patients [40].

Debate continues concerning the increased risk of thrombotic and infectious complications with femoral vein catheterization versus its alternatives [41]. In a randomized controlled trial performed in eight ICUs in France, 289 patients were assigned to have femoral vein or subclavian vein catheters placed [42]. Femoral catheterization was associated with significantly higher overall thrombotic complications (21.5% versus 1.9%, respectively) and complete thrombosis of the vessel (6% versus 0%, respectively). The femoral route was also related with a higher incidence of overall infectious complications (19.8% versus 4.5%, respectively) but not major infectious complications, such as clinical sepsis with or without blood stream infection (4.4% versus 1.5%, respectively). A longer duration of catheterization, insertion in two sites, and

Table 3
Factors associated with an increased risk of central venous catheter–related thrombosis and mechanical complications

Technical factors	Host factors
Material: polyvinyl and polyurethane > silicone, silastic, and coated polyurethane	No prophylactic or therapeutic heparin use
Non–heparin-bonded catheters	More than one central venous catheter simultaneously
Placement of catheter during the night	Extremes of age (preterm neonates and age >64 years)
Site: femoral and internal jugular > subclavian veins and axillary veins	Comorbidities (cancer, dehydration, and impaired tissue perfusion)
Duration of canulation (>6 days)	Thrombophilic states

placement during the night all led to an increased risk of mechanical complications.

Heparin-bonded catheters have been correlated with significantly fewer thrombotic complications and possibly with a decreased incidence of positive CVC-related blood culture in critically ill pediatric patients [25]. In a double-blind controlled trial, 209 critically ill children (aged 0 to 16 years) were randomly assigned to receive heparin-bonded venous catheters (HB-CVC) or non–heparin-bonded venous catheters (NHB-CVC) [43]. The investigators evaluated the risk of infection and thrombosis using an intensive protocol consisting of blood cultures performed at baseline and every 3 days and screening ultrasonography until the catheters had been removed. Heparin bonding was associated with a significant reduction in infections, with a hazards ratio of 0.11. The incidence of infection was 4% and 33% in the HB-CVC and NHB-CVC groups, respectively, and the incidence of thrombosis 0% and 8% in these groups, respectively.

Complications in 265 internal jugular vein and subclavian vein catheterizations were prospectively evaluated in an observational study of adult patients [37]. CVC-related thrombosis was independently associated with the internal jugular vein route (relative risk [RR], 4.13) and age greater than 64 years (RR, 2.44) and negatively correlated with therapeutic heparin use (RR, 0.47). Moreover, the risk for CVC-related sepsis was approximately threefold higher when thrombosis occurred. Randolph and co-workers [44] conducted a meta-analysis to evaluate the effect of heparin on thrombus formation and infection associated with CVC. The prophylactic use of heparin significantly decreased CVC-related thrombosis (RR, 0.43) and bacterial colonization of the CVC (RR, 0.26), with a trend toward decrease of CVC-related bacteremia (RR, 0.26).

Taken together, these data suggest that the development of thrombosis might negatively affect the CVC-related infectious complications in critically ill children and adults. The use of an HB-CVC with or without heparin has consistently been associated with less thrombus formation around the CVC and a trend toward less CVC-related infections. Whether mechanical methods of VTE prophylaxis have effects comparable with those of heparin on blood stream infections is still unknown.

Deep venous thrombosis of the upper extremity

Upper-extremity DVT is common in patients with systemic illness and in those with venous catheters [45]. Although, traditionally, upper-extremity DVT has been thought to cause few complications and offer a small risk for PE, this concept has been challenged recently. Thrombosis of the deep venous system of the upper body is likely to be missed because imaging of these vessels is not usually part of the investigation for PE. In a review of 329 cases of axillary or subclavian vein thrombosis, PE was reported in 9.4% of patients [36]. Monreal and colleagues [46] showed that CVC-related, upper-extremity DVT resulted in PE in 15% of patients studied with a ventilation–perfusion scintigraphy scan. More recently, Prandoni and co-workers [20] studied 58 consecutive patients with clinically suspected upper-extremity DVT using three ultrasound techniques and venography. Symptomatic upper-extremity DVT was associated with a CVC, thrombophilic state, or previous leg vein thrombosis. In patients with positive results for DVT of the upper extremities, a ventilation–perfusion scan with or without pulmonary angiography was performed and PE documented or highly probable in 36% of patients.

Complications from upper-extremity DVT are less frequent than after lower-extremity DVT; however, they are not trivial and should not be overlooked in patients with underlying cardiopulmonary compromise.

Prophylaxis for venous thromboembolism

Routine DVT prophylaxis (Table 4) is the most efficient and cost-effective way to prevent fatal and nonfatal VTE [47,48]; however, recent studies have shown that, even in high-risk critically ill patients, prophylactic measures are frequently underused [49,50]. Goldhaber [51] showed in a mixed medical–surgical ICU that DVT prophylaxis was applied to one-third of patients. Likewise, Keane et al [49] reported that, although 87% of their medical ICU patients had at least one risk factor for thrombosis, VTE prophylaxis was only prescribed to 32.9% of the patients with a mean delay of 2 days. Computerized order entry sets and intensive education have been shown to improve the rate of VTE prophylaxis [52]. Nevertheless, there is increasing concern about VTE occurring in the setting of (failed) prophylaxis [53,54].

The Sixth ACCP Consensus Conference on Antithrombotic Therapy [6] compiled an extensive review of available literature on VTE prophylaxis including 630 references. A large body of evidence in this review suggests the efficacy and safety of low-dose unfractionated heparin (LDUH) and low molecular weight heparin (LMWH) as DVT prophylaxis in surgical patients. Mechanical devices have proved useful as VTE prophylaxis in some surgical populations [50,55,56]. Less data are available in

Table 4
Recommended venous thromboembolism prophylaxis for intensive care unit patients

Intensive care population	Recommended prophylaxis
Medical patients	
Medical intensive care (including cancer, bedrest, heart failure, severe lung disease)	LDUH q12h or q8h, or LMWH ES or SCD if anticoagulation is contraindicated
Acute myocardial infarction	Prophylactic anticoagulation with SC LDUH, 5000 U q12h or q8h, or therapeutic SC UFH, or IV UFH
Acute ischemic stroke	LDUH, LMWH, or danaparoid; consider combination with mechanical prophylaxis with ES or SCD ES or SCD if anticoagulation is contraindicated
Hemorrhagic stroke	SCD
Acute spinal cord injury	LMWH preferred; consider mechanical prophylaxis with ES or SCD in combination with LMWH or LDUH ES or SCD if anticoagulation is contraindicated early after injury
Surgical patients	
Trauma	LMWH, ES, and/or SCD if LDWH is delayed or contraindicated early after trauma
Neurosurgery	SCD with or without ES; consider combination of mechanical method with LDUH or LMWH postoperatively
High-risk general surgery (non-major surgery and age >60 years or additional risk factors, or major surgery and age >40 years or additional risk factors)	LDUH, LMWH, or SCD; consider mechanical prophylaxis with ES or SCD in combination with LMWH or LDUH ES or SCD if anticoagulation is contraindicated early after surgery
Major orthopedic surgery (hip replacement, knee replacement, hip fracture)	LMWH or adjusted-dose warfarin; consider mechanical prophylaxis with ES or SCD in combination with LMWH or warfarin; LDUH not recommended

Abbreviations: ES, elastic stockings; IV, intravenous, LDUH, low-dose unfractionated heparin; LMWH, low molecular weight heparin; SC, subcutaneous; SCD, sequential compression devices; UFH, unfractionated heparin.

medical patients and even less in critically ill patients [57]. Based on the extrapolation of data from surgical and medical noncritically ill patients, the committee suggested the use of LDUH or LMWH for prophylaxis in the critically ill population. Elastic stockings or compression devices were suggested for patients with a high risk for bleeding.

Balancing the risk of thrombosis and bleeding

When compared with other ICU patients, critically ill medical patients frequently have chronic underlying illness and present with hematologic failure as a result of malignancy or sepsis [19]; consequently, they may be prone to bleeding complications, causing concerns about the safety of antithrombotic drugs in these patients. Overt bleeding and thrombocytopenia are usually considered contraindications for pharmacologic VTE prophylaxis and treatment with anticoagulants. When deciding about appropriate management of VTE in critically ill patients, intensivists must carefully balance the risks of thrombophilia and bleeding. Nevertheless, the objective assessment of risk factors is rarely performed, and the presumed

propensity for bleeding may lead physicians to avoid heparins as VTE prophylaxis and to opt for no prophylaxis instead. In a retrospective study of the choice of VTE prophylaxis in a medical ICU, the presence of one or more risk factors for bleeding was associated with underuse of prophylaxis, including mechanical methods (Rocha AT, Tapson VF. 2002.).

One of the feared complications in the ICU is gastrointestinal bleeding. In one respiratory ICU, gastrointestinal bleeding occurred in 20% of patients. Risk factors were the diagnosis of adult respiratory distress syndrome, an increasing number of days on a ventilator, the number of days in the ICU, and the development of thrombocytopenia [58]. Nevertheless, the use of heparin therapy was not associated with an increased risk of gastrointestinal hemorrhage. Supporting this observation are abundant data from meta-analyses and placebo-controlled, randomized studies demonstrating either no increase or a small increase in the absolute rate of major bleeding with the prophylactic use of LDUH or LMWH [59–61]. The results of three meta-analyses of the therapeutic use of heparins also suggest that LMWH drugs are as safe as unfractionated heparin with respect to major bleeding complications and seem to be slightly more effective in preventing thromboembolic recurrences [62–64].

Heparin-induced thrombocytopenia with or without thrombosis is another underrecognized problem that may occur in 1% to 2% of heparin recipients and in rare instances may result in limb amputation. The pathophysiology of this immune-mediated condition implicates the heparin–platelet factor 4 complex as the culprit antigen in most patients [65]. Heparin-induced thrombocytopenia may have a delayed onset (6–10 days); therefore, awareness and frequent platelet counts are required for early diagnosis and treatment [66]. Unfractionated heparin is approximately eight to ten times more likely to cause heparin-induced thrombocytopenia than is LMWH [67]. LMWH is not recommended as treatment for heparin-induced thrombocytopenia, because approximately 50% of patients may have persistence or worsening of the condition [68]. Because of the increased risk for thrombosis, an alternative intravenous anticoagulant (lepirudin or argatroban) should be used to treat heparin-induced thrombocytopenia until platelet count recovery [69].

A careful evaluation of the risk for thrombosis and bleeding is recommended in all critically ill patients. In a mail survey of 44 ICUs in Canada, the directors of the units answered that decisions about the type of VTE prophylaxis employed were made for the most part on a case-by-case basis (62.1%), rather than by preprinted orders (17.2%), institutional policies (20.7%), or formal practice guidelines (6.9%) [70]. The best way to accomplish adequate patient assessment and to improve the implementation of methods of VTE prophylaxis remains to be determined. Whether any particular approach leads to better use of resources and, more importantly, to improvement of patient outcome are unanswered questions.

Pharmacologic methods of venous thromboembolism prophylaxis

Venous thromboembolism prophylaxis with either LDUH or LMWH given subcutaneously is the preferred option and should be offered to most critically ill patients. One large randomized controlled trial showed a significant reduction in the incidence of DVT in critically ill patients using LDUH when compared with placebo (11% and 31%, respectively) [71]. The MEDical patients with ENOXaparin (MEDENOX) trial [5] also established a reduction in the risk for VTE among 1102 acutely ill medical patients when a placebo was compared with a LMWH (enoxaparin) (14.9% and 5.5%, respectively). Never-

theless, these trials excluded mechanically ventilated patients and patients with severe sepsis. In one of the few randomized controlled trials among mechanically ventilated patients, Fraisse and co-workers [15] evaluated 223 patients with acute decompensated chronic obstructive pulmonary disease (COPD). They demonstrated a 45% decreased incidence of DVT with another LMWH (nadroparin) when compared with placebo. The rates of adverse events, particularly hemorrhage, were similar in both groups.

Recent data suggest that LMWH is more effective than LDUH for VTE prophylaxis in critically ill trauma patients [72], and that high-dose LMWH is more effective than placebo or low-dose LMWH in seriously ill medical patients [6]. LMWH also seems superior to LDUH for the prevention of venographically proven lower-extremity DVT in acute stroke patients [6]. Mismetti and co-workers [73] performed a meta-analysis based on data for several heparins used in internal medicine, excluding patients sustaining acute myocardial infarction or stroke. A significant decrease in DVT and clinical PE was observed with heparin in a comparison with controls (RR, 56% and 58%, respectively; $P < 0.001$) without a significant difference in the incidence of major bleeding or death. Nine trials comparing LMWH with LDUH (4669 patients) were also included and showed no significant difference in DVT, clinical PE, or mortality; however, the use of LMWH seemed to reduce the risk of major hemorrhage by 52% in a comparison with LDUH.

Attia et al [9] have systematically reviewed the literature on different methods of DVT prophylaxis in patients admitted to ICUs and patients sustaining trauma, neurosurgery, or spinal cord injury. The use of subcutaneous LDUH reduced the rate of VTE by 50% when compared with no prophylaxis. Overall, the use of LDUH decreased the incidence of DVT by 20%, whereas the use of LMWH decreased the incidence by a further 30%. These investigators urged caution regarding the interpretation of results of combined trials, because methods of prophylaxis proven in one group do not necessarily generalize to other critically ill patient groups.

Mechanical methods of venous thromboembolism prophylaxis

Mechanical prophylaxis with sequential compression devices (SCD), also referred to as IPC, is an attractive form of VTE prophylaxis owing to the lack of bleeding risk and proven efficacy in postoperative circumstances [50,74]. These devices have been suggested to have a hemodynamic action (increase of blood flow velocity) and to stimulate endogenous fibrinolytic activity via the production of tissue-type plasminogen activator by the vascular endothelium, which might contribute to their antithrombotic properties [75]. In most surgical studies, the investigators have used devices that compressed the legs and thighs intraoperatively and for 1 to 5 days after operation. Even when IPC devices are applied to the arms during and after surgery, they may reduce the incidence of leg DVT to half the incidence in control patients, and blood fibrinolytic activity is maintained at preoperative values [76].

In a nonrandomized study, the use of graded compression stockings, LDUH, and aspirin was associated with a statistically significant reduction in DVT when compared with no prophylaxis in high-risk pulmonary patients [12]. Marik and co-workers [13] studied 102 critically ill medical–surgical patients using screening Doppler ultrasonography during the first week of ICU stay. DVT was detected in 25% of the patients receiving no prophylaxis, in 7% receiving LDUH, and in 19% receiving SCD. The difference between the SCD and LDUH groups did not reach significance, but the study lacked power to detect statistical differences. In a meta-analysis of five controlled trials of moderate- and high-risk surgical patients, the incidence of DVT detected by fibrinogen uptake test was 9.9% with SCD and 20.3% in control patients [59]. Wells and colleagues [74] performed a meta-analysis showing that mechanical prophylaxis was efficacious for moderate-risk postoperative patients with a pooled OR of 0.28 in five randomized trials. More recently, a different group of investigators documented similar findings for critically ill surgical patients [9]. They found that mechanical devices led to a 68% risk reduction of VTE; however, they were unable to evaluate thromboprophylaxis with mechanical methods for medical–surgical patients owing to a lack of sufficient information.

Although encouraging, not all of the available data favor mechanical methods of prophylaxis. In a small prospective trial of multiple trauma patients with severe head injury, similar rates of DVT and angiographically proven PE were found in patients receiving SCD (29%) or no prophylaxis (22%) [22]. Recently, Jimenez and co-workers [77] demonstrated that IPC devices failed to decrease the incidence of DVT in critically ill patients with a contraindication for heparin.

Controversy continues regarding the proper indication and compliance with the use of mechanical devices [23,53,78]. The presence of leg ulcers or peripheral arterial occlusive disease may preclude the use of SCD. Nevertheless, the combination of prolonged immobility and the high nursing-to-patient ratio in the ICU seems to be an ideal setting for improved compliance with mechanical devices.

Combination of prophylactic methods

The concomitant use of bilateral SCD and other forms of prophylaxis has been studied in a few patient groups. In a randomized trial of 2551 consecutive cardiac surgical patients, SCD in combination with LDUH led to a 62% reduction in postsurgical PE in comparison with prophylaxis with LDUH alone (1.5% and 4%, respectively) [55]. Kamran et al [79] reported a 40-fold reduction in the risk for DVT in nonhemorrhagic stroke patients when SCD were combined with LDUH versus LDUH alone. In neurosurgical patients, the use of LMWH as an adjunct to mechanical prophylaxis has been favorable, with a pooled OR of 0.59 when compared with SCD alone [60]. It seems logical to consider the combination of SCD with pharmacologic prophylaxis in high-risk ICU patients, but data continue to be sparse.

Heparins are beneficial in the prevention of VTE in critically ill medical and surgical patients and should be considered the first-line prophylaxis for most ICU patients, unless there is a significant risk of bleeding. Although SCD are not associated with bleeding risks and are generally recommended as an alternative in patients in whom the risk of bleeding is high, little is known about their efficacy as the sole method of VTE prophylaxis for critically ill medical patients. SCD may be most beneficial when used in conjunction with pharmacologic methods in a subgroup of high-risk patients. More research is needed to define the overall efficacy, risk-to-benefit ratios, and cost-effectiveness of the different methods of VTE prevention in critically ill patients.

Diagnosis of deep venous thrombosis and pulmonary embolism in the intensive care unit

Investigation for VTE happens infrequently in ICU patients owing to several factors. First, ICU patients frequently have underlying systemic illnesses that may mask common presenting signs and symptoms of VTE. Second, an increasing number of ICU patients now receive VTE prophylaxis as part of general ICU care and are assumed to be fully protected. Third, the presence of relative contraindications, such as renal impairment, mechanical ventilation, and hemodynamic compromise, makes definitive testing for PE more difficult. Furthermore, some of the current diagnostic tools perform less well in the critically ill, impairing efforts to diagnose VTE.

Clinical features

Diagnosing PE in ICU patients represents a significant challenge. In patients with respiratory failure, the usual clinical manifestations of PE are often already present owing to severe underlying pulmonary disease, and any superimposed manifestations of PE become less apparent [17]. Furthermore, signs and symptoms, such as dyspnea, tachypnea, hypoxia, chest pain, tachycardia, fever, hypotension, and hemoptysis, are common in the ICU but nonspecific for PE. Most patients with cardiopulmonary disease have an elevated alveolar–arterial difference of more than 20 mm Hg during acute PE. Nevertheless, as many as one third of patients with acute PE who are younger than 40 years and who do not have pre-existing cardiopulmonary disease may have a PaO_2 greater than 80 mm Hg and a normal alveolar–arterial difference [80]. Lightheadedness and syncope can be caused by PE with a large clot burden but are seen less often in the ICU. Abnormalities in the chest radiograph occur in most patients with PE. Radiographic findings such as atelectasis, pleural effusions, and infiltrates are common but may be secondary to coexisting cardiopulmonary processes; therefore, a high index of suspicion is necessary in patients with risk factors, because fatalities following PE usually occur within hours of the initial event [10].

Massive PE is a devastating clinical entity often undiscovered until autopsy. An unexplained drop in systolic blood pressure of more than 40 mm Hg or a systolic blood pressure of less than 90 mm Hg for 15 minutes is associated with respiratory decompensation in most cases [81]. Acute right ventricular failure may progress to death within minutes to hours after the embolic event, and prompt diagnostic and therapeutic intervention are imperative. Although clinical suspicion is crucial, objective testing is required to confirm or exclude the presence of PE and should be carried out thoroughly once the suspicion is raised. Hemodynamic instability may hinder a standard diagnostic evaluation, giving bedside tests a paramount role in guiding therapeutic interventions.

Diagnostic algorithms

Standardized diagnostic approaches to VTE are designed to obviate the need for invasive procedures and their associated morbidity in an already severely ill group of patients. Clinical assessment protocols have been developed and tested in the emergency room and in inpatient settings [20,30,35,82–86]. Using a clinical model in 1239 patients with suspected PE, Wells and colleagues [83] showed that the pretest probability was low in 3.4%, moderate in 27.8%, and high in 78.4% of patients with PE. Only 0.5% of patients with a low- to-moderate pretest probability and a non–high-probability scan who were considered negative for PE actually had PE or DVT during 90-day follow-up. A combined strategy using negative D-dimer results and a simplified "Wells model" safely excluded PE in a large proportion of patients [87]. This strategy had a negative predictive value of 99.5% by including the following seven variables: clinical symptoms of DVT, no alternative diagnosis, heart rate greater than 100 beats/minute, immobilization or surgery in the previous 4 weeks, previous DVT or PE, hemoptysis, and malignancy. Perrier and colleagues [88] showed that, in 1034 emergency room patients with low clinical probability of PE by empiric assessment and nondiagnostic ventilation–perfusion scans plus a negative lower-limb venous compression ultrasonography, the 3-month risk for VTE was low (1.7%). This approach eliminated the need for pulmonary angiography in 21.5% of the patients.

Ideally, the coupling of reliable clinical assessment and noninvasive imaging techniques would be preferred when evaluating the ICU patient with suspected VTE. Unfortunately, none of the clinical models described previously have been validated in the ICU. Nevertheless, it appears logical to incorporate a preclinical probability of PE based on the knowledge of risk factors and presenting signs and symptoms into diagnostic algorithms in an attempt to guide further diagnostic and therapeutic decisions.

In Figs. 1 and 2, the authors propose diagnostic algorithms for suspected PE in hemodynamically stable and unstable critically ill patients, respectively.

Electrocardiography

Electrocardiography is of limited diagnostic utility in suspected PE [89]. Nonspecific electrocardiographic abnormalities may develop in acute PE, including T-wave changes, ST-segment abnormalities, and left or right axis deviation. Occasionally, electrocardiographic changes occur that are more suggestive of PE, including the S1Q3T3 pattern, right bundle branch block, P-wave pulmonale, and right axis deviation [90]. In patients with massive acute PE, an increase in the amplitude of the negative T wave in precordial leads after thrombolytic therapy has been shown to reflect improvement in cardiopulmonary hemodynamics [91].

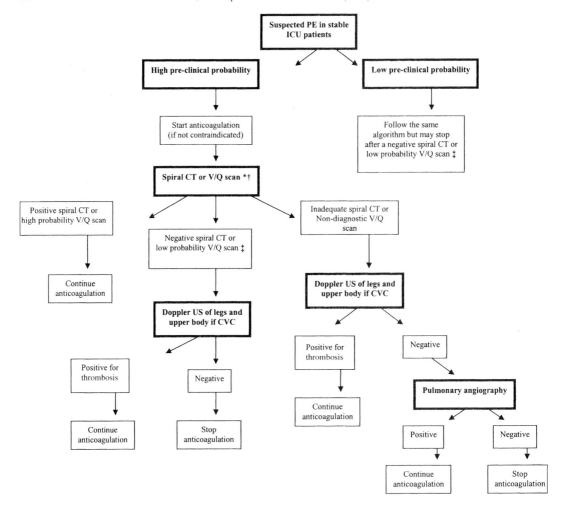

Fig. 1. Diagnostic algorithm for suspected pulmonary embolism in hemodynamically stable patient. CVC, central venous catheterization; ICU, intensive care unit; PE, pulmonary embolism; US, ultrasonography; V/Q scan, ventilation–perfusion lung scan. Notes: * Decision about spiral CT versus V/Q scan will depend on local availability, reader's experience, and presence of contraindications for intravenous contrast. † If a ventilation scan cannot be performed, an isolated perfusion scan can be useful if the scan reveals significant perfusion defects in the absence of radiographic explanation, or if it is near normal or normal. ‡ Consider stopping work-up at this point if there is low preclinical probability of pulmonary embolism.

End-tidal CO$_2$

An increase in dead space and a decrease in end-tidal CO$_2$ are known to occur in embolism that involves more than 25% of the pulmonary vasculature [42,43,92,93]. In one study, Johanning and colleagues [94] evaluated the value of negative D-dimer testing and changes in dead space from baseline to exclude PE in critically ill patients. A statistically significant increase in dead space from baseline was found in patients with PE and a decrease in patients without PE. Continuous monitoring of end-tidal CO$_2$ tension has been used to monitor the trends in mean pulmonary

artery pressure and cardiac index during thrombolytic therapy in mechanically ventilated patients with massive PE [95]. In this small study, recurrent embolism was detected in two patients by sudden reduction of the end-tidal CO$_2$. Nevertheless, there is a great deal of overlap among absolute values of end-tidal CO$_2$ in patients with COPD, and several other cardiopulmonary conditions may alter the difference between the PaCO$_2$ and end-tidal CO$_2$, decreasing its specificity for PE. High respiratory rates lower mixed–expired CO$_2$ because of increased sampling of the anatomic dead space. Variation in CO$_2$ production affects mixed–expired CO$_2$, and, in many patients with large emboli,

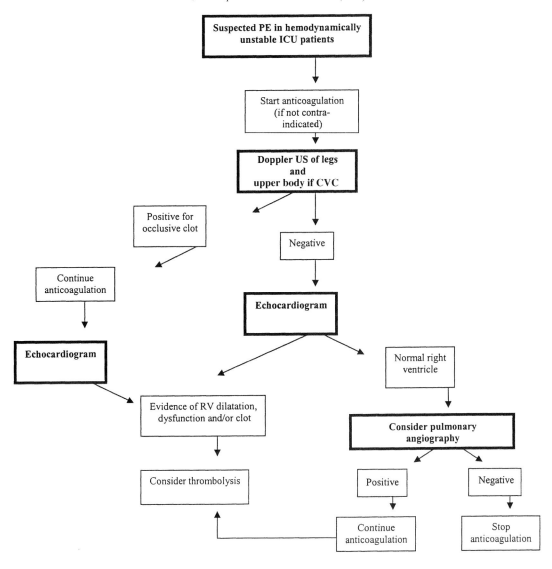

Fig. 2. Diagnostic algorithm for suspected pulmonary embolism in hemodynamically unstable patient. CVC, central venous catheterization; ICU, intensive care unit; PE, pulmonary embolism; RV, right ventricular; US, ultrasonography. * If spinal computed tomography scan or portable perfusion scan can be performed, then one of these should be the initial test.

it is extremely difficult to obtain a steady-state end-tidal CO_2 [93]. Moreover, the measurement of dead space can be normal in as many as one third of patients with PE. For these reasons, the utility of end-tidal CO_2 and the difference between the $PaCO_2$ and end-tidal CO_2 measurements as part of the diagnostic armamentarium in patients with suspected PE remains limited.

D-dimer levels

D-dimer levels are sensitive to the process of fibrin formation and dissolution occurring with ongoing thrombosis. Several D-dimer assays have been tested owing to their good negative predictive value for VTE. Currently available assays are based on latex agglutination, immunofixation techniques, or ELISA. The latter assay is the gold standard for measuring D-dimer levels; however, virtually all D-dimer assays have variable negative predictive value and lack specificity, because they are influenced by the presence of comorbid conditions, such as cancer, myocardial infarction, congestive heart failure, surgery, and infectious diseases, which are frequently found in critically ill patients. In a study of more than 1000 patients, a normal D-dimer test result was useful in excluding PE in patients with a low pretest probability of PE or a nondiagnostic ventilation–perfusion lung scan [96]. On the other hand, in patients with cancer, a negative D-dimer test does not reliably exclude DVT, because it has a significantly lower negative predictive value in these patients when they are compared with patients without cancer [52]. Furthermore, the accuracy of a rapid quantitative D-dimer assay is dependent on embolus location [97]. The sensitivity is 93% for larger emboli versus 50% for smaller subsegmental emboli.

The choice of the cutoff value for D-dimer testing is dependent on the method and the patient population studied. In the outpatient setting, a plasma D-dimer concentration below 500 μg/L allows the exclusion of PE in 29% of suspected cases [98]. Withholding anticoagulation from such patients is associated with a conservative 1% risk of VTE during follow-up. It is not yet known whether it is safe to withhold anticoagulation for suspected VTE in hospitalized individuals, particularly ICU patients, on the basis of negative D-dimer levels [99]. More solid recommendations about the utility of D-dimer levels for the diagnosis and management of VTE cannot be made at this time. Prospective management studies validating the utility of D-dimer measurement for the diagnosis of VTE in the ICU setting are needed.

Contrast venography

Venography remains the gold standard for the diagnosis of DVT; however, less invasive methods such as venous ultrasound have become the standard of care [100]. Because of its invasive nature and the availability of adequate alternatives, venography can be reserved for patients with nondiagnostic Doppler ultrasonography or in whom clinical suspicion is high despite negative serial ultrasonography.

Impedance plethysmography

Impedance plethysmography allows portable and noninvasive evaluation of DVT. It measures changes in the electrical impedance of the venous system during sequential inflation and deflation of a blood pressure cuff [101]. The sensitivity ranges from 75% to 96% and is higher among high-prevalence groups and very low in asymptomatic patients [102]. The specificity ranges from 45% to 84%. Impedance plethysmography can be problematic, especially in pregnant and obese patients, and in patients with heart failure, chronic DVT, or severe peripheral vascular disease. The sensitivity and specificity depend largely on

adhering to the validated protocol. Because of these limitations, impedance plethysmography has largely been supplanted by tests using ultrasonography.

Ultrasonography

Venous ultrasonography is the preferred noninvasive test for the diagnosis of a first symptomatic proximal DVT owing to its high accuracy [103]. Inability to compress the common femoral or popliteal vein is diagnostic of DVT in symptomatic patients with a positive predictive value of about 97%. Full compressibility of both of these sites excludes proximal DVT in symptomatic patients with a negative predictive value of about 98% [104]. Venous ultrasonography is much less reliable for the diagnosis of asymptomatic, isolated distal, and recurrent DVT than for the diagnosis of proximal DVT in symptomatic patients. Doppler ultrasonography may also miss pelvic venous clots when compared with venous phase spiral CT imaging [105]. For symptomatic DVT in the upper extremities, compression ultrasonography and color flow Doppler imaging are accurate methods of detection [20]. Doppler ultrasonography is required for the evaluation of subclavian vein thrombosis, because the clavicle precludes adequate compression of this vein. Routine diagnostic screening with ultrasonography is expensive and cannot be recommended for high-risk ICU patients [106].

Echocardiography

Right ventricular failure is the ultimate cause of death in patients who die of acute PE [107]. Transthoracic echocardiography has been suggested as a rapid, more readily available, and less invasive diagnostic technique for PE [108]. Hypokinesis and dilation of the right ventricle often accompany massive PE, and as many as 80% of patients with documented PE have imaging or Doppler evidence of right ventricular enlargement or dysfunction, which may suggest the diagnosis [109,110]. Echocardiography is useful in identifying substantial pulmonary hypertension with or without right ventricular dysfunction during acute cor pulmonale, but neither of these conditions is specific for the diagnosis of PE [111]. Transesophageal echocardiography may also identify intracardiac and main pulmonary artery clots, as shown in 12 of 24 patients with unexplained shock and distended neck veins in one study [108]. Because transesophageal echocardiography may miss clots in the left pulmonary artery, lobar, and segmental arteries, it has a relatively low sensitivity (58%) in identifying PE in patients with cor pulmonale [112].

Transesophageal echocardiography may clarify the diagnosis of PE within minutes without the need for further testing in ICU patients; however, a negative study does not exclude left proximal or lobar PE. Some echocardiographic findings, such as moderate-to-severe right ventricular hypokinesis, persistent pulmonary hypertension, a patent foramen ovale, and a free-floating right-sided heart thrombus, are markers of an increased risk of death or recurrent thromboembolism [113].

Echocardiography is not recommended as a routine imaging technique to diagnose suspected PE; however, it can be considered in patients presenting with suspected acute PE associated with hemodynamic instability, because it can be performed at the bedside to identify acute PE with right ventricular failure and to guide therapy with thrombolysis or embolectomy in addition to anticoagulation.

Ventilation–perfusion scintigraphy

Ventilation–perfusion scintigraphy scans are noninvasive and have an overall sensitivity of 96% for PE, making them an attractive screening technique. Nevertheless, only a minority of patients have diagnostic scans, and 33% of the patients with nondiagnostic scans ultimately have angiographically proven PE [114]. The test has important limitations in complex critically ill patients with other concomitant pulmonary derangements owing to frequent matched ventilation–perfusion defects. In one study, the ventilation–perfusion scans correlated poorly with pulmonary angiography results and with examinations at autopsy; the scan generally was inadequate to rule in or rule out PE [17]. Data from the Prospective Investigation of Pulmonary Embolism Diagnosis (PIOPED) [114] showed that intermediate-probability scans occurred in 43% of patients with prior cardiopulmonary disease and in 60% of patients with more complex underlying disease (ie, COPD). These findings were most likely the result of the distortion of ventilation and perfusion by the underlying pulmonary disease. A retrospective analysis of the PIOPED data demonstrated that the sensitivity of a high-probability, ventilation–perfusion scan in critically ill patients (only 33%) did not differ from that in non-critically ill medical patients [115]. Nevertheless, of the 850 subjects included in the study, only 46 were mechanically ventilated, and, as was true in the non-critically ill patients, most of the ventilation–perfusion scans had intermediate probability. If a ventilation scan cannot be performed, a perfusion scan with one or more segmental perfusion defects can be considered diagnostic of PE [116]. A positive perfusion scan has a positive predictive value of 95% and a negative scan a negative predictive value of 81%.

Dealing with the nondiagnostic scans is troublesome, particularly in the critical care arena. Combining the preclinical assessment with the results of the imaging test becomes crucial in determining the need for further testing and management. The combination of clinical assessment and lower-extremity studies using ultrasonography or impedance plethysmography can be useful when the lung scan is nondiagnostic. Perrier and colleagues [88] showed that, in the emergency room setting, anticoagulant treatment could be safely withheld in patients with a low clinical probability of PE and a nondiagnostic ventilation–perfusion scan provided that Doppler ultrasonography of the lower extremities was normal. Pulmonary angiography is recommended, particularly for hemodynamically unstable patients, as well as the consideration of serial noninvasive venous studies for stable patients. Because this strategy has not yet been tested in the ICU setting, additional evaluation for patients with nondiagnostic scans should be individualized.

Spiral computed tomography

The use of a spiral CT angiogram for the diagnosis of acute PE has received a great deal of attention over the past decade [80]. Spiral CT seems particularly attractive as the initial diagnostic test for patients with suspected PE and associated lung disease, because in approximately 50% of these patients, ventilation–perfusion scans are nondiagnostic. Another advantage of spiral CT is the ability to evaluate the thorax for other disease processes potentially causing the patient's symptoms [17,18]. According to a systematic review of 15 studies, the sensitivity of spiral CT ranges from 53% to 100% and the specificity from 81% to 100% [117]. Nevertheless, most high-quality studies with adequate gold standards have excluded critically ill and ventilated patients. In one of the few studies in ICU patients, Velmahos and colleagues [118] evaluated 22 critically ill surgical patients with marked pulmonary parenchymal disease using spiral CT and pulmonary angiography. They reported a sensitivity of 45% for all PEs and a sensitivity of 60% for central PEs in a comparison with angiography. The wide variation in sensitivity among studies probably reflects variable readers and institutional experience, technical factors, and the populations studied. Currently, the literature indicates that spiral CT may not be sufficiently sensitive in identifying subsegmental clots to permit its use as a screening test. Whether clots found in the peripheral pulmonary arteries significantly affect the outcomes of critically ill patients remains to be established. The ongoing PIOPED II study is being performed with the goal of analyzing state-of-the-art spiral CT (including pelvic/leg views) for the diagnosis of PE versus pulmonary angiography and the integration of ventilation–perfusion scans, lower-extremity ultrasonography, standard clinical assessment, and 3-month follow-up. This large multicenter study should resolve some of the issues involving the role of spiral CT for the diagnosis of PE. Unfortunately, the trial excludes critically ill and mechanically ventilated patients; therefore, future studies focusing on this patient population will be needed.

Frequently, it is desirable to image the deep venous system of the lower extremities as part of the evaluation of PE. Spiral CT venography has the potential of evaluating the pelvis and upper thighs for DVT without any additional intravenous contrast, minimal added study time, and radiation. Spiral CT venography was as effective as ultrasonography for femoropopliteal DVT in one study, showing a sensitivity of 100% and specificity of 100% [119]. In an investigation of 116 patients undergoing spiral CT venography and venous ultrasonography, 15 patients with DVT were diagnosed by both tests, but spiral CT venography also detected four pelvic DVTs not depicted by ultrasonography [105]. Spiral CT venography increased the detection of VTE by 18% because of the detection of DVT in patients with negative spiral CT angiography for PE.

Spiral CT may be considered as part of the diagnostic evaluation of PE; however, the utility of spiral CT for the diagnosis of VTE needs to be clarified in the ICU population. Spiral CT should probably not be used alone for suspected PE but could replace pulmonary angiography in combined strategies that include preclinical assessment, spiral CT venography, and ultrasound of the extremities.

Magnetic resonance imaging

Recent advances in MRI permit the evaluation of both lungs, simultaneous bilateral lower-extremity imaging, and excellent resolution of the inferior vena cava and pelvic veins. In a study of 101 patients with suspected DVT, the sensitivity and specificity of MRI were maintained below the knee when MRI was compared with venography [120]. MRI seems to be sensitive in detecting acute DVT, offering an accurate noninvasive alternative to venography, and may accurately distinguish acute DVT from chronic DVT [121].

Small studies have supported the potential use of MRI, particularly with gadolinium, in diagnosing PE [122,123]. The technique seems to be rapid and accurate, avoids nephrotoxic contrast, and is fre-

quently more acceptable to patients than pulmonary angiography. Potential disadvantages for critically ill patients include contraindications to MRI, the need for transportation to the radiology suite (a problem for mechanically ventilated patients), and the lack of sensitivity for subsegmental emboli. MRI has been compared with spiral CT in patients with proven PE by angiography or by high-probability, ventilation–perfusion scans plus a high clinical suspicion [124]. The average sensitivity and specificity of MRI for two expert readers were 71% and 97%, respectively, versus 73% and 97%, respectively, for spiral CT scanning. This pilot study was somewhat limited by the small number of patients and the small number of angiographic correlations. Larger studies employing more readily available equipment used by skilled readers are needed for confirmation of these encouraging results.

Pulmonary angiography

Currently, pulmonary angiography remains the most reliable technique to confirm or exclude PE in patients with respiratory failure. Angiography is not without risk, but serious morbidity and mortality are limited to 1% and 0.5% of cases, respectively [114]. Serious complications associated with pulmonary angiography include respiratory failure (0.4%), renal failure (0.3%), and bleeding requiring transfusion (0.2%) [125]. Although pulmonary angiography is considered the gold standard for the diagnosis of PE, interobserver agreement on the presence of PE in the PIOPED study was 92%, which suggests that even angiography can be difficult to interpret in some cases. Since the advent of less invasive diagnostic techniques, pulmonary angiography has been used with less frequency and is now generally reserved for patients with nondiagnostic ventilation–perfusion scans or technically inadequate spiral CT and a high clinical suspicion of PE.

Treatment

Standard unfractionated heparin is being increasingly replaced by LMWH for therapy and prophylaxis of VTE. Heparins and derivatives do not directly cause lysis of the thrombus but inhibit further clot formation while allowing the endogenous fibrinolytic system to dissolve the thrombi. For the treatment of acute VTE in ICU patients, unfractionated heparin is administered intravenously to achieve an activated partial thromboplastin time that is 1.5 to 2.0 times the control value. The short half-life and the easy reversibility of unfractionated heparin are ideal in treating patients who frequently need invasive procedures. Weight-based normograms for initial unfractionated heparin dosing should be applied, because they lead to more reliable therapeutic levels within 24 hours [126]. Failure to achieve full anticoagulation within 24 hours of the thrombotic event has been shown to increase the risk for recurrent thrombosis [127]. The platelet count should be monitored between days 3 and 5. Once the physician decides that is appropriate to convert anti-coagulation to an oral regimen, warfarin should be initiated and overlapped until the international nor-malized ratio (INR) is therapeutic for two consecutive days before UFA (or LMWH) is discontinued. For most patients, anticoagulation should be continued for greater than 3 months with the goal of reaching an international normalized ratio (INR) of 2.5 (range, 2.0–3.0) [128]. Recently published guidelines specify the INR goal and the duration of anticoagulation in special circumstances [128].

Subcutaneous administration of LMWH once or twice daily for VTE prophylaxis and treatment has been evaluated in many randomized trials among dif-ferent patient populations [129–132]. Currently, dal-teparin, enoxaparin and ardeparin have been approved for DVT prophylaxis, whereas enoxaparin and tinza-parin have been approved for the treatment of acute VTE in the United States, only enoxaparin is FDA-approved for use in medically ill patients as prophy-laxis. It is convenient to use LMWH from the patient and nursing viewpoint, particularly for the prophy-laxis of VTE. No monitoring is required with LMWH, except in special therapeutic circumstances, but its much longer half-life may be disadvantageous for ICU patients.

Central venous catheter–related thrombosis should generally be treated in a similar fashion as other uncomplicated DVTs with a caveat of prompt CVC removal after the diagnosis. The risk for chronic thrombotic complications and potential infection out-weighs the risk of inducing embolization of the thrombus with catheter removal.

In the setting of massive PE, initial efforts should focus on stabilizing blood pressure, enhancing cor-onary artery blood flow, and minimizing right ven-tricular ischemia. Supplemental oxygen must be administered, and, when necessary, intubation and mechanical ventilation should not be delayed. Intra-venous fluids should be administered cautiously. If hypotension persists after the administration of 500 to 1000 mL of isotonic saline, vasoactive medications are appropriate. Norepinephrine is preferred when there is a marked decrease of cardiac output. Dobutamine may be used to increase flow when a moderate decrease in

cardiac output complicates an increase in right ven-tricular afterload [133]. Therapeutic options aimed directly at reducing the embolic burden include sys-temic thrombolytic therapy, surgical embolectomy, and the use of intrapulmonary arterial catheter tech-niques. Thrombolytic therapy continues to be reserved for severe, life-threatening, acute PE. In the absence of contraindications, thrombolytic therapy is indicated in hypotensive patients. Surgical embolectomy for acute PE is controversial, but this modality seems to have a role in select patients. Various intrapulmonary arterial catheter techniques, with or without low-dose throm-bolytic therapy, have been used successfully to reduce the embolic burden, although no particular technique has clear advantages over others. Placement of an inferior vena cava filter may prevent additional poten-tially fatal emboli and seems appropriate in select patients with massive emboli [81]. Special aspects of therapy for VTE, including thrombolytic therapy, and embolectomy are discussed elsewhere in this issue.

Summary

Venous thromboembolism frequently complicates the management of patients with severe medical and surgical illnesses. Because the diagnosis of VTE is especially challenging in critically ill patients, the focus of intensivists should be on characterization of risk factors and the appropriate choice of VTE prophylaxis. LDUH or LMHW is the preferred choice for VTE prophylaxis in ICU patients. Mechanical methods of prophylaxis should be reserved for patients with a high risk for bleeding. The effective-ness of mechanical methods and of combined strat-egies of prevention and the clinically important outcomes of therapy need to be explored further in critically ill patients.

Few diagnostic strategies have been assessed in ICU patients with suspected PE. Ventilation–per-fusion lung scans remain a pivotal diagnostic test but retain the same limitations in critically ill patients as seen in other patient populations. Newer non-invasive techniques, such as spiral CT associated with imaging of the extremities, are gaining more wide-spread use, but, thus far, pulmonary angiogra-phy remains the most reliable technique to confirm or exclude PE in patients with respiratory failure. A consensus must be reached regarding the most appro-priate combination of tests for adequate and cost-effective diagnosis of VTE. Further investigation of diagnostic strategies that include adequate considera-tion of clinical diagnosis using standardized models and noninvasive imaging are warranted.

References

[1] Rubinstein I, Murray D, Hoffstein V. Fatal pulmonary emboli in hospitalized patients: an autopsy study. Arch Intern Med 1988;148(6):1425–6.

[2] Sandler DA, Martin JF. Autopsy proven pulmonary embolism in hospital patients: are we detecting enough deep vein thrombosis? J R Soc Med 1989;82(4): 203–5.

[3] Davidson BL. Risk assessment and prophylaxis of venous thromboembolism in acutely and/or critically ill patients. Haemostasis 2000;30(Suppl 2):77–81.

[4] Silverstein MD, Heit JA, Mohr DN, Petterson TM, O'Fallon WM, Melton III LJ. Trends in the incidence of deep vein thrombosis and pulmonary embolism: a 25-year population-based study. Arch Intern Med 1998;158(6):585–93.

[5] Turpie AG. Thrombosis prophylaxis in the acutely ill medical patient: insights from the prophylaxis in MEDical patients with ENOXaparin (MEDENOX) trial. Am J Cardiol 2000;86(12B):48M–52M.

[6] Geerts WH, Heit JA, Clagett GP, Pineo GF, Colwell CW, Anderson Jr FA, et al. Prevention of venous thromboembolism. Chest 2001;119(1 Suppl): 132S–75S.

[7] Collins R, Scrimgeour A, Yusuf S, Peto R. Reduction in fatal pulmonary embolism and venous thrombosis by perioperative administration of subcutaneous heparin: overview of results of randomized trials in general, orthopedic, and urologic surgery. N Engl J Med 1988;318(18):1162–73.

[8] Geerts WH, Code KI, Jay RM, Chen E, Szalai JP. A prospective study of venous thromboembolism after major trauma. N Engl J Med 1994;331(24):1601–6.

[9] Attia J, Ray JG, Cook DJ, Douketis J, Ginsberg JS, Geerts WH. Deep vein thrombosis and its prevention in critically ill adults. Arch Intern Med 2001;161(10): 1268–79.

[10] Moser KM, LeMoine JR, Nachtwey FJ, Spragg RG. Deep venous thrombosis and pulmonary embolism: frequency in a respiratory intensive care unit. JAMA 1981;246(13):1422–4.

[11] Cade JF. High risk of the critically ill for venous thromboembolism. Crit Care Med 1982;10(7):448–50.

[12] Ibarra-Perez C, Lau-Cortes E, Colmenero-Zubiate S, Arevila-Ceballos N, Fong JH, Sanchez-Martinez R, et al. Prevalence and prevention of deep venous thrombosis of the lower extremities in high-risk pulmonary patients. Angiology 1988;39(6): 505–13.

[13] Marik PE, Andrews L, Maini B. The incidence of deep venous thrombosis in ICU patients. Chest 1997; 111(3):661–4.

[14] Hirsch DR, Ingenito EP, Goldhaber SZ. Prevalence of deep venous thrombosis among patients in medical intensive care. JAMA 1995;274(4):335–7.

[15] Fraisse F, Holzapfel L, Couland JM, Simonneau G, Bedock B, Feissel M, et al. Nadroparin in the prevention of deep vein thrombosis in acute decompensated COPD: the Association of Non-University Affiliated Intensive Care Specialist Physicians of France. Am J Respir Crit Care Med 2000;161(4 Pt 1):1109–14.

[16] Cook D, Attia J, Weaver B, McDonald E, Meade M, Crowther M. Venous thromboembolic disease: an observational study in medical–surgical intensive care unit patients. J Crit Care 2000;15(4):127–32.

[17] Neuhaus A, Bentz RR, Weg JG. Pulmonary embolism in respiratory failure. Chest 1978;73(4):460–5.

[18] Gray HH, Firoozan S. The pulmonary physician and critical care. 5. Management of pulmonary embolism. Thorax 1992;47(10):825–32.

[19] Jain M, Schrader A. VTE: prevention and prophylaxis. Semin Respir Crit Care Med 1997;18:79–90.

[20] Prandoni P, Polistena P, Bernardi E, Cogo A, Casara D, Verlato F, et al. Upper-extremity deep vein thrombosis: risk factors, diagnosis, and complications. Arch Intern Med 1997;157(1):57–62.

[21] Ryskamp RP, Trottier SJ. Utilization of venous thromboembolism prophylaxis in a medical–surgical ICU. Chest 1998;113(1):162–4.

[22] Gersin K, Grindlinger GA, Lee V, Dennis RC, Wedel SK, Cachecho R. The efficacy of sequential compression devices in multiple trauma patients with severe head injury. J Trauma 1994;37(2):205–8.

[23] Bouthier J. The venous thrombotic risk in nonsurgical patients. Drugs 1996;52(Suppl 7):16–28.

[24] Eldor A. Applying risk assessment models in nonsurgical patients: effective risk stratification. Blood Coagul Fibrinolysis 1999;10(Suppl 2):S91–7.

[25] Krafte-Jacobs B, Sivit CJ, Mejia R, Pollack MM. Catheter-related thrombosis in critically ill children: comparison of catheters with and without heparin bonding. J Pediatr 1995;126(1):50–4.

[26] Chastre J, Cornud F, Bouchama A, Viau F, Benacerraf R, Gibert C. Thrombosis as a complication of pulmonary artery catheterization via the internal jugular vein: prospective evaluation by phlebography. N Engl J Med 1982;306(5):278–81.

[27] Bona RD. Thrombotic complications of central venous catheters in cancer patients. Semin Thromb Hemost 1999;25(2):147–55.

[28] Joynt GM, Kew J, Gomersall CD, Leung VY, Liu EK. Deep venous thrombosis caused by femoral venous catheters in critically ill adult patients. Chest 2000;117(1):178–83.

[29] di Costanzo J, Sastre B, Choux R, Kasparian M. Mechanism of thrombogenesis during total parenteral nutrition: role of catheter composition. JPEN J Parenter Enteral Nutr 1988;12(2):190–4.

[30] Borow M, Crowley JG. Prevention of thrombosis of central venous catheters. J Cardiovasc Surg (Torino) 1986;27(5):571–4.

[31] Harter C, Salwender HJ, Bach A, Egerer G, Goldschmidt H, Ho AD. Catheter-related infection and thrombosis of the internal jugular vein in hematologic-oncologic patients undergoing chemotherapy: a prospective comparison of silver-coated and uncoated catheters. Cancer 2002;94(1):245–51.

[32] Trottier SJ, Veremakis C, O'Brien J, Auer AI. Femoral deep vein thrombosis associated with central venous catheterization: results from a prospective, randomized trial. Crit Care Med 1995;23(1):52–9.

[33] Martin C, Viviand X, Saux P, Gouin F. Upper-extremity deep vein thrombosis after central venous catheterization via the axillary vein. Crit Care Med 1999; 27(12):2626–9.

[34] Brismar B, Hardstedt C, Jacobson S. Diagnosis of thrombosis by catheter phlebography after prolonged central venous catheterization. Ann Surg 1981;194(6): 779–83.

[35] Bozzetti F, Scarpa D, Terno G, Scotti A, Ammatuna M, Bonalumi MG, et al. Subclavian venous thrombosis due to indwelling catheters: a prospective study on 52 patients. JPEN J Parenter Enteral Nutr 1983; 7(6):560–2.

[36] Becker DM, Philbrick JT, Walker FB. Axillary and subclavian venous thrombosis: prognosis and treatment. Arch Intern Med 1991;151(10):1934–43.

[37] Timsit JF, Farkas JC, Boyer JM, Martin JB, Misset B, Renaud B, et al. Central vein catheter-related thrombosis in intensive care patients: incidence, risks factors, and relationship with catheter-related sepsis. Chest 1998;114(1):207–13.

[38] Gemma M, Beretta L, De Vitis A, Mattioli C, Calvi MR, Antonino A, et al. Complications of internal jugular vein retrograde catheterization. Acta Neurochir Suppl (Wien) 1998;71:320–3.

[39] Lucas JW, Berger AM, Fitzgerald A, Winfield B. Nosocomial infections in patients with central catheters. J Intraven Nurs 1992;15(1):44–8.

[40] Raad II, Luna M, Khalil SA, Costerton JW, Lam C, Bodey GP. The relationship between the thrombotic and infectious complications of central venous catheters. JAMA 1994;271(13):1014–6.

[41] Durbec O, Viviand X, Potie F, Vialet R, Albanese J, Martin C. A prospective evaluation of the use of femoral venous catheters in critically ill adults. Crit Care Med 1997;25(12):1986–9.

[42] Merrer J, De Jonghe B, Golliot F, Lefrant JY, Raffy B, Barre E, et al. Complications of femoral and subclavian venous catheterization in critically ill patients: a randomized controlled trial. JAMA 2001;286(6): 700–7.

[43] Pierce CM, Wade A, Mok Q. Heparin-bonded central venous lines reduce thrombotic and infective complications in critically ill children. Intensive Care Med 2000;26(7):967–72.

[44] Randolph AG, Cook DJ, Gonzales CA, Andrew M. Benefit of heparin in central venous and pulmonary artery catheters: a meta-analysis of randomized controlled trials. Chest 1998;113(1):165–71.

[45] Marinella MA, Kathula SK, Markert RJ. Spectrum of upper-extremity deep venous thrombosis in a community teaching hospital. Heart Lung 2000;29(2): 113–7.

[46] Monreal M, Raventos A, Lerma R, Ruiz J, Lafoz E, Alastrue A, et al. Pulmonary embolism in patients with upper extremity DVT associated to venous central lines–a prospective study. Thromb Haemost 1994;72(4):548–50.

[47] Hull RD, Hirsh J, Sackett DL, Stoddart GL. Cost-effectiveness of primary and secondary prevention of fatal pulmonary embolism in high-risk surgical patients. Can Med Assoc J 1982;127(10):990–5.

[48] Velmahos GC, Oh Y, McCombs J, Oder D. An evidence-based cost-effectiveness model on methods of prevention of posttraumatic venous thromboembolism. J Trauma 2000;49(6):1059–64.

[49] Keane MG, Ingenito EP, Goldhaber SZ. Utilization of venous thromboembolism prophylaxis in the medical intensive care unit. Chest 1994;106(1):13–4.

[50] Hull RD, Pineo GF. Intermittent pneumatic compression for the prevention of venous thromboembolism. Chest 1996;109(1):6–9.

[51] Goldhaber SZ. Venous thromboembolism in the intensive care unit: the last frontier for prophylaxis. Chest 1998;113(1):5–7.

[52] Lee AY, Julian JA, Levine MN, Weitz JI, Kearon C, Wells PS, et al. Clinical utility of a rapid whole-blood D-dimer assay in patients with cancer who present with suspected acute deep venous thrombosis. Ann Intern Med 1999;131(6):417–23.

[53] Velmahos GC, Nigro J, Tatevossian R, Murray JA, Cornwell III EE, Belzberg H, et al. Inability of an aggressive policy of thromboprophylaxis to prevent deep venous thrombosis (DVT) in critically injured patients: are current methods of DVT prophylaxis insufficient? J Am Coll Surg 1998;187(5):529–33.

[54] Goldhaber SZ, Dunn K, MacDougall RC. New onset of venous thromboembolism among hospitalized patients at Brigham and Women's Hospital is caused more often by prophylaxis failure than by withholding treatment. Chest 2000;118(6):1680–4.

[55] Ramos R, Salem BI, De Pawlikowski MP, Coordes C, Eisenberg S, Leidenfrost R. The efficacy of pneumatic compression stockings in the prevention of pulmonary embolism after cardiac surgery. Chest 1996; 109(1):82–5.

[56] Spain DA, Bergamini TM, Hoffmann JF, Carrillo EH, Richardson JD. Comparison of sequential compression devices and foot pumps for prophylaxis of deep venous thrombosis in high-risk trauma patients. Am Surg 1998;64(6):522–5.

[57] Geerts W, Cook D, Selby R, Etchells E. Venous thromboembolism and its prevention in critical care. J Crit Care 2002;17(2):95–104.

[58] Harris SK, Bone RC, Ruth WE. Gastrointestinal hemorrhage in patients in a respiratory intensive care unit. Chest 1977;72(3):301–4.

[59] Clagett GP, Anderson Jr FA, Geerts W, Heit JA, Knudson M, Lieberman JR, et al. Prevention of venous thromboembolism. Chest 1998;114(5 Suppl): 531S–60S.

[60] Nurmohamed MT, Rosendaal FR, Buller HR, Dekker E, Hommes DW, Vandenbroucke JP, et al. Low-molecular-weight heparin versus standard heparin in

general and orthopaedic surgery: a meta-analysis. Lancet 1992;340(8812):152–6.

[61] Jorgensen LN, Wille-Jorgensen P, Hauch O. Prophylaxis of postoperative thromboembolism with low molecular weight heparins. Br J Surg 1993;80(6): 689–704.

[62] Gould MK, Dembitzer AD, Doyle RL, Hastie TJ, Garber AM. Low-molecular-weight heparins compared with unfractionated heparin for treatment of acute deep venous thrombosis: a meta-analysis of randomized, controlled trials. Ann Intern Med 1999; 130(10):800–9.

[63] Lensing AW, Prins MH, Davidson BL, Hirsh J. Treatment of deep venous thrombosis with low-molecular-weight heparins: a meta-analysis. Arch Intern Med 1995;155(6):601–7.

[64] Siragusa S, Cosmi B, Piovella F, Hirsh J, Ginsberg JS. Low-molecular-weight heparins and unfractionated heparin in the treatment of patients with acute venous thromboembolism: results of a meta-analysis. Am J Med 1996;100(3):269–77.

[65] Brieger DB, Mak KH, Kottke-Marchant K, Topol EJ. Heparin-induced thrombocytopenia. J Am Coll Cardiol 1998;31(7):1449–59.

[66] Guidry JR, Raschke RA, Morkunas AR. Toxic effects of drugs used in the ICU: anticoagulants and thrombolytics. Risks and benefits. Crit Care Clin 1991; 7(3):533–54.

[67] Warkentin TE, Sheppard JA, Horsewood P, Simpson PJ, Moore JC, Kelton JG. Impact of the patient population on the risk for heparin-induced thrombocytopenia. Blood 2000;96(5):1703–8.

[68] Ranze O, Ranze P, Magnani HN, Greinacher A. Heparin-induced thrombocytopenia in paediatric patients – a review of the literature and a new case treated with danaparoid sodium. Eur J Pediatr 1999; 158(Suppl 3):S130–3.

[69] Warkentin TE. Heparin-induced thrombocytopenia and its treatment. J Thromb Thrombolysis 2000; 9(Suppl 1):S29–35.

[70] Cook D, McMullin J, Hodder R, Heule M, Pinilla J, Dodek P, et al. Prevention and diagnosis of venous thromboembolism in critically ill patients: a Canadian survey. Crit Care 2001;5(6):336–42.

[71] Kupfer Y, Anwar J. Prophylaxis with subcutaneous heparin significantly reduces the incidence of deep venous thrombophlebitis in the critically ill [abstract]. Am J Respir Crit Care Med 1999;159(Suppl):A519.

[72] Geerts WH, Jay RM, Code KI, Chen E, Szalai JP, Saibil EA, et al. A comparison of low-dose heparin with low-molecular-weight heparin as prophylaxis against venous thromboembolism after major trauma. N Engl J Med 1996;335(10):701–7.

[73] Mismetti P, Laporte-Simitsidis S, Tardy B, Cucherat M, Buchmuller A, Juillard-Delsart D, et al. Prevention of venous thromboembolism in internal medicine with unfractionated or low-molecular-weight heparins: a meta-analysis of randomised clinical trials. Thromb Haemost 2000;83(1):14–9.

[74] Wells PS, Lensing AW, Hirsh J. Graduated compression stockings in the prevention of postoperative venous thromboembolism: a meta-analysis. Arch Intern Med 1994;154(1):67–72.

[75] Christen Y, Wutschert R, Weimer D, de Moerloose P, Kruithof EK, Bounameaux H. Effects of intermittent pneumatic compression on venous haemodynamics and fibrinolytic activity. Blood Coagul Fibrinolysis 1997;8(3):185–90.

[76] Knight MT, Dawson R. Effect of intermittent compression of the arms on deep venous thrombosis in the legs. Lancet 1976;2(7998):1265–8.

[77] Jimenez R, Kupfer Y, Tessler S. Pneumatic stockings do not decrease the incidence of deep venous thrombophlebitis in the critically ill [abstract]. Crit Care Med 2001;29(Suppl 12):A98.

[78] Comerota AJ, Katz ML, White JV. Why does prophylaxis with external pneumatic compression for deep vein thrombosis fail? Am J Surg 1992;164(3):265–8.

[79] Kamran SI, Downey D, Ruff RL. Pneumatic sequential compression reduces the risk of deep vein thrombosis in stroke patients. Neurology 1998;50(6):1683–8.

[80] Tapson VF, Carroll BA, Davidson BL, Elliott CG, Fedullo PF, Hales CA, et al. The diagnostic approach to acute venous thromboembolism: clinical practice guideline. Am J Respir Crit Care Med 1999;160(3): 1043–66.

[81] Tapson VF, Witty LA. Massive pulmonary embolism: diagnostic and therapeutic strategies. Clin Chest Med 1995;16(2):329–40.

[82] Wicki J, Perneger TV, Junod AF, Bounameaux H, Perrier A. Assessing clinical probability of pulmonary embolism in the emergency ward: a simple score. Arch Intern Med 2001;161(1):92–7.

[83] Wells PS, Ginsberg JS, Anderson DR, Kearon C, Gent M, Turpie AG, et al. Use of a clinical model for safe management of patients with suspected pulmonary embolism. Ann Intern Med 1998;129(12): 997–1005.

[84] Wells PS, Anderson DR, Rodger M, Stiell I, Dreyer JF, Barnes D, et al. Excluding pulmonary embolism at the bedside without diagnostic imaging: management of patients with suspected pulmonary embolism presenting to the emergency department by using a simple clinical model and d-dimer. Ann Intern Med 2001;135(2):98–107.

[85] Bozzetti F, Scarpa D, Terno G, Scotti A, Ammatuna M, Bonalumi MG, et al. Subclavian venous thrombosis due to indwelling catheters: a prospective study on 52 patients. JPEN J Parenter Enteral Nutr 1983; 7(6):560–2.

[86] Prandoni P, Villalta S, Bagatella P, Rossi L, Marchiori A, Piccioli A, et al. The clinical course of deep-vein thrombosis: prospective long-term follow-up of 528 symptomatic patients. Haematologica 1997;82(4): 423–8.

[87] Wells PS, Anderson DR, Rodger M, Ginsberg JS, Kearon C, Gent M, et al. Derivation of a simple clinical model to categorize patients' probability of pul-

monary embolism: increasing the model's utility with the SimpliRED D-dimer. Thromb Haemost 2000; 83(3):416–20.

[88] Perrier A, Miron MJ, Desmarais S, de Moerloose P, Slosman D, Didier D, et al. Using clinical evaluation and lung scan to rule out suspected pulmonary embolism: is it a valid option in patients with normal results of lower-limb venous compression ultrasonography? Arch Intern Med 2000;160(4):512–6.

[89] Rodger M, Makropoulos D, Turek M, Quevillon J, Raymond F, Rasuli P, et al. Diagnostic value of the electrocardiogram in suspected pulmonary embolism. Am J Cardiol 2000;86:807–9.

[90] The urokinase pulmonary embolism trial: a national cooperative study. Circulation 1973;47(2 Suppl): II1–108.

[91] Yoshinaga T, Ikeda S, Nishimura E, Shioguchi K, Shikuwa M, Miyahara Y, et al. Serial changes in negative T wave on electrocardiogram in acute pulmonary thromboembolism. Int J Cardiol 1999;72(1): 65–72.

[92] Randolph AG, Cook DJ, Gonzales CA, Andrew M. Benefit of heparin in peripheral venous and arterial catheters: systematic review and meta-analysis of randomised controlled trials. BMJ 1998;316(7136): 969–75.

[93] Weg JG. A new niche for end-tidal CO2 in pulmonary embolism. Crit Care Med 2000;28(11):3752–4.

[94] Johanning JM, Veverka TJ, Bays RA, Tong GK, Schmiege SK. Evaluation of suspected pulmonary embolism utilizing end-tidal CO2 and D-dimer. Am J Surg 1999;178(2):98–102.

[95] Wiegand UK, Kurowski V, Giannitsis E, Katus HA, Djonlagic H. Effectiveness of end-tidal carbon dioxide tension for monitoring thrombolytic therapy in acute pulmonary embolism. Crit Care Med 2000;28(11): 3588–92.

[96] Ginsberg JS, Wells PS, Kearon C, Anderson D, Crowther M, Weitz JI, et al. Sensitivity and specificity of a rapid whole-blood assay for D-dimer in the diagnosis of pulmonary embolism. Ann Intern Med 1998;129(12):1006–11.

[97] De Monye W, Sanson BJ, Mac Gillavry MR, Pattynama PM, Buller HR, van den Berg-Huysmans AA, et al. Embolus location affects the sensitivity of a rapid quantitative D-dimer assay in the diagnosis of pulmonary embolism. Am J Respir Crit Care Med 2002; 165(3):345–8.

[98] Perrier A, Desmarais S, Goehring C, de Moerloose P, Morabia A, Unger PF, et al. D-dimer testing for suspected pulmonary embolism in outpatients. Am J Respir Crit Care Med 1997;156(2 Pt 1):492–6.

[99] Janssen MC, Wollersheim H, Verbruggen B, Novakova IR. Rapid D-dimer assays to exclude deep venous thrombosis and pulmonary embolism: current status and new developments. Semin Thromb Hemost 1998; 24(4):393–400.

[100] Graziano JN, Charpie JR. Thrombosis in the intensive care unit: etiology, diagnosis, management, and pre-

vention in adults and children. Cardiol Rev 2001; 9(3):173–82.

[101] Patterson RB, Fowl RJ, Keller JD, Schomaker W, Kempczinski RF. The limitations of impedance plethysmography in the diagnosis of acute deep venous thrombosis. J Vasc Surg 1989;9(5):725–9.

[102] Legere BM, Dweik RA, Arroliga AC. Venous thromboembolism in the intensive care unit. Clin Chest Med 1999;20(2):367–84.

[103] Kearon C, Julian JA, Newman TE, Ginsberg JS. Noninvasive diagnosis of deep venous thrombosis: McMaster Diagnostic Imaging Practice Guidelines Initiative. Ann Intern Med 1998;128(8):663–77.

[104] Kearon C, Ginsberg JS, Hirsh J. The role of venous ultrasonography in the diagnosis of suspected deep venous thrombosis and pulmonary embolism. Ann Intern Med 1998;129(12):1044–9.

[105] Cham MD, Yankelevitz DF, Shaham D, Shah AA, Sherman L, Lewis A, et al. Deep venous thrombosis: detection by using indirect CT venography. The Pulmonary Angiography-Indirect CT Venography Cooperative Group. Radiology 2000;216(3):744–51.

[106] Meyer CS, Blebea J, Davis Jr K, Fowl RJ, Kempczinski RF. Surveillance venous scans for deep venous thrombosis in multiple trauma patients. Ann Vasc Surg 1995;9(1):109–14.

[107] Tapson VF. Pulmonary embolism–new diagnostic approaches. N Engl J Med 1997;336(20):1449–51.

[108] Krivec B, Voga G, Zuran I, Skale R, Pareznik R, Podbregar M, et al. Diagnosis and treatment of shock due to massive pulmonary embolism: approach with transesophageal echocardiography and intrapulmonary thrombolysis. Chest 1997;112(5):1310–6.

[109] Come PC. Echocardiographic evaluation of pulmonary embolism and its response to therapeutic interventions. Chest 1992;101(4 Suppl):151S–62S.

[110] Wolfe MW, Lee RT, Feldstein ML, Parker JA, Come PC, Goldhaber SZ. Prognostic significance of right ventricular hypokinesis and perfusion lung scan defects in pulmonary embolism. Am Heart J 1994; 127(5):1371–5.

[111] Jardin F, Dubourg O, Bourdarias JP. Echocardiographic pattern of acute cor pulmonale. Chest 1997; 111(1):209–17.

[112] Vieillard-Baron A, Qanadli SD, Antakly Y, Fourme T, Loubieres Y, Jardin F, et al. Transesophageal echocardiography for the diagnosis of pulmonary embolism with acute cor pulmonale: a comparison with radiological procedures. Intensive Care Med 1998;24(5): 429–33.

[113] Goldhaber SZ. Echocardiography in the management of pulmonary embolism. Ann Intern Med 2002;136(9): 691–700.

[114] The PIOPED Investigators. Value of the ventilation/ perfusion scan in acute pulmonary embolism: results of the prospective investigation of pulmonary embolism diagnosis (PIOPED). JAMA 1990;263(20): 2753–9.

[115] Henry JW, Stein PD, Gottschalk A, Relyea B, Leeper

Jr RM. Scintigraphic lung scans and clinical assessment in critically ill patients with suspected acute pulmonary embolism. Chest 1996;109(2):462–6.

[116] Invasive and noninvasive diagnosis of pulmonary embolism: preliminary results of the Prospective Investigative Study of Acute Pulmonary Embolism Diagnosis (PISA-PED). Chest 1995;107(1 Suppl): 33S–8S.

[117] Rathbun SW, Raskob GE, Whitsett TL. Sensitivity and specificity of helical computed tomography in the diagnosis of pulmonary embolism: a systematic review. Ann Intern Med 2000;132(3):227–32.

[118] Velmahos GC, Vassiliu P, Wilcox A, Hanks SE, Salim A, Harrel D, et al. Spiral computed tomography for the diagnosis of pulmonary embolism in critically ill surgical patients: a comparison with pulmonary angiography. Arch Surg 2001;136(5):505–11.

[119] Loud PA, Katz DS, Klippenstein DL, Shah RD, Grossman ZD. Combined CT venography and pulmonary angiography in suspected thromboembolic disease: diagnostic accuracy for deep venous evaluation. AJR Am J Roentgenol 2000;174(1):61–5.

[120] Fraser DG, Moody AR, Morgan PS, Martel AL, Davidson I. Diagnosis of lower-limb deep venous thrombosis: a prospective blinded study of magnetic resonance direct thrombus imaging. Ann Intern Med 2002;136(2):89–98.

[121] Evans AJ, Sostman HD, Witty LA, Paulson EK, Spritzer CE, Hertzberg BS, et al. Detection of deep venous thrombosis: prospective comparison of MR imaging and sonography. J Magn Reson Imaging 1996;6(1):44–51.

[122] Meaney JF, Weg JG, Chenevert TL, Stafford-Johnson D, Hamilton BH, Prince MR. Diagnosis of pulmonary embolism with magnetic resonance angiography. N Engl J Med 1997;336(20):1422–7.

[123] Gupta A, Frazer CK, Ferguson JM, Kumar AB, Davis SJ, Fallon MJ, et al. Acute pulmonary embolism: diagnosis with MR angiography. Radiology 1999; 210(2):353–9.

[124] Sostman HD, Layish DT, Tapson VF, Spritzer CE, DeLong DM, Trotter P, et al. Prospective comparison of helical CT and MR imaging in clinically suspected acute pulmonary embolism. J Magn Reson Imaging 1996;6(2):275–81.

[125] Stein PD, Athanasoulis C, Alavi A, Greenspan RH, Hales CA, Saltzman HA, et al. Complications and validity of pulmonary angiography in acute pulmonary embolism. Circulation 1992;85(2):462–8.

[126] Raschke RA, Reilly BM, Guidry JR, Fontana JR, Srinivas S. The weight-based heparin dosing nomogram compared with a "standard care" nomogram: a randomized controlled trial. Ann Intern Med 1993; 119(9):874–81.

[127] Hull RD, Raskob GE, Hirsh J. The diagnosis of clinically suspected pulmonary embolism: practical approaches. Chest 1986;89(5 Suppl):417S–25S.

[128] Hyers TM, Agnelli G, Hull RD, Morris TA, Samama M, Tapson V, et al. Antithrombotic therapy for venous thromboembolic disease. Chest 2001;119(1 Suppl): 176S–93S.

[129] Hull RD, Raskob GE, Pineo GF, Green D, Trowbridge AA, Elliott CG, et al. Subcutaneous low-molecular-weight heparin compared with continuous intravenous heparin in the treatment of proximal vein thrombosis. N Engl J Med 1992;326(15):975–82.

[130] Simonneau G, Charbonnier B, Decousus H, Planchon B, Ninet J, Sie P, et al. Subcutaneous low-molecular-weight heparin compared with continuous intravenous unfractionated heparin in the treatment of proximal deep vein thrombosis. Arch Intern Med 1993; 153(13):1541–6.

[131] The Columbus Investigators. Low-molecular-weight heparin in the treatment of patients with venous thromboembolism. N Engl J Med 1997;337(10): 657–62.

[132] Merli G, Spiro TE, Olsson CG, Abildgaard U, Davidson BL, Eldor A, et al. Subcutaneous enoxaparin once or twice daily compared with intravenous unfractionated heparin for treatment of venous thromboembolic disease. Ann Intern Med 2001;134(3): 191–202.

[133] Prewitt RM. Hemodynamic management in pulmonary embolism and acute hypoxemic respiratory failure. Crit Care Med 1990;18(1 Pt 2):S61–9.

CLINICS
IN CHEST
MEDICINE

Clin Chest Med 24 (2003) 123–137

Prevention and management of venous thromboembolism in pregnancy

Ian A. Greer, MD, FRCP (Glas)(Ed)(Lond), FRCOG MFFP

Division of Developmental Medicine, Department of Obstetrics and Gynaecology, University of Glasgow,
Glasgow Royal Infirmary, 10 Alexandra Parade, Glasgow, G31 2ER, Scotland, UK

Pulmonary thromboembolism (PTE) remains a major cause of maternal mortality in the developed world. In the United Kingdom [1], one of the few countries that comprehensively collect, review, and publish data on maternal deaths (http://www.cemd.org.uk/), PTE has been the most common direct cause of maternal mortality for many years. PTE arises from deep venous thrombosis (DVT), but many DVTs are not recognized before the occurrence of PTE. DVT also is associated with a significant risk of recurrent thrombosis, especially if there is an underlying thrombophilia, and deep venous insufficiency manifests as the postthrombotic syndrome. PTE carries a risk of subsequent pulmonary hypertension. Pregnancy-related venous thromboembolism (VTE) may identify women with an underlying thrombophilia that may be associated with an increased risk of pregnancy complications. Many of the maternal deaths from PTE are associated with substandard care [1], including failures to recognize risk factors for VTE, failures to provide appropriate thromboprophylaxis for those persons at risk, failures to diagnose VTE objectively, and failures to provide appropriate treatment.

Epidemiology of venous thromboembolism in pregnancy

The incidence of antenatal DVT varies with age. It has been estimated to be 0.615 event per 1000 maternities in women less than 35 years of age and

1.216 events per 1000 maternities in women more than 35 years of age [2]. The incidence of postpartum DVT has been estimated to be 0.304 event per 1000 maternities in women less than 35 years of age and 0.72 event per 1000 maternities in women more than 35 years of age. Although antenatal DVT is more common than postpartum DVT [2], the event rate is higher in the 6 weeks of the puerperium. Almost 40% of postpartum DVTs present following the woman's discharge from hospital. Complete data on postpartum DVT are difficult to obtain, because many cases present to nonobstetric services. The United Kingdom Confidential Enquiries provide accurate data for fatal PTE. Overall, the incidence of fatal PTE has fallen substantially from the early 1950s. The greatest reduction has occurred in the number of deaths following vaginal delivery. This decrease is probably related to the "demedicalization" of childbirth, with shorter stays inhospital, more rapid mobilization, and shorter labors. Nonetheless, in recent years, there has been no further reduction in fatalities after vaginal delivery [1], and the number of deaths during the antenatal period has changed little from the early 1950s despite major advances in the identification of risk, thromboprophylaxis, diagnosis, and therapeutics over this same period. The total number of deaths following cesarean section seems to have fallen sharply since the widespread introduction of specific thromboprophylaxis to United Kingdom clinical obstetric practice in the mid-1990s.

The major risk factors for VTE are increasing maternal age (particularly over 35 years), operative vaginal delivery, cesarean section (especially if carried out as an emergency in labor), a high body mass index, previous VTE (especially idiopathic or throm-

E-mail address: I.A.Greer@clinmed.gla.ac.uk

bophilia associated), thrombophilia, and a family history of thrombosis suggestive of an underlying thrombophilia [3] (Table 1). The risk of VTE associated with ovarian hyperstimulation for assisted conception therapy is often overlooked. Hyperstimulation provokes procoagulant changes in the hemostatic and fibrinolytic systems. These changes can result in venous and arterial thrombosis, although the overall rate of thrombosis in assisted conception is low. When VTE occurs, it is usually in the internal jugular vein and presents with neck pain and swelling. A risk assessment for thrombosis should be undertaken in women undergoing assisted conception therapy and appropriate thromboprophylaxis provided for those at high risk.

Following DVT, there is a risk of deep venous insufficiency. A recent study found that more than 60% of women had objectively confirmed deep venous insufficiency following a treated DVT, and almost 80% experienced postthrombotic syndrome. The odds ratio for developing venous insufficiency after a DVT has been estimated at 10.9 (95% confidence interval [CI], 4.2–28.0) versus 3.8 (95% CI, 1.2–12.3) after a PTE [4]. The difference may be ex-

Table 1
Common risk factors for venous thromboembolism in pregnancy

Patient factors	Pregnancy/obstetric factors
Age over 35 years	Ovarian hyperstimulation
Obesity (BMI > 29 kg/m^2) in early pregnancy	Cesarean section, particularly as an emergency in labor
Thrombophilia	Operative vaginal delivery
Past history of VTE (especially if idiopathic or thrombophilia associated)	Major obstetric hemorrhage
Gross varicose veins	Hyperemesis gravidarum
Significant current medical problem (eg, nephrotic syndrome)	Pre-eclampsia
Current infection or inflammatory process (eg, active inflammatory bowel disease or urinary tract infection)	
Immobility (eg, bed rest or lower limb fracture)	
Paraplegia	
Recent long distance travel	
Dehydration	
Intravenous drug abuse	

Abbreviations: BMI, body mass index; VTE, venous thromboembolism.

Table 2
Subjective complaints in women followed up after pregnancy-associated deep venous thrombosis (DVT)

Parameter	DVT in pregnancy	DVT in puerperium
Number of women studied	61	33
Follow-up time (median)	10 years (range, 7–21)	11 years (range, 7–26)
Leg swelling	59%	48%
Varicose veins	36%	30%
Skin discoloration	28%	27%
Regular use of compression bandage	21%	3%
Leg ulcer	6.5%	0%

From Bergqvist D, Bergqvist A, Lindhagen A, et al. Long-term outcome of patients with venous thromboembolism during pregnancy. In: Greer IA, Turpie AGG, Forbes CD, editors. Haemostasis and thrombosis in obstetrics and gynaecology. London: Chapman and Hall; 1992. p. 349–59; with permission.

plained by thrombus clearing from the legs in women with PTE, leading to less extensive damage to the deep venous system. Another study has also illustrated the frequency of symptoms associated with the postthrombotic syndrome following DVT in pregnancy (Table 2) [5]. The risk of pulmonary hypertension has not been quantified for pregnancy-associated VTE.

Pathogenesis of venous thromboembolism in pregnancy

Virchow's classic triad of factors underlying VTE, that is, hypercoagulability, venous stasis, and endothelial damage, occur in the course of normal pregnancy and delivery. Hypercoagulability results from the increased levels of coagulation factors, such as von Willebrand factor, factor VIII, and fibrinogen; from an acquired resistance to the endogenous anticoagulant, activated protein C, found in almost 40% of normal pregnancies; from a reduction in protein S, the cofactor for activated protein C [6]; and from impaired fibrinolysis through increases in plasminogen activator inhibitors 1 and 2, the latter being placentally derived [7]. High factor VIII levels and resistance to activated protein C are independently associated with an increased risk of VTE. Venous flow in the lower limbs is reduced by approximately 50% by the end of the second trimester, reaching a nadir at 36 weeks [8] and returning to normal nonpregnant flow rates at approximately 6 weeks postpartum. Endothelial damage to pelvic vessels can occur during the course of vaginal delivery or cesarean section.

More than 70% of DVTs in pregnancy are iliofemoral in contrast to their location in the nonpregnant situation, when the majority are calf vein thrombosis, with approximately 9% of DVTs being iliofemoral. Iliofemoral DVTs are more likely to embolize than are isolated calf vein thromboses. Almost 90% of DVTs affect the left side in pregnancy versus 55% in nonpregnant women [3,9]. This difference may be the result of compression of the left iliac vein by the right iliac artery and the ovarian artery, which cross the vein on the left side only.

Thrombophilia and venous thromboembolism in pregnancy

Thrombophilia is found in approximately 50% of women with a VTE during pregnancy. The major heritable forms of thrombophilia include deficiencies of the endogenous anticoagulant proteins, that is, antithrombin, protein C, and protein S; abnormalities of procoagulant factors, particularly factor V Leiden; and the prothrombin gene variant, prothrombin 20210A.

Hyperhomocysteinemia is associated with VTE in nonpregnant women [10] and may reflect underlying homozygosity for a variation in the methylenetetrahydrofolate reductase gene (MTHFR C677T), which occurs in approximately 10% of Western populations. This genotype is not directly linked to VTE and requires an interaction with dietary deficiency of B vitamins. In contrast to the nonpregnant situation, this genotype has not been associated with an increased risk of pregnancy-related VTE [11–13]. The lack of association in pregnancy may reflect the physiologic decrease in homocysteine levels seen in normal pregnancy or the effects of folic acid supplements.

Quantitative or qualitative deficiencies of the anticoagulant proteins antithrombin, protein C, and protein S [14] have a combined prevalence of less than 10 in 1000 in European populations (the true prevalence of protein S deficiency has not yet been clearly established), and, collectively, such deficiencies are found in less than 10% of cases of VTE.

Factor V Leiden produces resistance to activated protein C, the endogenous anticoagulant directed against factors Va and VIIIa. Activated protein C inhibits coagulation by proteolytic cleavage of these factors. With factor V Leiden, resistance to the activity of protein C is caused by a single point mutation in the factor V gene at the cleavage site where activated protein C acts. This defect results in a potentially hypercoagulable effect. Factor V Leiden has a prevalence of approximately 2% to 7% in Western Europeans [14] (the prevalence is much lower in other populations such as the Chinese) and can be identified in 20% to 40% of patients with VTE [15]. Activated protein C resistance can be caused by problems other than factor V Leiden, including antiphospholipid antibody syndrome and other genetic defects in the factor V molecule. It also can be acquired in pregnancy [6], possibly owing to increases in factors V and VIII. The prothrombin gene variant (prothrombin G20210A) is present in approximately 2% of the population. It is associated with elevated plasma prothrombin levels and increases the risk for VTE by threefold [16]. This variant is found in approximately 6% of patients with VTE and in 18% of patients with a family history of VTE [16]. It has been found in pregnancy-associated VTE [13,17]. Although factor V Leiden is associated with an increased risk for VTE, this risk is largely an increase in DVT. The prevalence of underlying factor V Leiden in PTE is approximately half of that in DVT. In contrast, in other thrombophilias such as prothrombin G20210A, there is no difference in the underlying prevalence of DVT and PTE. Factor V Leiden may be associated with a more adherent and stable thrombus, possibly owing to increased local thrombin generation, reducing the likelihood of embolization. Whether this effect occurs in pregnant women with factor V Leiden is not clear.

Heritable causes [18,19] are present in at least 15% of Western populations and underlie approximately 50% of episodes of VTE in pregnancy (Table 3). Nonetheless, the incidence of VTE in pregnancy is only 1 in 1000. The presence of a thrombophilia, even when combined with the prothrombotic changes in coagulation and venous flow found in pregnancy, does not usually result in VTE. VTE in women with thrombophilia reflects a multicausal event resulting from the interaction between congenital and acquired risk factors [19]. The level of risk depends on the underlying thrombophilic defects, the history of thrombotic events, and addi-

Table 3

Typical prevalence rates for congenital thrombophilia in European populations

Thrombophilic defect	Prevalence (%)
Antithrombin deficiency	0.25–0.55
Protein C deficiency	0.20–0.33
Factor V Leiden heterozygotes	2–7
Prothrombin G20210A heterozygotes	2
MTHFR C677T homozygotes	10

Abbreviations: MTHFR, methylene-tetrahydrofolate reductase.

tional risk factors (see Table 1). One must establish the risk of thrombosis in pregnant women with thrombophilia to guide thromboprophylaxis.

Initial estimates of the risk for VTE in pregnant women with thrombophilia without thromboprophylaxis were high. The rates were estimated to be as high as 60% in antithrombin-deficient women [14,20], 3% to 10% in protein C deficiency, and 0% to 6% in protein S deficiency [14,20]; however, these data were obtained from observational studies of symptomatic thrombophilic kindreds. This type of study overestimates the risk in asymptomatic kindreds. Factor V Leiden has been found in as many as 46% of women investigated for VTE in pregnancy [21], but, again, this finding reflects the investigation of symptomatic women. Recent studies have provided estimates of the risk for VTE in pregnancy in women with the more common thrombophilias. Gerhardt et al [12] reported a relative risk for VTE in pregnancy after adjusting for other key variables of 6.9 (95% CI, 3.3–15.2) with factor V Leiden, 9.5 (95% CI, 2.1–66.7) with prothrombin G20210A, and 10.4 (95% CI, 2.2–62.5) with antithrombin deficiency. Combined defects (including homozygous thrombophilias) substantially increased the risk, with an odds ratio estimated at 107 for the combination of factor V Leiden and prothrombin G20210A in pregnancy. Additional risk factors, such as obesity, were

present in 25% of the cases versus 11% of controls. Women with recurrent VTE were more likely to have underlying combined thrombophilic defects, protein C or antithrombin deficiency, or prothrombin G20210A. The study by Gerhardt and co-workers also provided a positive predictive value for each thrombophilia, assuming an underlying rate of VTE of 0.66 per 1000 pregnancies, consistent with estimates from Western populations [18]. These values were 1 in 500 for factor V Leiden, 1 in 200 for prothrombin G20210A, and 4.6 in 100 for these defects combined. These data are supported by a retrospective study of 72,000 pregnancies in women with VTE who were assessed for thrombophilia [4] and in whom the underlying prevalence of these defects in the population was known. The risk of thrombosis was 1 in 437 for factor V Leiden, 1 in 113 for protein C deficiency, 1 in 2.8 for type 1 (quantitative) antithrombin deficiency, and 1 in 42 for type 2 (qualitative) antithrombin deficiency. This study was recently extended [13], reporting an odds ratio of 4.4 (95% CI, 1.2–16) for prothrombin G20210A, 4.5 (95% CI, 2.1–14.5) for factor V Leiden, 282 (95% CI, 31–2532) for antithrombin deficiency type 1 (quantitative deficiency), and 28 (95% CI, 5.5–142) for antithrombin deficiency type 2 (qualitative deficiency). More recently, Martinelli et al [22] reported a case–control study of 119 women with a

Table 4
Risk of venous thromboembolism in pregnant women with thrombophilia

Thrombophilia	Odds ratio (95% CI) for VTE in pregnancy[a]	Relative risk (95% CI) for VTE in pregnancy[b]	Relative risk (95% CI) for VTE in pregnancy or puerperium[c]
AT deficiency type 1 (quantitative deficiency)	282 (31–2532)	NA	NA
AT deficiency type 2 (qualitative deficiency)	28 (5.5–142)	NA	NA
AT deficiency (activity <80%)	NA	10.4 (2.2–62.5)	NA
Factor V Leiden heterozygotes	4.5 (2.1–14.5)	6.9 (3.3–15.2)	8.7 (3.4–22.5)
Prothrombin G20210A heterozygotes	4.4 (1.2–16)	9.5 (2.1–66.7)	1.8 (0.6–5.4)
MTHFR C677T homozygotes	0.45 (0.13–1.58)	No increase in risk (relative risk not reported)	NA
Any thrombophilia	NA	NA	9.0 (4.7–17.1)
Antithrombin, protein C, or protein S deficiency (not adjusted for parity)	NA	NA	13.1 (5.0–34.5)

Abbreviations: AT, antithrombin; CI, confidence interval, MTHFR, methylenetetrahydrofolate reductase; NA, not available; VTE, venous thromboembolism.

[a] Based on a retrospective study of 93,000 pregnancies in which the odds ratios were calculated by screening women with VTE in pregnancy for thrombophilia and relating this to the known prevalence of these defects in the population [12].

[b] Based on a study of 119 women with thromboembolism in pregnancy and 233 controls for the presence of congenital thrombophilia [12]. Relative risk was calculated after logistic regression to adjust for age, body mass index, oral contraceptive use, protein C and S activity, factor V Leiden, prothrombin G20210A, MTHFR 677TT, and antithrombin activity.

[c] Based on a case–control study of 119 women who had a first episode of objectively confirmed VTE in pregnancy or the puerperium and 232 controls. Relative risk was adjusted for parity. No difference was noted between relative risk in pregnancy or puerperium [22].

first episode of VTE during pregnancy or the puerperium. The relative risk for VTE was 10.6 (95% CI, 5.6–20.4) for heterozygotes of factor V Leiden, 2.9 (95% CI, 1.0–8.6) for prothrombin G20210A heterozygotes, and 13.1 (95% CI, 5.0–34.2) for protein C, protein S, and antithrombin deficiency grouped together. These data are valuable in evaluating risk and in advising women whether to use thromboprophylaxis in pregnancy (Table 4).

Currently, there is no evidence to support a policy of routine universal screening for thrombophilia in pregnancy. The natural history of many of these conditions, particularly in asymptomatic women, has not been fully established, and the need for and the type of intervention are not established. The author and his colleagues have recently assessed the cost-effectiveness of screening for factor V Leiden in pregnancy and have found that universal screening is not cost-effective (Table 5) [23]. There is a stronger argument for selective screening of women with a personal or family history of VTE, because a thrombophilia will be found in approximately 50% of cases [18]. There is a consensus that women with a personal history of VTE and an underlying thrombophilia should receive specific thromboprophylaxis during pregnancy, particularly in the puerperium [24]. Screening for thrombophilia in patients with problems such as recurrent miscarriage, intrauterine death, severe and recurrent intrauterine growth restriction, or pre-eclampsia should also be considered in view of the evidence linking thrombophilia with these pregnancy complications [18]. If screening

is to be employed in these situations, appropriate interventions must be identified.

Recurrent venous thromboembolism in pregnancy

There is a consensus that women with more than one previous VTE should receive antenatal thromboprophylaxis. The management of the woman with a single previous VTE has been more controversial because of the wide variation in reported risk, ranging from 1% to 13% [24–28], and the side effects of unfractionated heparin in pregnancy. Nevertheless, these studies have the following limitations: objective testing was not used in all of the cases; some of the studies were retrospective; and the prospective studies had relatively small sample sizes. Brill-Edwards et al [29] recently provided valuable data for the management of such women. They prospectively studied 125 pregnant women with a single previous objectively diagnosed VTE. No heparin was given antenatally, but anticoagulant therapy, usually warfarin following an initial short course of heparin or low molecular weight heparin (LMWH), was given for 4 to 6 weeks postpartum. The overall antenatal recurrence rate was 2.4% (95% CI, 0.2–6.9). There were no episodes of recurrent VTE in the 44 women (95% CI, 0–8.0) who did not have an underlying thrombophilia and whose previous VTE had been associated with a temporary risk factor. The temporary risk factors were pregnancy in 35%, oral contraceptive use in 23%, surgery in 18%, trauma in 14%,

Table 5
Cost-effectiveness of screening for factor V Leiden in pregnancy

	No screening (n = 967)	Selective screening (n = 113)	Universal screening (n = 967)
Cost of screening for mutation	0	£1305.31	£11,543.29
Cost of prophylactic postpartum LMWH for those positive for FVL	0	£595.48	£5959.80
Cost of prophylactic LMWH (from 12–40 weeks' gestation) for those positive for FVL	0	£2774.94	£27,787.20
Averted costs of treating vascular events (assumes 50% reduction with prophylaxis)	0	£908.13	£5448.81
Net cost of treatment for whole cohort	£158,013.4	£157,105.3	£152,566.6
Total cost of management strategy	£158,013.4	£161,781.0	£197,856.9
Number of women identified with FVL	0	3	30
Number of women with complications possibly associated with FVL	87	1	6
Events prevented by screening (assumes 50% reduction with prophylaxis)	0	0.5	3

Abbreviations: FVL, factor V Leiden; LMWH, low molecular weight heparin.
From Clark P, Twaddle S, Walker ID, Scott L, Greer IA. Screening for the factor V Leiden mutation in pregnancy is not cost effective. Lancet 2002;359:1919–20; with permission.

immobility in 4%, and chemotherapy in 1%. In contrast, women who were found to have an underlying thrombophilia or whose previous VTE was idiopathic had an antepartum recurrence rate of 5.9% (95% CI, 1.2–16). These data suggest that women with a single previous event associated with a temporary risk factor and who do not have identifiable thrombophilia should not routinely receive heparin or LMWH antenatally. Nonetheless, given the wide confidence intervals and the implications of a further event, this decision should be discussed with the patient and her wishes taken into account. In women with an underlying thrombophilia or in whom VTE is idiopathic, there is a much stronger argument for pharmacologic thromboprophylaxis.

Diagnostic issues regarding venous thromboembolism in pregnancy

The clinical features of DVT include leg pain or discomfort (especially on the left side), swelling, tenderness, increased temperature and edema, lower abdominal pain, mild pyrexia, and an elevated white blood cell count. Women presenting with abdominal pain, leukocytosis, and pyrexia can be misdiagnosed as sustaining intra-abdominal pathology such as appendicitis. Features suggestive of PTE include dyspnea, collapse, chest pain, hemoptysis, faintness, raised jugular venous pressure, and focal signs in the chest, sometimes combined with the symptoms and signs of DVT. As is true in the nonpregnant patient, the clinical diagnosis of VTE during pregnancy is unreliable, particularly because problems such as leg swelling and discomfort are common features of normal pregnancy. In a study of consecutive pregnant women presenting with a clinical suspicion of DVT, the diagnosis was confirmed in less than 10% [24]. In contrast, approximately 25% of diagnoses are confirmed in the nonpregnant patient [30–32]. Approximately 30% of nonpregnant patients presenting with possible PTE have the diagnosis confirmed [33,34], but the number of positive results following investigation seems to be substantially lower in pregnancy [24], reflecting a low threshold for investigation. An objective diagnosis of VTE in pregnancy is essential, because the failure to identify a VTE will endanger the mother, and unnecessary treatment will expose her to the hazards of anticoagulation.

Real-time or duplex ultrasound venography is the main diagnostic tool [35] to detect DVT. If DVT is confirmed, anticoagulant treatment should be commenced or continued. In nonpregnant subjects, the pretest clinical probability of DVT modifies the positive predictive value and the negative predictive value of objective diagnostic tests [36,37]. Applying this principle to pregnancy, a negative ultrasound result with a low level of clinical suspicion suggests that anticoagulant treatment can be discontinued or withheld. In the presence of a negative ultrasound report and a high level of clinical suspicion, the woman should be anticoagulated and ultrasound repeated in 1 week, or alternative imaging techniques such as x-ray venography or MRI should be considered. If repeat testing is negative, anticoagulant treatment should be discontinued [38].

In the woman with suspected PTE, a ventilation–perfusion lung scan and bilateral duplex ultrasound leg examinations should ideally be performed. In the nonpregnant woman, a normal perfusion scan has a negative predictive value of over 99% and a high-probability lung scan a positive predictive value of over 85%. When there is a strong clinical suspicion of PTE, the positive predictive value of a high-probability lung scan increases to over 95%, whereas with low clinical probability, it decreases to under 60%.

The greatest diagnostic problem is when the ventilation–perfusion scan is in the medium range. In practical terms, when the scan suggests a "medium" or "high" probability of PTE, or when there is a "low" probability of PTE on a ventilation–perfusion scan but a positive result on ultrasound for DVT, anticoagulant treatment should be continued. When a ventilation–perfusion scan suggests a low risk for PTE and there are negative leg ultrasound examinations in a patient in whom there is a high level of clinical suspicion, anticoagulant treatment should be continued with repeat testing in 1 week (ventilation–perfusion scan and leg ultrasound examination), or alternative imaging techniques such as pulmonary angiography, MRI, or helical CT should be employed [38]. Similarly, if the chest radiograph reveals abnormalities that lead to difficulties in the diagnosis of PTE using ventilation–perfusion scanning, alternative imaging techniques are warranted. Helical CT scanning is likely to be of particular value. As the test becomes more widely available, it may threaten the role of ventilation–perfusion scans in the diagnosis of PTE. Helical CT can rapidly image the whole thorax within the time of a single breath hold with good visualization of the pulmonary arterial tree down to the level of the segmental arteries. Technical advances are likely to allow even greater resolution and faster image acquisition times. It may be useful to employ echocardiography of the right side of the heart, particularly when performed transesophageally, when PTE is suspected. This modality may allow direct visualization of thrombus in the pulmonary arteries or right side of the heart. Indirect signs of PTE include a dilated hypokinetic right ventricle, tricuspid regurgitation, and high pulmonary artery pressures as measured with Doppler ultrasound. The radiation dose from investigations such as ventilation–perfusion scanning, chest radiography, helical CT, and even limited venography is modest [39] and is considered to pose a negligible risk to the fetus, particularly when set in the context of the risk from PTE. Objective diagnostic testing should not be withheld because of concern regarding fetal radiation exposure.

Assays for D-dimer are now used as a screening test for VTE in the nonpregnant patient, in whom they have a high negative predictive value [35]. A low level of D-dimer suggests the absence of VTE, and further objective tests are not performed. An increased level of D-dimer leads to an objective diagnostic test for VTE. In pregnancy, the level of D-dimer can be increased owing to the physiologic changes in the coagulation system, particularly if there is a concomitant problem such as pre-eclampsia or hemorrhage (conditions that are themselves risk factors for VTE). A positive D-dimer test in pregnancy is not necessarily consistent with VTE, and objective diagnostic testing is required. A low level of D-dimer in pregnancy and in the nonpregnant patient suggests that there is no VTE. Nonetheless, there is limited information on the efficacy and safety of D-dimer screening for VTE in pregnancy, and, until more information is available, firm guidance cannot be given.

The following thrombophilia screening performed at the time of presentation and before starting anticoagulant therapy can be useful in women with VTE:

- Activated partial thromboplastin time (may identify anticardiolipin antibodies)
- Prothrombin time (aids in interpretation of low protein C or S)
- Thrombin time (can identify problems such as dysfibrinogenemia or heparin contamination)
- Activated protein C resistance (genetic testing for factor V Leiden; only required when there is evidence of activated protein C resistance on the modified test for this resistance that predilutes the test sample with factor V deficient plasma)
- Protein C deficiency
- Protein S deficiency
- Antithrombin deficiency
- Prothrombin G20210A mutation
- Lupus anticoagulant
- Anticardiolipin antibodies (IgG and IgM)

This screening should include a family history of thrombosis. Although the results of a thrombophilia screen will not influence immediate management, they may influence the duration and intensity of anticoagulation, such as when antithrombin deficiency is identified. One must be aware of the effects of pregnancy and thrombus on the results of a thrombophilia screen. For example, protein S levels fall in normal pregnancy, making it extremely difficult to make a diagnosis of protein S deficiency. Activated protein C resistance occurs in approximately 40% of pregnancies, and anticardiolipin antibodies can influence the result of this test. Antithrombin may be reduced when thrombus is present. In liver disease, protein C and protein S will be reduced. Genotyping for the presence of factor V Leiden and prothrombin G20210A is not influenced by pregnancy or thrombosis. Thrombophilia screens must be interpreted by clinicians with specific expertise in the area. As noted previously, factor V Leiden is associated with an increase in the risk for VTE largely owing to DVT rather than PTE [40]. This observation may reflect a more adherent and stable thrombus with factor V Leiden, reducing the likelihood of embolization. Whether this effect applies in pregnancy is not yet established.

Antithrombotic therapy in pregnancy

Low molecular weight heparins are the anticoagulants of choice in pregnancy owing to the fetal hazards of coumarin [41] and side effects of unfractionated heparin. Warfarin is not secreted in breast milk in clinically significant amounts and is safe to use during lactation but crosses the placenta and is a teratogen. Warfarin embryopathy (midface hypoplasia, stippled chondral calcification, scoliosis, short proximal limbs, and short phalanges) can occur in approximately 4% to 5% [41] of fetuses exposed between 6 and 9 weeks' gestation. Substitution of heparin for warfarin during the first trimester can prevent this side effect. The risk of embryopathy may be dose dependent, with an increased risk when the dose of warfarin is greater than 5 mg/day [42]. In addition to warfarin embryopathy, there is the possibility of problems arising owing to fetal bleeding. Because the fetal liver is immature and levels of vitamin K–dependant coagulation factors low, maternal warfarin therapy maintained in the therapeutic range will be associated with excessive anticoagulation and potential bleeding problems in the fetus. Warfarin should be avoided beyond 36 weeks' gestation [41] because of the excessive bleeding risk to the mother and fetus in the peripartum period. In addition, recent data suggest that prenatal exposure to coumarin is associated with an increased risk of disturbance in development manifest as minor neurologic dysfunction or a low intelligence quotient in school-aged children, with a relative risk of 7.6 for two or more of these minor abnormalities [43].

In contrast to warfarin, unfractionated heparin [44] and LMWH do not cross the placenta [45,46] as determined by measuring heparin activity in fetal blood, and there is no evidence of teratogenesis or risk of fetal hemorrhage. Based on a systematic review, these agents seem to be safe for the fetus [47]. Heparins are not secreted in breast milk and can be used during breast feeding. Prolonged use of unfractionated heparin can be associated with symptomatic osteoporosis (approximately 2% incidence of osteoporotic fractures), allergy, and heparin-induced thrombocytopenia [48]. LMWHs are associated with substantially less risk of osteoporosis. A recent study randomized women to receive unfractionated heparin or dalteparin for thromboprophylaxis in pregnancy and measured bone mineral density in the lumbar spine for up to 3 years after delivery [49]. Bone density did not differ in the healthy controls and dalteparin group but was significantly lower in the unfractionated heparin group when compared with the controls and dalteparin-treated women. Multiple logistic regression revealed that the type of heparin therapy was the only independent factor associated with reduced bone mass. Heparin-induced thrombocytopenia is a rare but life-threatening side effect. It is an idiosyncratic immune-mediated reaction associated with extensive VTE that usually occurs between 5 and 15 days after the institution of heparin. The risk has been estimated to be 1% to 3% with unfractionated heparin and is substantially lower with LMWH [50]. Allergic reactions usually take the form of itchy erythematous lesions at the injection sites. Switching heparin preparations may be helpful; however, a degree of cross-reactivity can still occur. Allergic reactions should be distinguished from faulty injection technique with associated bruising. Almost 1500 cases of prophylaxis or treatment of VTE in pregnancy with enoxaparin and dalteparin, the two most commonly reported LMWHs in pregnancy, have been reported in the literature. The risk for recurrent VTE has been approximately 1.2% and the risk for symptomatic osteoporotic fracture, 0.007% (Greer IA, 2002). LMWH is now the heparin of choice in pregnancy because of its better side-effect profile, good safety record for the mother and fetus, and once daily dosing [47,51–56].

Dextran should be avoided in pregnancy and alternative thromboprophylactic measures employed because of the risk for maternal anaphylactoid reactions, which have been associated with uterine hypertonus, profound fetal distress, and a high incidence of fetal death or profound neurologic damage [57].

Graduated elastic compression stockings are effective in the nonpregnant patient and, in view of the pregnancy-related changes in the venous system, could be of considerable value in pregnancy. They may act by preventing overdistension of veins, preventing endothelial damage and exposure of subendothelial collagen [58]. They also can be employed in acute DVT. Other mechanical techniques, such as intermittent pneumatic compression, are of value during cesarean section and immediately postpartum for prophylaxis.

Hirudin, a direct thrombin inhibitor used in the nonpregnant patient for the treatment of heparin-induced thrombocytopenia, is also used for postoperative prophylaxis. Because this agent crosses the placenta, it should not be used in pregnancy. It has been used in a lactating mother because of heparin-induced thrombocytopenia and was not detectable in breast milk [59].

Aspirin has been found in a meta-analysis to have a beneficial effect in the prevention of DVT. Its effectiveness in pregnancy in comparison with heparin remains to be established, but it is likely to offer some benefit. Its effectiveness is likely to be less than that of LMWH [60]. In women who are unable to take heparin, or in whom the balance of risk is not considered sufficient to merit heparin, aspirin may be useful in combination with compression stockings. Low-dose aspirin (60–75 mg daily) is not associated with an adverse pregnancy outcome in the second and third trimesters [61,62].

Management of acute venous thromboembolism in pregnancy

When DVT or PTE is suspected clinically, treatment with unfractionated heparin or LMWH should be given until the diagnosis is excluded by objective testing, unless anticoagulation is contraindicated. Thromboembolic deterrent stockings should be employed along with leg elevation for DVT. Analgesia for pleuritic pain and oxygen are often required in patients with PTE. Traditionally, unfractionated heparin has been used in the initial management of VTE when such treatment reduces the risk for further thromboembolism when compared with no treatment [63–66]. Failure to achieve the lower limit of the target therapeutic range of the aPTT ratio is associated with a 10 to 15 fold increase in the risk for recurrent VTE [67]. Frequently, use of the aPTT to monitor unfractionated heparin is poorly performed and is technically problematic, particularly in late pregnancy when an apparent heparin resistance occurs owing to increased fibrinogen and factor VIII. This effect can lead to unnecessarily high doses of heparin with subsequent hemorrhagic problems. When such problems are considered to exist, it may be useful to determine the anti-Xa level as a measure of heparin dose (target range, 0.35–0.7 U/mL) [63]. Alternatively, LMWH could be employed. Two meta-analyses of randomized controlled trials have compared LMWH with unfractionated heparin in the initial treatment of DVT in nonpregnant subjects [68,69]. LMWH was found to be more effective than unfractionated heparin with lower mortality and was associated with a lower risk of hemorrhagic complications. LMWH has been as effective as unfractionated heparin in the initial treatment of PTE in studies carried out in nonpregnant subjects [70]. LMWH has been used for the initial management of VTE in pregnancy [53,71,72] and has been recommended for this purpose [24]. Occasionally, thrombolytic therapy may be required for life-threatening PTE or when a massive DVT threatens limb viability. Experience is limited, and there is a risk of major hemorrhage if systemic thrombolysis is used around the time of delivery or postpartum.

Unfractionated heparin can be given by continuous intravenous infusion or by subcutaneous injection. Unfractionated heparin is preferred to LMWH by some authorities in the initial management of massive PTE because of its rapid effect and the extensive experience in this situation. The dose is adjusted by monitoring the aPTT, with a therapeutic target ratio of 1.5 to 2.5 times the mean laboratory control value. The aPTT should be performed 6 hours after the loading dose and then on a daily basis. Protocols for heparin dose adjustment according to aPTT ratio results can be useful [63,73], and each laboratory should standardize its own target range for the aPTT ratio [63,72]. If anti-Xa measurements are used to monitor heparin, the target range is 0.35 to 0.70 IU/mL. Subcutaneous unfractionated heparin is an effective alternative to intravenous administration. In a meta-analysis of randomized controlled trials, 12 hourly subcutaneous unfractionated heparin was as effective and at least as safe as intravenous unfractionated heparin in the prevention of VTE in nonpregnant patients with acute DVT [74]. When administered subcutaneously, unfractionated heparin is given in subcutaneous injections of 15,000 to

20,000 IU, 12 hourly, after an initial intravenous bolus of 5000 IU. The dose should be adjusted to maintain the midinterval aPTT between 1.5 and 2.5 times the control [72].

In nonpregnant patients, once daily administration with LMWH is recommended for acute treatment of VTE (enoxaparin, 1.5 mg/kg body weight once daily; dalteparin, 10,000–18,000 U once daily depending on body weight). In view of the alterations in the pharmacokinetics of dalteparin and enoxaparin during pregnancy [75,76], the author recommends a twice daily dosage regimen for these LMWHs in the treatment of VTE in pregnancy (enoxaparin, 1 mg/kg twice daily; dalteparin, 100 U/kg twice daily up to a maximum of 18,000 U/24 hours). These doses are also used to treat VTE in the nonpregnant patient. The regimen for the administration of a LMWH (enoxaparin) in the immediate management of VTE in pregnancy is shown in Table 6 [72]. The initial dose of enoxaparin is 1 mg/kg twice daily, based on the early pregnancy weight, because LMWH does not cross the placenta. Enoxaparin is available in syringes of 40, 60, 80 100 and 120 mg. The dose closest to the patient's weight should be employed and should be continued 12 hourly until objective testing has been performed. If the diagnosis of VTE is confirmed, treatment is continued. Peak anti-Xa activity (3 hours postinjection) can be measured by a chromogenic substrate assay to confirm that an appropriate dose has been given. A suitable target therapeutic range is 0.6 to 1.2 U/mL. If the peak anti-Xa level is above the upper limit of the therapeutic target range, the dose of LMWH should be reduced and peak anti-Xa activity reassessed. The author's experience indicates that satisfactory anti-Xa levels are obtained using this regimen, and further monitoring of these levels can be deferred until the next routine working day [71]. Indeed, the experience suggests that this dose regimen rarely requires adjustment, and monitoring with assays for anti-Xa is probably unnecessary except at extremes of body weight. Care must be taken in women with a very high body mass index, in whom it is critical to ensure that an appropriate dose of heparin is used [1].

Table 6
Initial dose of enoxaparin for acute treatment of venous thromboembolism

Early pregnancy weight (kg)	Initial dose of enoxaparin
< 50	40 mg twice daily
50–69	60 mg twice daily
70 89	80 mg twice daily
≥ 90	100 mg twice daily

With heparin therapy, the platelet count should be monitored 4 to 8 days after treatment commences, followed by testing on a monthly basis to detect heparin-induced thrombocytopenia. Pregnant women in whom heparin-induced thrombocytopenia develops and who require ongoing anticoagulant therapy should be managed with the heparinoid [77] danaparoid sodium.

Because coumarin is contraindicated in pregnancy, subcutaneous LMWH is usually used for maintenance treatment of VTE for the remainder of the pregnancy [71,78,79]. Women can be taught to self-inject and can be managed as outpatients once the acute event has been dealt with. Arrangements should be made to allow for safe disposal of needles and syringes. Evidence suggests that therapeutic doses of heparin should be employed for maintenance therapy, because a high recurrence rate of VTE was reported (47%) in a prospective randomized controlled trial in nonpregnant patients when thromboprophylactic doses of unfractionated heparin (5000 IU every 12 hours) were employed after initial management with intravenous unfractionated heparin [79]. The duration of therapeutic anticoagulant treatment in the nonpregnant situation is usually 6 months. Because pregnancy is associated with prothrombotic changes in the coagulation system and venous flow, it would seem logical to apply this duration of therapy to pregnancy. If the VTE occurs early in the pregnancy, and if there are no additional risk factors, the dose of LMWH could be reduced to prophylactic levels (40 mg of enoxaparin once per day or 5000 IU of dalteparin). Following delivery, treatment should continue for at least 6 weeks. Coumarin therapy can be used following delivery. If the woman chooses to use coumarin postpartum, it can usually be initiated on the second or third postnatal day. The international normalized ratio (INR) should be checked on day 2 and subsequent warfarin doses titrated to maintain the INR between 2.0 and 3.0 [80]. Heparin treatment should be continued until the INR is greater than 2.0 on 2 successive days.

Considerations for labor and delivery

The woman receiving anticoagulants should be advised that, once she is established in labor or thinks that she is in labor, she should not inject any further heparin until she has been assessed. Further doses should be prescribed by medical staff on an individualized basis. Generally, when the induction of labor is planned, the dose of heparin should be reduced to a thromboprophylactic level on the day before delivery.

Graduated elastic compression stockings can be worn to provide some thromboprophylaxis. The treatment dose (twice daily administration) should be recommenced following delivery. Because of the small risk for epidural hematoma formation during spinal instrumentation in anticoagulated patients, epidural anesthesia should be sited only after a discussion with a senior anesthetist. There must be a degree of caution in the concomitant use of LMWH and neuraxial anesthesia, with vigilance for signs of cord compression. The combination must be avoided in patients undergoing therapeutic anticoagulation. In women receiving prophylactic doses of heparin and LMWH, neuraxial anesthesia should be avoided around the time of peak heparin levels. The timing of anesthesia and heparin administration need to be adjusted. Generally, regional techniques are not used until at least 12 hours after the previous prophylactic dose of LMWH. When a woman presents during a therapeutic regimen of LMWH (ie, twice daily regimen), regional techniques should not be employed for at least 24 hours after the last dose of LMWH. LMWH should not be given for at least 3 hours after the epidural catheter has been removed, and the cannula should not be removed within 10 to 12 hours of the most recent injection [81–83].

For elective cesarean section, the woman should receive a thromboprophylactic dose of LMWH on the day before delivery. On the day of delivery, the morning dose of LMWH should be omitted and the operation performed as soon as possible thereafter. Graduated elastic compression stockings can be worn or mechanical methods used to provide some thromboprophylaxis intraoperatively. A thromboprophylactic dose of LMWH should be given by 3 hours postoperatively and after removal of the epidural catheter. The treatment dose should be recommenced that evening. This practice reflects the general principles of management, and individualized management plans are often required with regard to anticoagulant treatment. There is an increased risk of wound hematoma following cesarean section with the use of unfractionated heparin and LMWH of approximately 2%. Consideration should be given to the use of drains (abdominal and rectus sheath) at cesarean section, and the skin incision should be closed with staples or interrupted sutures to allow for drainage of any hematoma that develops [84].

If there is a high risk for hemorrhage in a patient in whom continued heparin treatment is considered essential, she should be treated with intravenous unfractionated heparin until the risk factors for hemorrhage have resolved. Intravenous unfractionated heparin has a short duration of action, and anticoagulation will reverse soon after cessation of the infusion should a hemorrhagic problem occur. Risk factors that should lead to the use of intravenous unfractionated heparin include recent major antepartum hemorrhage or coagulopathy, progressive wound hematoma, suspected intra-abdominal bleeding, and postpartum hemorrhage [84].

Thromboprophylaxis in pregnancy

In the woman with a previous VTE associated with a risk factor that is no longer present and with no additional risk factor or underlying thrombophilia, antenatal LMWH should not be prescribed routinely. This strategy must be discussed with the woman and her views taken into account, especially in view of the wide confidence intervals reported by Brill-Edwards et al (rate of recurrence, 0%; 95% CI, 0–8.0) [29]. Graduated elastic compression stockings with or without low-dose aspirin can be employed antenatally in these women. Postpartum, the patient should receive anticoagulant therapy for at least 6 weeks (eg, 40 mg of enoxaparin or 5000 IU of dalteparin daily, or coumarin [target INR, 2–3] with LMWH overlap until the INR is $\geq$ 2.0) with or without wearing graduated elastic compression stockings (Table 7).

In women with a single previous VTE and an underlying thrombophilia, in women in whom the VTE was idiopathic, or in women who have additional risk factors such as obesity, there is a stronger argument for pharmacologic prophylaxis antenatally, although this regimen will depend in part on the severity of the previous event and the type of thrombophilia. Antenatally, these women should be considered for prophylactic doses of LMWH (eg, 40 mg of enoxaparin or 5000 IU of dalteparin daily) with or without wearing graduated elastic compression stockings. More intense LMWH prophylaxis in the presence of antithrombin deficiency is usually prescribed (eg, enoxaparin, 0.5–1 mg/kg 12 hourly, or dalteparin, 50–100 IU/kg 12 hourly) [85], although many women with previous VTE and antithrombin deficiency are maintained on long-term anticoagulant therapy. Postpartum anticoagulant prophylaxis for at least 6 weeks (eg, 40 mg of enoxaparin or 5000 IU of dalteparin daily, or coumarin [target INR, 2–3] with LMWH overlap until the INR is $\geq$ 2.0) with or without wearing graduated elastic compression stockings is recommended.

For the woman with multiple previous VTE and no identifiable thrombophilia who is not receiving long-term anticoagulant therapy, there is a consensus that she should receive antenatal LMWH thromboprophylaxis and wear graduated elastic compression stockings. Postpartum, she should receive at least 6 weeks of pharmacologic prophylaxis with either LMWH or warfarin. If she is switched to coumarin postpartum, the target INR is 2 to 3, and LMWH should be continued until the INR is 2 or greater. A longer duration of postpartum prophylaxis may be required for women with additional risk factors.

The woman with previous episodes of VTE receiving long-term anticoagulants (eg, with underlying thrombophilia) should be switched from oral anticoagulants to LMWH by 6 weeks' gestation and be fitted with graduated elastic compression stockings. These women should be considered at very high risk for antenatal VTE and should receive anticoagulant prophylaxis throughout pregnancy. They should be advised, ideally pre-pregnancy, of the need to switch from warfarin to LMWH as soon as pregnancy is confirmed. The dose of LMWH given should be closer to that used for the treatment of VTE rather than that used for prophylaxis (eg, enoxaparin, 0.5–1 mg/kg 12 hourly, or dalteparin, 50–100 IU/kg 12 hourly. It should be noted that 12 hourly injections may be preferable to once daily injections in view of the increased clearance of LMWH in pregnancy]) based on the early pregnancy weight [85]. The platelet count should be checked before and 1 week after the introduction of LMWH, followed by monthly checks. Postpartum, the patient should resume long-term oral anticoagulants with LMWH overlap until the INR is in the pre-pregnancy therapeutic range and wear graduated elastic compression stockings.

In the woman who has a heritable thrombophilia diagnosed on laboratory testing, such as a woman with a positive family history, but who has no prior VTE, surveillance or prophylactic LMWH with or without graduated elastic compression stockings can be used antenatally. In antithrombin-deficient women, there is a strong argument for antenatal LMWH. Similarly, in a symptomatic kindred, antenatal LMWH is recommended. Postpartum, these women should receive anticoagulant therapy for at least 6 weeks (eg, 40 mg of enoxaparin or 5000 IU of dalteparin daily, or coumarin [target INR, 2–3] with LMWH overlap until the INR is $\geq$ 2.0) with or without wearing graduated elastic compression stockings. These women usually require specialized and individualized advice from clinicians with expertise in the area.

Women undergoing cesarean section or vaginal delivery should undergo a risk assessment for VTE [52]. In the patient undergoing cesarean section, thromboprophylaxis (eg, 40 mg of enoxaparin or

Table 7
Suggested management strategies for prophylaxis in various clinical situations

Clinical situation	Suggested management
Single previous VTE associated with a temporary risk factor that is no longer present and no additional current risk factors such as obesity	Antenatal: Surveillance or prophylactic doses of LMWH are indicated (eg, 40 mg of enoxaparin or 5000 IU of dalteparin daily) $\pm$ graduated elastic compression stockings. Discuss decision regarding antenatal LMWH with the woman. Postpartum: Anticoagulant therapy is indicated for at least 6 weeks (eg, 40 mg of enoxaparin or 5000 IU of dalteparin daily or coumarin [target INR, 2–3] with LMWH overlap until the INR is ≥ 2.0.) $\pm$ graduated elastic compression stockings.
Single previous idiopathic VTE or single previous VTE with underlying thrombophilia and not on long-term anticoagulant therapy, or single previous VTE and additional current risk factor(s) (eg, obesity, nephrotic syndrome)	Antenatal: Prophylactic doses of LMWH are indicated (eg, 40 mg of enoxaparin or 5000 IU of dalteparin daily) $\pm$ graduated elastic compression stockings. Note that there is strong support for more intense LMWH therapy in antithrombin deficiency (eg, enoxaparin, 0.5–1 mg/kg 12 hourly or dalteparin, 50–100 IU/kg 12 hourly). Postpartum: Anticoagulant therapy is indicated for at least 6 weeks (eg, 40 mg of enoxaparin or 5000 IU of dalteparin daily or coumarin [target INR, 2–3] with LMWH overlap until the INR is ≥ 2.0.) $\pm$ graduated elastic compression stockings.
More than one previous episode of VTE, with no thrombophilia and not on long-term anticoagulant therapy	Antenatal: Prophylactic doses of LMWH are indicated (eg, 40 mg of enoxaparin or 5000 IU of dalteparin daily) + graduated elastic compression stockings. Postpartum: Anticoagulant therapy is indicated for at least 6 weeks (eg, 40 mg of enoxaparin or 5000 IU of dalteparin daily or coumarin [target INR, 2–3] with LMWH overlap until the INR is ≥ 2.0.) + graduated elastic compression stockings.
Previous episode(s) of VTE in women receiving long-term anticoagulants (eg, with underlying thrombophilia)	Antenatal: A switch should be made from oral anticoagulants to LMWH therapy (eg, enoxaparin, 0.5–1 mg/kg 12 hourly or dalteparin, 50–100 IU/kg 12 hourly) by 6 weeks' gestation + graduated elastic compression stockings. Postpartum: Long-term oral anticoagulants should be resumed with LMWH overlap until the INR is in the pre-pregnancy therapeutic range + graduated elastic compression stockings.
Thrombophilia (confirmed laboratory abnormality) but no prior VTE	Antenatal: Surveillance or prophylactic LMWH is indicated $\pm$ graduated elastic compression stockings. The indication for pharmacologic prophylaxis in the antenatal period is stronger in AT-deficient women than in the other thrombophilias, in symptomatic kindreds when compared with asymptomatic kindreds, and also when additional risk factors are present. Postpartum: Anticoagulant therapy is indicated for at least 6 weeks (eg, 40 mg of enoxaparin or 5000 IU of dalteparin daily or coumarin [target INR, 2–3] with LMWH overlap until the INR is ≥ 2.0.) $\pm$ graduated elastic compression stockings.
Following cesarean section or vaginal delivery	Carry out risk assessment for VTE. If additional risk factors such as emergency section in labor, age over 35 years, or a high BMI present, consider LMWH thromboprophylaxis (eg, 40 mg of enoxaparin or 5000 IU of dalteparin) $\pm$ graduated elastic compression stockings.

Specialist advice for individualized management of patients is advisable in many of these situations.
Abbreviations: AT, antithrombin; BMI, body mass index; INR, international normalized ratio; LMWH, low molecular weight heparin; VTE, venous thromboembolism.

5000 IU of dalteparin) should be prescribed if she has one or more additional risk factors, such as emergency section in labor, age greater than 35 years, or a high body mass index. In patients at high risk, graduated elastic compression stockings should also be used. Stockings can also be employed if heparin is contraindicated. In the woman undergoing vaginal delivery, a similar strategy can be used, with LMWH prescribed if there are two or more additional risk factors [1] or one major risk factor such as morbid obesity.

Summary

Pulmonary thromboembolism is a major cause of maternal mortality. DVT causes significant morbidity in pregnancy and in later life owing to the post-thrombotic syndrome. Obstetricians must have an understanding of the risk factors for VTE, the appropriate use of prophylaxis, the need for objective diagnosis in women with suspected VTE, and the appropriate use of anticoagulant therapy. Greater use of prophylaxis is needed after vaginal delivery. Because acute VTE is relatively uncommon, greater use of proposed guidelines [24,84,85] may be of value in improving management, but the involvement of clinicians with expertise in the management of these cases is also important.

References

[1] Department of Health, Welsh Office, Scottish Home and Health Department, and Department of Health and Social Services Northern Ireland. Confidential enquiries into maternal deaths in the United Kingdom, 1997–99. London: TSO; 2001.

[2] Macklon NS, Greer IA. Venous thromboembolic disease in obstetrics and gynaecology: the Scottish experience. Scot Med J 1996;41:83–6.

[3] McColl M, Ramsay JE, Tait RC, Walker ID, McCall F, Conkie JA, et al. Risk factors for pregnancy associated venous thromboembolism. Thromb Haemost 1997;78: 1183–8.

[4] McColl M, Ellison J, Greer IA, Tait RC, Walker ID. Prevalence of the post-thrombotic syndrome in young women with previous venous thromboembolism. Br J Haematol 2000;108:272–4.

[5] Bergqvist D, Bergqvist A, Lindhagen A, et al. Long-term outcome of patients with venous thromboembolism during pregnancy. In: Greer IA, Turpie AGG, Forbes CD, editors. Haemostasis and thrombosis in obstetrics and gynaecology. London: Chapman and Hall; 1992. p. 349–59.

[6] Clarke P, Brennand J, Conkie JA, McCall F, Greer IA, Walker ID. Activated protein C sensitivity, protein C, protein S and coagulation in normal pregnancy. Thromb Haemost 1998;79:1166–70.

[7] Greer IA. Haemostasis and thrombosis in pregnancy. In: Bloom AL, Forbes CD, Thomas DP, Tuddenham EGD, editors. Haemostasis and thrombosis. Churchill Livingstone: Edinburgh; 1994. p. 987–1015.

[8] Macklon NS, Greer IA, Bowman AW. An ultrasound study of gestational and postural changes in the deep venous system of the leg in pregnancy. Br J Obstet Gynaecol 1997;104:191–7.

[9] Lindhagen A, Bergqvist A, Bergqvist D, Hallbook T. Late venous function in the leg after deep venous thrombosis occurring in relation to pregnancy. Br J Obstet Gynaecol 1986;93:348–52.

[10] Den Heijer M, Koster T, Blom HJ, Bos GMJ, Briet E, Reitsma PH, et al. Hyperhomocysteinemia as a risk factor for deep vein thrombosis. N Engl J Med 1998; 334:759–62.

[11] Greer IA. The challenge of thrombophilia in maternal-fetal medicine. N Engl J Med 2000;342:424–5.

[12] Gerhardt A, Scharf RE, Beckman MW, et al. Prothrombin and factor V mutations in women with thrombosis during pregnancy and the puerperium. N Engl J Med 2000;342:374–80.

[13] McColl MD, Ellison J, Reid F, et al. Prothrombin 20210GA, MTHFR C677T mutations in women with venous thromboembolism associated with pregnancy. Br J Obstet Gynaecol 2000;107:567–9.

[14] Walker ID. Congenital thrombophilia. In: Greer IA, editor. Bailliere's clinical obstetrics and gynaecology—thromboembolic disease in obstetrics and gynaecology. London: Bailliere Tindall; 1997. p. 431–45.

[15] Zoller B, Holm J, Dahlback B. Resistance to activated protein C due to a factor V gene mutation: the most common inherited risk factor of thrombosis. Trends Cardiovasc Med 1996;6:45–9.

[16] Poort SR, Rosendaal FR, Reitsma PH, Bertina RM. A common genetic variation in the three untranslated region of the prothrombin gene is associated with elevated plasma prothrombin levels and an increase in venous thrombosis. Blood 1996;88:3698.

[17] McColl MD, Walker ID, Greer IA. A mutation in the prothrombin gene contributing to venous thrombosis in pregnancy. Br J Obstet Gynaecol 1998;105: 923–5.

[18] Greer IA. Thrombosis in pregnancy: maternal and fetal issues. Lancet 1999;353:1258–65.

[19] Rosendaal FR. Venous thrombosis: a multicausal disease. Lancet 1999;353:1167–73.

[20] Conard J, Horellou MH, van Dreden P, Le Compte T, Samama M. Thrombosis in pregnancy and congenital deficiencies in AT III, protein C or protein S: study of 78 women. Thromb Haemost 1990;63:319–20.

[21] Bokarewa MI, Bremme K, Blomback M. Arg 506-Gln mutation in factor V and risk of thrombosis during pregnancy. Br J Haematol 1996;92:473–8.

[22] Martinelli I, de Stefano V, Taioli E, et al. Inherited

thrombophilia and first venous thromboembolism during pregnancy and puerperium. Thromb Haemost 2002;87:791–5.

[23] Clark P, Twaddle S, Walker ID, Scott L, Greer IA. Screening for the factor V Leiden mutation in pregnancy is not cost effective. Lancet 2002;359: 1919–20.

[24] Ginsberg J, Greer IA, Hirsh J. Sixth ACCP consensus conference on antithrombotic therapy: use of antithrombotic agents during pregnancy. Chest 2001;119: 122S–31S.

[25] Howell R, Fidler J, Letsky E, et al. The risk of antenatal subcutaneous heparin prophylaxis: a controlled trial. Br J Obstet Gynecol 1983;90:1124–8.

[26] Badaracco MA, Vessey M. Recurrent venous thromboembolic disease and use of oral contraceptives. BMJ 1974;1:215–7.

[27] Tengborn L. Recurrent thromboembolism in pregnancy and puerperium: is there a need for thromboprophylaxis? Am J Obstet Gynecol 1989;160:90–4.

[28] De Swiet M, Floyd E, Letsky E. Low risk of recurrent thromboembolism in pregnancy [letter]. Br J Hosp Med 1987;38:264.

[29] Brill-Edwards P, Ginsberg JS, for the Recurrence Of Clot In This Pregnancy (ROCIT) Study Group. Safety of withholding antepartum heparin in women with a previous episode of venous thromboembolism. N Engl J Med 2000;343:1439–44.

[30] Hull RD, Raskob GF, Carter CJ. Serial IPG in pregnancy patients with clinically suspected DVT: clinical validity of negative findings. Ann Intern Med 1990; 112:663–7.

[31] Hull RD, Hirsh J, Sackett D, et al. Diagnostic efficacy of IPG in suspected venous thrombosis: an alternative to venography. N Engl J Med 1977;296:1497–500.

[32] Lensing AWA, Prandoni P, Brandjes D, et al. Detection of DVT by real-time B-mode ultrasonography. N Engl J Med 1989;320:342–5.

[33] PIOPED Investigators. Value of the ventilation/perfusion scan in acute pulmonary embolism: results of the prospective investigation of pulmonary embolism diagnosis (PIOPED). JAMA 1990;263:2753–9.

[34] Hull RD, Hirsh J, Carter CJ, et al. Diagnostic value of ventilation-perfusion lung scanning in patients with suspected pulmonary embolism. Chest 1985;88:819–28.

[35] Macklon NS. Diagnosis of deep venous thrombosis and pulmonary embolism. In: Bailliere's clinical obstetrics and gynaecology—thromboembolic disease in obstetrics and gynaecology. London: Bailliere Tindall; 1997. p. 463–77.

[36] Wheeler HB, Hirsh J, Wells P, Anderson Jr FA. Diagnostic tests for deep vein thrombosis: clinical usefulness depends on probability of disease. Arch Intern Med 1994;154:1921–8.

[37] Wells PS, Anderson DR, Bormanis J, et al. Value of assessment of pretest probability of deep vein thrombosis in clinical management. Lancet 1997;350:1795–8.

[38] Thomson AJ, Greer IA. Nonhaemorrhagic obstetric shock. Baillieres Clin Obstet Gynaecol 2000;14:19–41.

[39] Ginsberg JS, Hirsh J, Rainbow AJ, et al. Risks to the fetus of radiological procedures used in the diagnosis of maternal venous thromboembolic disease. Thromb Haemost 1989;61:189–96.

[40] Bounameaux H. Factor V Leiden paradox: risk of deep vein thrombosis but not of pulmonary embolism. Lancet 2000;356:182–3.

[41] Bates SM, Ginsberg JS. Anticoagulants in pregnancy: fetal defects. In: Bailliere's clinical obstetrics and gynaecology—thromboembolic disease in obstetrics and gynaecology. London: Bailliere Tindall; 1997. p. 479–88.

[42] Vitale N, De Feo M, De Santo LS, Pollice A, Tedesco N, Contrufo M. Dose-dependent fetal complications of warfarin in pregnant women with mechanical heart valves. J Am Coll Cardiol 1999;33:1642–5.

[43] Wesseling J, van Driel D, Heymans HAS, et al. Coumarins during pregnancy: long term effects on growth and development in school age children. Thromb Haemost 2001;85:609–13.

[44] Flessa HC, Klapstrom AB, Glueck MJ, et al. Placental transport of heparin. Am J Obstet Gynecol 1965;93: 570–3.

[45] Forestier F, Daffos F, Capella-Pavlovsky M. Low molecular weight heparin (PK 10169) does not cross the placenta during the second trimester of pregnancy: study by direct fetal blood sampling under ultrasound. Thromb Res 1984;34:557–60.

[46] Forestier F, Daffos F, Rainaut M, et al. Low molecular weight heparin (CY 216) does not cross the placenta during the third trimester of pregnancy. Thromb Haemost 1987;57:234.

[47] Sanson BJ, Lensing AWA, Prins MH, et al. Safety of low-molecular-weight heparin in pregnancy: a systematic review. Thromb Haemost 1999;81:668–72.

[48] Nelson-Piercy C. Hazards of heparin: allergy, heparin-induced thrombocytopenia and osteoporosis. In: Bailliere's clinical obstetrics and gynaecology—thromboembolic disease in obstetrics and gynaecology. London: Bailliere Tindall; 1997. p. 489–509.

[49] Pettila V, Leinonen P, Markkola A, Hiilesmaa V, Kaaja R. Postpartum bone mineral density in women treated for thromboprophylaxis with unfractionated heparin or LMW heparin. Thromb Haemost 2002;87:182–6.

[50] Warkentin TE, Levine MN, Hirsh J, Horsewood P, Roberts RS, Gent M, et al. Heparin-induced thrombocytopenia in patients treated with low molecular weight heparin or unfractionated heparin. N Engl J Med 1995;332:1330–5.

[51] Nelson-Piercy C, Letsky EA, de Swiet M. Low-molecular-weight heparin for obstetric thromboprophylaxis: experience of sixty-nine pregnancies in sixty-one women at high risk. Am J Obstet Gynecol 1997;176:1062–8.

[52] Greer IA. Epidemiology, risk factors and prophylaxis of venous thromboembolism in obstetrics and gynaecology. In: Bailliere's clinical obstetrics and gynaecology—thromboembolic disease in obstetrics and gynaecology. London: Bailliere Tindall; 1997. p. 403–30.

[53] Ellison J, Walker ID, Greer IA. Antifactor Xa profiles in pregnant women receiving antenatal thromboprophylaxis with enoxaparin for prevention and treatment of thromboembolism in pregnancy. Br J Obstet Gynaecol 2000;107:1116–21.

[54] Lepercq J, Conard J, Borel-Derlon A, et al. Venous thromboembolism during pregnancy: a retrospective study of enoxaparin safety in 624 pregnancies. Br J Obstet Gynaecol 2001;108:1134–40.

[55] Hunt BJ, Doughty HA, Majumdar G, Copplestone A, Kerslake S, Buchanan N, et al. Thromboprophylaxis with low molecular weight heparin (Fragmin) in high risk pregnancies. Thromb Haemost 1997;77:39–43.

[56] Blomback M, Bremme K, Hellgren M, Siegbahn A, Lindberg H. Thromboprophylaxis with low molecular mass heparin, "Fragmin" (dalteparin), during pregnancy—longitudinal safety study. Blood Coagul Fibrinolysis 1998;9:1–9.

[57] Barbier P, Jongville AP, Autre TE, Coureau C. Fetal risks with dextran during delivery. Drug Saf 1992;7: 71–3.

[58] Macklon NS, Greer IA. Technical note: compression stockings and posture—a comparative study of their effects on the proximal deep veins in the leg at rest. Br J Radiol 1995;68:515–8.

[59] Lindoff-Last E, Willeke A, Thalhammer C, Nowak G, Bauersachs R. Hirudin treatment in a breastfeeding woman. Lancet 2000;355:467–8.

[60] Clagett GP, Anderson FA, Geerts W, et al. Prevention of venous thromboembolism. Chest 1998;114:521S–60S.

[61] CLASP Collaborative Group. CLASP: a randomised trial of low dose aspirin for the prevention and treatment of pre-eclampsia among 9364 pregnant women. Lancet 1994;343:619–29.

[62] Imperiale TF, Petrulis AS. A meta-analysis of low-dose aspirin for prevention of pregnancy-induced hypertensive disease. JAMA 1991;266:260–4.

[63] Hirsh J. Heparin. N Engl J Med 1991;324:1565–74.

[64] Barritt DV, Jordan SC. Anticoagulant drugs in the treatment of pulmonary embolism: a controlled trial. Lancet 1960;1:1309–12.

[65] Kanis JA. Heparin in the treatment of pulmonary thromboembolism. Thromb Diath Haemorrh 1974;32: 519–27.

[66] Carson JL, Kelley MA, Duff A, et al. The clinical course of pulmonary embolism. N Engl J Med 1992; 326:1240–5.

[67] Hyers TM, Hull RD, Weg JG. Antithrombotic therapy for venous thromboembolic disease. Chest 1995;108: 335S–51S.

[68] Dolovich L, Ginsberg JS. Low molecular weight heparin in the treatment of venous thromboembolism: an updated meta-analysis. Vessels 1997;3:4–11.

[69] Gould MK, Dembitzer AD, Doyle RL, et al. Low molecular weight heparins compared with unfractionated heparin for treatment of acute deep venous thrombosis: a meta-analysis of randomized, controlled trials. Ann Intern Med 1999;130:800–9.

[70] Simmoneau G, Sors H, Charbonnier B, et al. A comparison of low-molecular weight heparin with unfractionated heparin for acute pulmonary embolism. N Engl J Med 1997;337:663–9.

[71] Thomson AJ, Walker ID, Greer IA. Low molecular weight heparin for the immediate management of thromboembolic disease in pregnancy. Lancet 1998;352:1904.

[72] Rodie VA, Thomson AJ, Stewart FM, et al. Low molecular weight heparin for the treatment of venous thromboembolism in pregnancy—a case series. Br J Obstet Gynaecol 2002;109:1020–4.

[73] Hirsh J, Raschke R, Warkentin TE, et al. Heparin: mechanism of action, pharmacokinetics, dosing considerations, monitoring, efficacy, and safety. Chest 1995; 108:258S–75S.

[74] Hommes DW, Bura A, Mazzolai L, et al. Subcutaneous heparin compared with continuous intravenous heparin administration in the initial treatment of deep venous thrombosis: a meta-analysis. Ann Intern Med 1992; 116:279–84.

[75] Blomback M, Bremme K, Hellgren M, Lindberg H. A pharmacokinetic study of dalteparin (Fragmin) during late pregnancy. Blood Coagul Fibrinolysis 1998;9: 343–50.

[76] Casele HL, Laifer SA, Woelkers DA, Venkataraman R. Changes in the pharmacokinetics of the low molecular weight heparin enoxaparin sodium during pregnancy. Am J Obstet Gynecol 1999;181:1113–7.

[77] Magnani HN. Heparin-induced thrombocytopenia (HIT): an overview of 230 patients treated with Organ (Org 10172). Thromb Haemost 1993;70:554–61.

[78] Monreal M. Long-term treatment of venous thromboembolism: the place of low molecular weight heparin. Vessels 1997;3:18–21.

[79] Hull RD, Delmore T, Carter C, et al. Adjusted subcutaneous heparin versus warfarin sodium in the long-term treatment of venous thrombosis. N Engl J Med 1982; 306:1676–81.

[80] British Society for Haematology. Guidelines on oral anticoagulation: third edition. Br J Haematol 1998; 101:374–87.

[81] Checketts MR, Wildsmith JAW. Central nerve block and thromboprophylaxis—is there a problem? Br J Anaesth 1999;82:164–7.

[82] Horlocker TT, Wedel DJ. Spinal and epidural blockade and perioperative low molecular weight heparin: smooth sailing on the Titanic. Anesth Analg 1998;86: 1153–6.

[83] Consensus statement on anticoagulants and neuraxial anaesthesia from the American Society of Regional Anesthesia. Available at: http://www.asra.com/ items_of_interest/consensus_statements/index.iphtml. Accessed January 2003.

[84] Thomson AJ, Greer IA. Thromboembolic disease in pregnancy and the puerperium: acute management. RCOG guideline. London: RCOG; 2001.

[85] Scottish Intercollegiate Guidelines Network. Prophylaxis of venous thromboembolism: a national clinical guideline. Edinburgh: Scottish Intercollegiate Guidelines Network; 2002, in press.

CLINICS
IN CHEST
MEDICINE

Clin Chest Med 24 (2003) 139–151

The evolution and impact of the American College of Chest Physicians consensus statement on antithrombotic therapy

Victor F. Tapson, MD, FCCP

Division of Pulmonary and Critical Care, Box 31175, Room 351, Bell Building, Duke University Medical Center,
Durham, NC 27710, USA

Venous thromboembolism (VTE) results in substantial morbidity and mortality worldwide. The risk for VTE is influenced by patient-related and clinical factors. Optimal management requires the institution of appropriate preventive measures and the timely recognition of established VTE followed by appropriate treatment. Much progress has been made over the past several decades in the diagnosis, prevention, and treatment of deep venous thrombosis (DVT) and pulmonary embolism (PE).

By 1985, an increasing number of randomized clinical trials involving antithrombotic therapy were focused on the prevention and treatment of VTE, coronary artery disease, and cerebral vascular disease. Nevertheless, the results of these studies were not always applied in a uniform manner clinically. The American College of Chest Physicians (ACCP), in conjunction with the National Heart, Lung, and Blood Institute (NHLBI), appointed a special working group to evaluate the studies and to make recommendations for appropriate antithrombotic therapy. The participants included cardiologists, pulmonary specialists, hematologists, neurologists, vascular and thoracic surgeons, and epidemiologists. Of the original 32 members, 25 were American, 5 were Canadian, and 2 were British. The project was led by James Dalen and Jack Hirsh, who worked with the group to formulate written recommendations regarding antithrombotic therapy based on a critical review

of the current literature and the collective expert experience. The working group was divided into eight task forces to examine the use of antithrombotic therapy in coronary artery disease, coronary artery bypass surgery, valvular heart disease, prosthetic heart valves, atrial fibrillation, VTE, and cerebral vascular disease. These first consensus conference recommendations, published in 1986 [1], have evolved over the last 15 years to become the premier evidence-based consensus statement on antithrombotic therapy. This article reviews the evolution of the ACCP consensus, specifically with regard to the prevention and treatment of VTE, and offers a perspective on the impact of the recommendations. Special circumstances such as pregnancy and heparin-induced thrombocytopenia are briefly addressed.

The initial critical review of antithrombotic therapy for VTE was a 10-page report with 120 references and reviewed the prophylaxis of VTE and the treatment of established disease [2]. This perspective, offered by three leading clinical investigators in the field of VTE, reviewed the use of anticoagulants, the optimal dosing and duration of parenteral and oral therapy, the complications and cost-effectiveness of therapy, and the available data on medical and surgical prophylaxis.

Rules of evidence

At the time of its inception, the ACCP consensus conference was unique because of its strict adherence

E-mail address: tapso001@mc.duke.edu

to an evidence-based approach. As the first conference was organized, rules of evidence were developed and used to generate the consensus guidelines [2]. The grading of data was based on the rigor with which the clinical studies were performed. Data based on randomized trials with low false-positive and false-negative rates were classified as level I, whereas data based on less rigorously designed studies were given lower levels of classification. When randomized trials or prospective cohort studies were not available, the opinions of experienced clinicians were sought to guide recommendations. It was emphasized that such recommendations that were not derived from properly designed studies were subject to change as new knowledge was generated. The levels of evidence that accompanied each recommendation ranged from level I to level V; the level V designation was reserved for case series without controls. Ultimate recommendations were based on three grades (A through C), which depended on the level of evidence available.

Over the past 15 years, the approach to grading recommendations has been refined continuously. By 1995, evidence from meta-analyses was included, and

Table 1
Current approach to grades of recommendations for the American College of Chest Physicians consensus on antithrombotic therapy (2001)

Grade of recommendation	Clarity of risk/benefit	Methodologic strength of supporting evidence	Implications
1A	Clear	Randomized trials without important limitations	Strong recommendation; can apply to most patients in most circumstances without reservation
1B	Clear	Randomized trials with important limitations (inconsistent results, methodologic flaws)[a]	Strong recommendations, likely to apply to most patients
1C+	Clear	No randomized controlled trials, but randomized controlled trial results can be unequivocally extrapolated, or overwhelming evidence from observation studies	Strong recommendation; can apply to most patients in most circumstances
1C	Clear	Observation studies	Intermediate-strength recommendation; may change when stronger evidence available
2A	Unclear	Randomized trials without important limitations	Intermediate-strength recommendation; best action may differ depending on circumstances or patients' or societal values
2B	Unclear	Randomized trials with important limitations (inconsistent results, methodologic flaws)	Weak recommendation; alternative approaches likely to be better for some patients under some circumstances
2C	Unclear	Observation studies	Very weak recommendations; other alternatives may be equally reasonable

Because studies in categories B and C are flawed, it is likely that most recommendations in these classes will be level 2. The designation of grade 1 or 2 will depend on the magnitude and precision of the treatment effect, patients' risk of the target event being prevented, the nature of the benefit, the magnitude of the risk associated with implementation, variability in patient preferences, regional resources and health care delivery practices, and cost considerations. Inevitably, weighing these considerations involves subjective judgment.

[a] These situations include randomized controlled trials with lack of blinding and subjective outcomes in which the risk of bias in measurement of outcomes is high and with large loss to follow-up.

From Guyatt GH, Schunemann H, Cook D, et al. Grades of recommendation for antithrombotic agents. Chest 2001;119(Suppl):3S–7S; with slight truncation of footnotes and permission from the American College of Chest Physicians.

the precision of study results was considered as expressed in the confidence interval around the treatment effect [3]. Refinements in grading recommendations included a separation of the methodologic quality from the magnitude and precision of the treatment effect, the inclusion of recommendations not to treat, and consideration of the trade-off between the benefit of a particular therapy and its potential risk or cost.

In 1998, the grading system was further tailored by Guyatt and colleagues [4] to better emphasize the concept of a clinically important difference and to incorporate the benefit–risk ratio of a specific therapy into the grading system. The levels of evidence used for making recommendations were reduced from five to three based on a modified scale (A1-2, B1-2, and C1-2). This approach to grading the strength of recommendations separately rated the methodologic rigor and the trade-off between benefit and risk [5]. The three categories of methodologic strength included (A) a meta-analysis or a large randomized trial with consistent results, (B) randomized trials with inconsistent results, and (C) observational studies. The trade-off between benefits and risks was graded in two categories: (1) the trade-off was considered clear enough that most patients, despite differences in values, would make the same choice; or (2) the trade-off was not as clear, and an individual patient's values or preferences would likely lead to different choices. Recommendations ranged from very strong (A1: methods strong; benefit–risk clear) to very weak (C2: methods weak; benefit–risk questionable) [4].

In 2001, an additional change involved placing the emphasis (and the number) denoting the clarity of the risk–benefit trade-off first, followed by the letter

Table 2
Number of recommendations in each grading category for treatment of acute venous thromboembolism

Year[a]	Grade A	Grade B	Grade C
1986	2	0	3
1989	3	0	1
1992	3	0	1
1995	3	0	1
1998	6 (5 = A1, 1 = A2)	0	1 (C2)
2001	6 (All = 1A)	1 (1B)	6 (2 = 1C+, 4 = 1C)

The classification system modifications that evolved from 1986 to 2001 are described in the footnote for Table 1.

[a] The year denotes the year of publication of each American College of Chest Physicians consensus conference (see text).

Table 3
Number of recommendations in each grading category for prevention of acute venous thromboembolism

Year[a]	Grade A	Grade B	Grade C
1986	4	0	0
1989	4	0	0
1992	12	2	6
1995	13	3	6
1998	14 (11 = A1, 3 = A2)	4 (All = B1)	8 (5 = C1, 3 = C2)
2001	18 (14 = 1A, 4 = 2A)	6 (4 = 1B, 2 = 2B)	19 (5 = 1C+, 12 = 1C, 2 = 2C)

In 1998, the classification system was modified (see text). In 2001, the number denoting the clarity of the risk–benefit trade-off was placed first, followed by the letter indicating the methodologic quality of the underlying evidence. Grade A indicates the highest methodologic quality. Also in 2001, grade C recommendations were modified to include grade 1C+.

[a] The year denotes the year of publication of each American College of Chest Physicians consensus conference (see text).

indicating the methodologic quality of the underlying evidence (eg, 1A, 1B, 1C+, 1C, 2A) [6]. This method emphasized the initial importance of the risk–benefit judgment (Table 1). Grade C recommendations, derived from observational studies and from generalization from randomized trials in one group of patients to a different group, were modified to include grade 1C+. The addition of the 1C+ grade denoted the finding that generalization from randomized trials was secure, or that data from observational studies were overwhelmingly compelling. In 2001, the 1C+ grade was employed five times in the VTE prevention chapter and twice in the VTE therapy section. From 1986 to 2001, based on increasing available data from randomized clinical trials, the number of total recommendations made for therapeutic strategies for VTE increased. For VTE prophylaxis, the number of total recommendations increased tenfold, with those in the grade A category increasing from four to 43 (Tables 2, 3).

This grading system with its progressive modification has served as the foundation of the ACCP consensus for antithrombotic therapy and has provided an avenue through which clinicians have reached a unified stand in the prevention and treatment of thrombotic disorders. These recommendations have been offered not as irrefutable dogma but as guidelines, and "they should not be construed as dictates by the readers, including clinicians, third-party payers, institutional review committees, and courts" [6]. In general, it was agreed that progressively greater weight should be placed on these expert recommendations as they move from 2C to 1A.

The evolution of the statement: antithrombotic therapy for venous thromboembolic disease

The initial VTE therapy statement was developed by Hyers, Hull, and Weg [7]. At the time of this 1986 statement, several clinical studies had already influenced the treatment of VTE substantially. Heparin had been used to treat VTE for more than 2 decades when Barritt and Jordan performed their randomized trial involving 35 patients with symptoms of acute PE [8]. Their landmark study, which was published in 1960, revealed that intravenous heparin given together with an oral vitamin K antagonist reduced mortality and recurrence when compared with no anticoagulant therapy. Barritt and Jordan justified the inclusion of an untreated control, stating that physicians were reluctant to use anticoagulants to treat patients with suspected PE because of the perceived risk of bleeding. The performance of the study was criticized by some physicians because they considered it to be unethical [9].

Initial heparin therapy and long-term oral anticoagulation

The results of the study by Barritt and Jordan in patients with PE were extrapolated to DVT. For both conditions, the standard of care was heparin during hospitalization and a vitamin K antagonist after discharge from the hospital. Subsequently, the strong clinical perception that the initial use of heparin was important in the management of DVT was proven by the results of a randomized trial [10].

By 1989, several developments led to expanded antithrombotic recommendations. Nevertheless, for some indications, such as the unequivocal effectiveness of aspirin in acute myocardial infarction, the recommendations did not influence VTE therapy. Several clinical trials published in the mid to late 1980s led to a change in the grade C recommendation for heparin overlapping with warfarin to a grade A recommendation for 5 to 10 days of heparin with 4 to 5 days of heparin/warfarin overlap [11–13]. The minimum duration of therapy was 3 months. In 1992, increased available data, particularly for VTE prophylaxis, necessitated that the antithrombotic therapy section of the ACCP statement be split into separate treatment and prophylaxis sections.

For decades before the first ACCP conference, the optimal therapeutic range for laboratory control had been debated [14]. The international normalized ratio (INR) concept was developed, and the 1992 statement underscored its importance as the most appropriate method of monitoring warfarin therapy. The variability in thromboplastins translated into substantial variability in INR values for a given prothrombin time. Because thromboplastins as well as different batches of the same brand of thromboplastins could vary, calculation of the INR was important in patients treated with warfarin. The INR should be calculated based on the formula, INR = (observed prothrombin time ratio)^{ISI}, where *ISI* is the index of sensitivity for the thromboplastin reagent used [15]. The introduction of the INR and the recommendation for its use and acceptance were credited with reducing bleeding complications. Sensitive thromboplastins with an ISI less than 1.5 (preferably < 1.2) were recommended [16].

An important concept that evolved was weight-based heparin therapy. Although early studies suggested the importance of keeping the activated partial thromboplastin time (aPTT) above 1.5 times control [11,17], evidence suggested that heparin was underdosed [18]. Clinical trials suggested that the daily maintenance dose of heparin should be greater than 31,000 U (> 1300 U/hour) [12,19,20]. The basic tenet that recurrent thromboembolism was clearly associated with subtherapeutic heparin dosing, whereas a less certain relationship existed with supratherapeutic heparin and bleeding, supported the use of a weight-based dosing algorithm. In the 1992 statement, an algorithm was recommended for heparin dosing in an attempt to encourage adequate dosing [20]. Subsequent statements included a weight-based regimen example that recommended an initial bolus of 80 U/kg followed by 18 U/kg/hour. Weight-based heparin regimens were the optimal means by which one could keep the aPTT in a range that corresponded to a plasma heparin level of 0.2 to 0.4 U/mL [21–23].

Despite a tremendous amount of research culminating in satisfactory recommendations for the use of unfractionated heparin, limitations of heparin remained evident, including its limited bioavailability, the frequent requirement for intravenous administration, and the importance of frequent monitoring in the setting of therapy.

Low–molecular-weight heparin

In 1976, two groups reported that low–molecular-weight heparin (LMWH) fractions prepared from standard heparin had progressively less effect on the aPTT but still inhibited activated factor X [24,25].

The difference in the anticoagulant profile between LMWH and unfractionated heparin was subsequently elucidated. For the 1986 ACCP statement, inadequate data existed for any recommendations involving the use of LMWH. By 1992, several clinical trials comparing unfractionated heparin and LMWH for the treatment of established VTE had been conducted. Although the results of the studies suggested that subcutaneously delivered LMWHs were as safe and effective as intravenous unfractionated heparin, and that outpatient therapy could be feasible and cost-effective, no graded therapeutic recommendations were made. Nevertheless, graded recommendations were suggested for the prophylactic use of LMWH preparations [26].

By 1995, although the use of LMWH for the treatment of acute VTE was increasing, particularly in Europe, none of the preparations had been approved for use in the United States. No graded recommendations were made for the therapeutic use of LMWH in the 1995 ACCP consensus statement. By the time the 1998 statement was published, LMWHs were replacing heparin for many indications in Europe and were increasingly used in North America, especially in Canada. A grade A1 recommendation was made, indicating that substituting LMWH for standard heparin for the treatment of DVT and stable patients with PE was appropriate [27]. None of the studies were conducted in the United States. The same recommendations were made for LMWH and unfractionated heparin with regard to overlapping with warfarin. When the 2001 statement was published, based on the major benefits of convenient dosing and facilitation of outpatient treatment with LMWH, as well as the evidence suggesting slightly less recurrent VTE and a possible survival benefit in cancer, a grade 2B recommendation was made favoring LMWH over unfractionated heparin [28].

Outpatient therapy with LMWH has revolutionized the treatment of DVT. Two landmark trials (Canada and Europe) comparing inpatient intravenous unfractionated heparin and outpatient LMWH therapy were published in 1996, indicating that the latter approach was at least as safe and effective as inpatient heparin therapy [29,30]. This approach has become more prevalent, and most large hospitals in North America and Europe now treat at least some selected patients with established VTE in the outpatient setting. The cost–benefit of this approach has been confirmed based on the outpatient approach [31]. PE has been treated in the outpatient setting by selected groups with experience in this setting [32]. A significant number of patients with proximal DVT have concomitant silent PE; therefore, outpatient therapy intended for DVT is, in fact, often used for PE in this setting [33]. No specific recommendations for outpatient PE therapy have been made by the ACCP to date. There is continuing discussion with regard to the superiority of various LMWH preparations.

Duration of oral anticoagulation therapy

From the beginning, the ACCP recommendations have indicated that the duration of therapy should be tailored to the individual patient but within some general guidelines. In 1986, a grade A recommendation was made for 3 months of therapy with warfarin for patients with uncomplicated acute VTE. For patients with recurrent VTE or a continuing risk factor such as thrombophilia or cancer, indefinite treatment was recommended (grade C). Over the next 15 years, recommendations for the latter category of patients evolved very little, and, in 2001, a treatment duration of 12 months or longer was recommended for these patients (grade 1C). These recommendations remained grade C, because there were inadequate controlled trials of the duration of therapy for most acquired or hereditary conditions. More robust data became available for patients with idiopathic VTE, indicating that therapy for more than 6 months reduced the risk of recurrence [34–36]. For this setting, the recommendation was upgraded from grade A2 in 1998 to 1A in 2001.

The need for an additional recommendation became evident with regard to long-term anticoagulation. The substitution of LMWH or adjusted-dose unfractionated heparin for long-term therapy was deemed appropriate (grade 1A) in settings in which oral anticoagulation was inconvenient or contraindicated.

Thrombolytic therapy

The recommendations for thrombolytic therapy in patients with acute VTE have been hampered by inadequately powered clinical trials. Although it is clear that thrombolytic therapy results in more rapid clot lysis than when heparin is used alone, clinical trials have not been large enough to assess mortality benefit adequately. No mention was made of thrombolysis for acute DVT or PE in 1986 despite the large Urokinase in Pulmonary Embolism Trial conducted more than a decade prior [37].

From 1989 through 1995, thrombolytic therapy for acute VTE was reviewed in detail in the ACCP statements. Although appropriate regimens were outlined, there was continued emphasis that the use of these agents should be highly individualized. It was eventually stated that, in general, patients with massive PE and iliofemoral DVT were the best candidates, but, even in the 2001 statement, no graded recommendations were made. In contrast, several grade A recommendations were made for thrombolytic therapy in patients with acute myocardial infarction [38]. Recent studies have begun to explore means to select appropriate candidates for thrombolytic therapy other than patients with systemic hypotension, in whom lytic agents have been classically administered. A recent prospective, randomized, double-blind clinical trial suggests that patients with proven PE but without hypotension may require "escalation of therapy" less often when receiving tissue plasminogen activator with heparin versus heparin alone [39]; however, because there was no difference in mortality, the uncertainty persists.

Placement of an inferior vena cava filter

Definitive indications for the placement of an inferior vena cava filter have changed little despite the fact that they have been used clinically for nearly 30 years [40]. Although the use of these devices was recommended in the first ACCP statement in 1986 as the only acceptable alternative when anticoagulation was contraindicated, no graded recommendations were made until 2001. At that time, filter placement in the inferior vena cava was given a grade 1C+ recommendation for patients with, or at high risk for, proximal DVT when a contraindication or complication of anticoagulation therapy was present. Other indications, such as the recurrence of VTE despite therapeutic anticoagulation, were graded 1C. The use of temporary filters that can be placed for 2 weeks and then removed or left in place is increasing. These devices may be appropriate in certain patients with VTE and a transient increased risk of hemorrhage, but no clinical trials completed to date permit clear recommendations.

Therapy for isolated calf vein thrombosis

The recommendations for isolated calf DVT have remained consistent over the 15-year history of the ACCP consensus, with the basic theme being heparin followed by oral anticoagulation for 6 to 12 weeks or serial impedance plethysmography. In 2001, the specific recommendations were for this anticoagulation plan (grade 1A). If the latter could not be done, serial impedance plethysmography was recommended over 10 to 14 days for isolated calf thrombosis and a negative plethysmographic study (grade 1C) [41]. In reality, impedance plethysmography is rarely performed, and serial compression ultrasound would be a more likely study. In fact, any serial diagnostic study protocol is difficult unless patients are willing and able to return for follow-up.

The evolution of the statement: prevention of venous thromboembolism

Because of the large number of indications for VTE prophylaxis and the increasing number of clinical trials in all areas of VTE prevention, the ACCP consensus statement has evolved considerably since 1986. At that time, there was no separate statement on prevention. One paragraph in the section on antithrombotic therapy was dedicated to prophylaxis, followed by four recommendations and 34 references related to prophylaxis [7]. Only a general overview of the evolving recommendations is discussed herein.

In 1986, some evidence suggested the efficacy of prophylaxis in patients undergoing general surgery, orthopedic surgery, or surgery of the thorax, abdomen, or extremities, as well as in patients with myocardial infarction, respiratory failure, acute paraplegia, quadriplegia, and stroke. The specific recommendations were (1) low-dose heparin (5000 U every 12 hours) or intermittent pneumatic compression (IPC) for moderate-risk patients; (2) IPC for neurosurgery, major knee surgery, and urologic surgery; (3) adjusted-dose heparin or moderate-dose warfarin for elective hip surgery; and (4) moderate-dose warfarin for surgery for fractured hips. All of these recommendations were grade A but were inadequate to characterize all patient populations or clinical scenarios [7]. The advent of LMWH preparations dramatically changed the approach to VTE prevention. The preparations began to be included in recommendations in the ACCP statement in 1992, although they were not available in many countries at that time, including the United States.

Dextran

Other means of prophylaxis were less frequently recommended as the number of clinical trials with LMWHs increased. In 1986, dextran was considered an effective means of prophylaxis and was thought be superior to heparin in very high-risk patients [7,42]. Disadvantages of dextran included the need for intravenous administration with potential fluid overload and the rare occurrence of severe allergic reactions. It was stated that, "it is probably best used for prophylaxis of the high-risk patient when subcutaneous heparin is contraindicated." No graded recommendation was given for the use of this drug until the 1992 statement, when it was given a grade A recommendation for higher-risk general surgery patients prone to wound complications such as hematoma or wound infection. Its use in combination with IPC was also a grade A recommendation for very high-risk general surgery patients. It was emphasized that dextran should not be used routinely in patients undergoing total hip replacement or with hip fractures (grade A). Because of the potential for a lower risk of wound hematomas, dextran remained an option (in combination with another method) in very high-risk general surgery patients in 1992. Because of the substantial increase in clinical trials evaluating LMWH preparations, dextran was not given a graded recommendation for any indication after 1995. In the 2001 statement, it was specifically stated that dextran should not be used in total hip replacement [41].

Aspirin

Although it has been proven efficacious in other areas, aspirin is not appropriate for use as VTE prophylaxis. Nevertheless, the controversy surrounding its use merits discussion. For medical and surgical (including orthopedic surgery) patients, a meta-analysis revealed that, although aspirin was more effective than no prophylaxis [43], it was not as effective as other prophylaxis regimens in high-risk patients [44–46]. In addition, none of the clinical trials included in this meta-analysis used routine contrast venography as an outcome measure. The use of antiplatelet agents in patients sustaining hip fracture has been encouraged by the reduction in the incidence of stroke and myocardial infarction with aspirin, events that are common causes of death after hip fracture surgery [43,47,48]. The results of the Pulmonary Embolism Prevention trial published in 2001 provided the focus for substantial discussion with regard to the use of aspirin as prophylaxis. In this clinical trial, 13,356 patients with hip fracture from 148 hospitals in five countries were randomized to treatment with 160 mg of enteric-coated aspirin or placebo (started before surgery in 82%) continued for 35 days [49]. Prophylaxis with low-dose unfractionated heparin, LMWH, or elastic stockings was also used in 18%, 26%, and 30% of patients, respectively. Fatal PE and DVT were significantly reduced by the addition of aspirin (each with an absolute risk reduction of 0.4%), whereas fatal and nonfatal arterial events (myocardial infarction or stroke) and all-cause mortality were not. Wound-related bleeding and gastrointestinal bleeding and transfusions were slightly and significantly more common in patients receiving

aspirin. When compared with a placebo, for every 1000 patients with hip fracture given perioperative aspirin prophylaxis, it was expected that nine fewer VTE events (including four fewer fatal PEs) would occur. One would also expect six more fatal or nonfatal cardiac events with or without ten more episodes of gastrointestinal bleeding, six more episodes of bleeding requiring transfusion, or six more episodes of wound hemorrhage. These clinical trial results were carefully scrutinized by the ACCP task force on VTE prevention. Based on their analysis, the routine use of aspirin as thromboprophylaxis in patients with hip fracture was not recommended [41]. Similarly, among 4088 hip and knee arthroplasty patients randomized to treatment with aspirin or placebo (with or without other thromboprophylactic measures), there was no benefit associated with aspirin use in regard to the number of venous or arterial thromboembolic events [49]. Aspirin has not received a graded recommendation for any VTE prophylactic indication. In fact, a grade 2A recommendation against using aspirin in the setting of hip fracture surgery was made in 2001 [41].

Heparin and low–molecular-weight heparin

Most progress has been made with regard to prophylactic indications with LMWH preparations. The evolution of the prophylaxis recommendations for heparin and warfarin is not reviewed in detail herein. The LMWH preparations are being used increasingly. In 2001, unfractionated heparin and LMWH received grade A recommendations for general surgery indications. Even in 2001, a few grade 1A recommendations remained that favored unfractionated heparin over LMWH [41]. These indications included major gynecologic surgery for benign disease (twice-daily heparin [grade 1A] versus LMWH once daily or IPC [grade 1C+]) and extensive surgery for gynecologic malignancy (heparin three times daily [grade 1A] versus higher-dose LMWH or combination prophylaxis [grade C]). In orthopedic surgery, adjusted-dose heparin is considered acceptable (grade 2A) but is inconvenient, and LMWH is clearly favored.

The use of prophylactic LMWH first appeared as a graded ACCP recommendation in 1992. At that time, graded recommendations were available for LMWH in eight settings [26]. By 2001, this number had increased to 17 (Table 4). In addition to specific pharmacologic and mechanical recommendations for DVT prevention, the evaluation of prophylaxis duration is now being investigated. Clinical trials have suggested that prolonged prophylaxis (approximately

Table 4
Use of low molecular weight heparin preparations for venous thromboembolism prophylaxis: graded recommendations

Year[a]	Grade A	Grade B	Grade C
1986	0	0	0
1989	0	0	0
1992	4	1	3
1995	6	2	1
1998	12 (10 = A1, 2 = A2)	3 (All = B1)	2 (1 = C1, 1 = C2)
2001	11 (9 = 1A, 2= 2A)	3 (All = 1B)	5 (1 = 1C+, 4 = 1C)

The letter denotes the methodologic quality of the underlying evidence with grade A being the highest. The number denotes the clarity of the risk–benefit trade-off. In 2001, the order of the letter and number was reversed. Also, in 2001, grade C recommendations were modified to include grade 1C+.

[a] The year denotes the year of publication of each American College of Chest Physicians consensus conference (see text).

4 weeks) with LMWH is safe and effective in the setting of total hip replacement and abdominal/pelvic cancer surgery, reducing venographically demonstrated thrombosis [50,51]. A grade 2A recommendation was made in 2001 for extended prophylaxis with LMWH in major orthopedic surgery, whereas the data for cancer surgery were not available at the time the ACCP conference met for the statement published in 2001. Based on the favorable bioavailability, the apparent lower incidence of heparin-induced thrombocytopenia [52], convenience, and increasing data on LMWH, prophylactic indications should continue to increase for these agents.

Mechanical prophylaxis

Intermittent pneumatic compression devices have been used for VTE prevention for decades based on early and continuing efficacy data and safety [53–55]. These devices have been recommended at the grade A level since 1986 (and still are) for moderate-risk patients scheduled for general surgery or neurosurgery. In 2001, other recommendations were made for the indications of higher-risk general surgery (grade 1A), higher-risk general surgery with bleeding risk (1C), and very high-risk general surgery as part of a combination regimen (grade 1C) [41]. Additional recommendations included the use of IPC devices in gynecologic surgery for benign disease (1C+), in extensive gynecologic surgery for malignancy (in combination [grade 1C]), in major open urologic surgery (1B), as adjuvant prophylaxis in elective hip

replacement (2C), and in elective knee replacement (1B), trauma (1C), and acute spinal cord injury (if anticoagulants are contraindicated early after injury [grade 2B]). In only a few of these grade 1C surgical indications is an anticoagulant given a more favorable grading. IPC prophylaxis is deemed appropriate for intensive care unit patients at high risk for bleeding (combined with elastic stockings) until the bleeding risk decreases [41]. No graded recommendation has been made for IPC use in critically ill medical patients or any other group of medical patient.

Although elastic stockings reduce the incidence of DVT and supplement the protection offered by parenteral anticoagulants, inadequate data are available to assess their effect on the rates of proximal DVT and PE [56]. The use of elastic stockings was first recommended by the ACCP in 1992 [26]. At that time, a grade A recommendation was given for their use in moderate-risk patients scheduled for general surgery (but also for low-dose heparin and IPC). In addition, the recommendation for elastic stockings was graded A for intracranial neurosurgery, but only if used together with IPC. A grade 1C recommendation was offered for elastic stockings in the setting of myocardial infarction and in ischemic stroke and lower-extremity paralysis, but other grade A recommendations existed at that time for these clinical settings. Although elastic stockings were included as a grade A recommendation for some indications through 2001 (1A), these recommendations were made by comparing the efficacy of this modality with no prophylaxis [41].

Patients in many high-risk conditions have not been evaluated sufficiently to permit conclusive recommendations regarding the efficacy of elastic stockings. In some of the randomized trials, high-risk patients were specifically excluded [57,58]. Although further clinical trials would be needed to assess the effectiveness of this method in these patients, it would seem unlikely that such individuals would be deemed appropriate for randomization, at least, against parenteral anticoagulation. Combination therapy with other modalities may offer the most benefit.

Perceptions and impact of the American College of Chest Physicians statement

The ACCP initiative has primarily been a North American effort. By 1998, there were 54 individuals contributing from the United States, 18 from Canada, and eight from Europe. Of the seven individuals on the VTE treatment task force, two were European and one Canadian. Of the eight persons in the VTE prevention group, only one was Canadian, with the rest from the United States. During a discussion of the 1998 ACCP report in Paris on January 21, 1999, French clinicians expressed some divergent views from the ACCP 1998 statement [59]. In June 2000, a European view of this statement was published by a working group (including one ACCP member) with extensive experience in patient care and research in the field of VTE [59]. Each section of the ACCP statement was addressed. The hope was that a more global consensus could be reached. The European group worked to update the recommendations based on new literature.

With regard to the treatment of established VTE, there were no perceived fundamental disagreements. It was emphasized that European practice was probably a step ahead of the United States Food and Drug Administration with regard to PE being an accepted indication for LMWH. European physicians have several choices of coumarin derivatives, and phenprocoumon and acenocoumarol are prescribed in addition to warfarin. Differing views have persisted among European experts with regard to the optimal duration of therapy for certain types of patients. Some clinicians believe that patients with acquired or inherited thrombophilias who sustain a first episode of VTE not precipitated by an additional transient risk factor should be treated indefinitely, whereas others believe that more cost–benefit data should be made available before making a definitive recommendation. Recent studies have offered more data on duration, indicating that more prolonged therapy offers treatment benefit but at the risk of increased bleeding [34]. An additional European concern was the ACCP recommendation suggesting the consideration of prolonged therapy with LMWH when oral anticoagulation is inconvenient or contraindicated. The European opinion has been that inadequate information is available to justify a grade A1 recommendation.

Although the treatment of VTE in pregnant patients is recommended until term by the ACCP, the European group believes this may not always be necessary, and that the VTE severity, its evolution during therapy, and the circumstances surrounding its development should be considered when treatment duration is decided. With regard to thrombolytic therapy, the flexible opinion offered by the ACCP that the use of thrombolysis should be highly individualized is deemed appropriate by the European contingent. Despite some disagreements among the experts, there is considerable consensus with regard to most recommendations. In fact, European experts have been involved in many sections of the ACCP statement.

The European consensus statement published in 1992 outlined appropriate prophylactic and therapeutic strategies based on the available data at that time [60]. Subsequently, a larger international conference was held, involving some of the same participants. An international VTE prevention statement, published in 1997, was developed from this meeting and reviewed the available clinical data using an evidence-based approach in exhaustive detail. There were 85 participants from 27 countries, including 20 from North America and 15 from the United Kingdom, and representatives from the rest of Europe, South America, Asia, Africa, and Australia [61]. This statement also used five levels of evidence and three grades of recommendation derived from the 1995 ACCP consensus statement [3]. The notable similarities to the ACCP statement were a positive finding in light of the worldwide participation.

Unfortunately, in clinical practice, the implementation of these guidelines may be inconsistent and inadequate [62–64]. Adherence to the 1995 ACCP consensus guidelines was recently evaluated [63]. A retrospective review of medical records in ten teaching or community-based hospitals in the United States was conducted between January 1996 and February 1997. The medical charts of 1907 patients were randomly selected for review from the population of patients who underwent high-risk major abdominal surgery, total hip or knee replacement, or hip fracture repair. Prophylaxis was administered to 89.3% of patients overall, including 93.7% of patients in the three orthopedic groups and 75.2% of patients in the high-risk major abdominal surgery group. The use of grade A preventive methods was highest in the hip replacement group (84.3%) and lowest in the hip fracture repair group (45.2%). In the abdominal surgery group, the rate of use of grade A recommendations was 50.3%. The findings indicated that, despite the availability of carefully researched guidelines, preventive measures were underused. Other studies have also emphasized that VTE prophylaxis is underused.

Another study attempted to identify the obstacles hindering the success of VTE prevention [65]. At a hospital with more than 600 beds in Montreal, Canada, a chart review of all patients with objectively diagnosed VTE was conducted between October 1996 and October 1997. The goal was to determine whether the 1995 ACCP consensus guidelines were followed. There were 253 cases of VTE in 245 patients. It was concluded that two of three cases of VTE for which thromboprophylaxis had been indicated could have potentially been prevented if physicians had followed the ACCP guidelines. A total of

44 cases were thought to be potentially preventable. Among the preventable cases, the most common reason for inadequacy of prophylaxis was the omission of prophylaxis (47.7%), followed by an inadequate duration of prophylaxis (22.7%) and an incorrect type of prophylaxis (20.5%).) Thrombosis was deemed preventable in patients having nonorthopedic surgery, pneumonia, or stroke with lower-limb paralysis. Underlying VTE risk factors included recent immobility, active cancer, and obesity. The inadequacy of prophylaxis was most commonly related to the actual omission of prophylaxis. Possible reasons for omission are a primary focus on the underlying disease or surgical procedure, concern about bleeding risk, and a lack of awareness of consensus guidelines such as the ACCP statement. For patients undergoing neurosurgery or having fresh strokes, the perceived risk of bleeding may dissuade physicians from ordering anticoagulant prophylaxis despite the fact that there are sufficient data to refute such concerns [66–68]. Despite the publication of exhaustive consensus statements, VTE prophylaxis must be used more widely and appropriately.

The future

The ACCP consensus conference on antithrombotic therapy has evolved into the most comprehensive resource for evidence-based recommendations regarding the prevention and treatment of venous thromboembolic disease and other areas of antithrombotic therapy. Over the past 15 years, six statements have been published. During this interval, the method of grading has evolved while using the same basic principles. Undoubtedly, the single most important factor leading to new recommendations and influencing the prevention and management of VTE has been the introduction of LMWH preparations. These preparations have led to the practical implementation of outpatient therapy for DVT (with clear cost–benefit implications), more convenient inpatient therapy for patients and nursing personnel, and more effective and safe prophylaxis for high-risk clinical settings such as total joint replacement.

The seventh ACCP consensus, now in preparation, will offer additional insight into the comprehensive approach to VTE prevention and therapy. Areas that require additional research include the precise indications for thrombolytic therapy, the appropriate duration and intensity of long-term anticoagulation (particularly for patients with certain thrombophilic disorders), and the framing of precise recommendations for LMWHs in obese patients and those with renal insufficiency. The increased use of temporary filters in the inferior vena cava mandates the development of supporting therapeutic (and prophylactic) guidelines. Ongoing clinical trials will enhance the knowledge base. Certain therapies, such as thrombolytic agents, should continue to be individualized, allowing clinicians some degree of flexibility, even as graded recommendations evolve.

With regard to prevention, the duration of prophylaxis in certain patient populations needs clarification. In patients undergoing total hip replacement and cancer surgery, extending prophylaxis with LMWH has proven to reduce the incidence of VTE [50,51]. Clarification of the appropriate duration of prophylaxis in other surgical populations and in medical patients is needed. Although prophylaxis in medical settings (such as cancer patients, bed rest, heart failure, or severe lung disease) with low-dose unfractionated heparin or LMWH has been given a grade 1A recommendation, several questions remain. Are some LMWHs more effective or safer than others? How can medical patients be better risk stratified? What constitutes the level of reduced mobility that places a medical patient at risk? How does the baseline severity of an underlying condition such as congestive heart failure factor into the severity of an acute exacerbation or additional superimposed risk factor? Is unfractionated heparin, 5000 U every 12 hours, as effective as when it is administered every 8 hours? Is either regimen as effective as LMWH prophylaxis? How do new agents such as pure anti–factor Xa inhibitors compare? Should certain individuals receive prophylaxis before prolonged travel? These questions will be answered by ongoing and subsequent large prospective randomized trials. It is hoped that these studies will eventually emulate the clinical trials conducted in patients with acute myocardial infarction by being powered to determine mortality endpoints in addition to VTE occurrence rates, recurrence rates, and bleeding rates. The introduction of new anticoagulants is also likely to impact on subsequent consensus statements.

Perhaps the most important recommendation made in the VTE prevention section of the ACCP statements to date (and first appearing in 2001) is the statement that, "We recommend that every hospital develop a formal strategy that addresses the prevention of thromboembolic complications. This should generally be in the form of a written thromboprophylaxis policy." This approach employed with an optimal adherence to evidence-based guidelines and the option of flexibility to practice medicine effectively would seem to be an effective strategy for the future.

Acknowledgments

This article was reviewed by Jack Hirsh, MD, FCCP, Director of the Hamilton Civic Hospital Research Center, Hamilton, Ontario, Canada.

References

[1] ACCP/NHLBI National Conference on Antithrombotic Therapy. Chest 1986;89(Suppl):1S–106S.

[2] Sackett DL. Rules of evidence and clinical recommendations on the use of antithrombotic agents. Chest 1986;89(2 Suppl):2S–3S.

[3] Cook DJ, Guyatt GH, Laupacis A, et al. Clinical recommendations using levels of evidence for antithrombotic agents. Chest 1995;108(Suppl):227S–30S.

[4] Guyatt GH, Cook DJ, Sackett DL, et al. Grades of recommendations for antithrombotic agents. Chest 1998;114(Suppl):441S–4S.

[5] Guyatt GH, Sackett DL, Sinclair J, et al. Users' guide to the medical literature: IX. A method for grading health-care recommendations. JAMA 1995;274:1800–4.

[6] Guyatt GH, Schunemann H, Cook D, et al. Grades of recommendation for antithrombotic agents. Chest 2001;119(Suppl):3S–7S.

[7] Hyers TM, Hull RD, Weg JG. Antithrombotic therapy for venous thromboembolic disease. Chest 1986;89(Suppl):26S–35S.

[8] Barritt DW, Jordan SC. Anticoagulant drugs in the treatment of pulmonary embolism: a controlled trial. Lancet 1960;1:1309–12.

[9] Hunter RB, Walker W. Anticoagulant drugs in the treatment of pulmonary embolism [letter]. Lancet 1960;2:206.

[10] Brandjes DP, Heijboer H, Buller HR, et al. Acenocoumarol and heparin compared with acenocoumarol alone in the initial treatment of proximal-vein thrombosis. N Engl J Med 1992;327:1485–9.

[11] Hull RD, Raskob GE, Hirsh J, et al. Continuous intravenous heparin compared with intermittent subcutaneous heparin in the initial treatment of proximal-vein thrombosis. N Engl J Med 1986;315:1109–14.

[12] Gallus A, Jackaman J, Tillett J, et al. Safety and efficacy of warfarin started early after submassive venous thrombosis or pulmonary embolism. Lancet 1986;2:1293–6.

[13] Holmgren K, Andersson G, Fagrell B, et al. One month versus six month therapy with oral anticoagulants after symptomatic deep vein thrombosis. Acta Med Scand 1985;218:279–84.

[14] Enger E, Boysen S. Long-term anticoagulant therapy in patients with cerebral infarction. Acta Med Scand 1965;178(Suppl):7–55.

[15] Hirsh J, Dalen JE, Deykin D, Poller L. Oral anticoagulants: mechanism of clinical action, clinical effec-

tiveness, and optimal therapeutic range. Chest 1992; 102(Suppl):312S–26S.

[16] Dalen JE, Hirsh J, Deykin D, et al. Oral anticoagulants: mechanism of clinical action, clinical effectiveness, and optimal therapeutic range. Chest 1995;108(Suppl): 231S–46S.

[17] Basu D, Gallus A, Hirsh J, et al. A prospective study of the value of monitoring heparin treatment with the activated partial thromboplastin time. N Engl J Med 1972;287:325–7.

[18] Wheeler AP, Jaquiss RD, Newman JH. Physician practices in the treatment of venous thromboembolism. Arch Intern Med 1988;148:1321–5.

[19] Hull RD, Raskob GE, Rosenbloom D, et al. Heparin for 5 days as compared with 10 days in the initial treatment of proximal venous thrombosis. N Engl J Med 1990;322:1260–4.

[20] Hull RD, Raskob GE, Lemaire J, et al. Optimal therapeutic level of heparin therapy in patients with venous thrombosis. Arch Intern Med 1992;152:1589–95.

[21] Brill-Edwards P, Ginsberg JS, Johnston M, et al. Establishing a therapeutic range for heparin therapy. Ann Intern Med 1993;119:104–9.

[22] Cruickshank MK, Levine MN, Hirsh J, et al. A standard heparin nomogram for the management of heparin therapy. Arch Intern Med 1991;151:333–7.

[23] Raschke RA, Gollihare B, Peirce JC. The effectiveness of implementing the weight-based heparin nomogram as a practice guideline. Arch Intern Med 1996;156:1645–9.

[24] Johnson EA, Kirkwood TBL, Stirling Y, et al. Four heparin preparations: anti-Xa potentiating effect of heparin after subcutaneous heparin after subcutaneous injection. Thromb Haemost 1976;35:586–91.

[25] Andersson LO, Barrowcliffe TW, Holmer E, et al. Anticoagulant properties of heparin fractionated by affinity chromatography on matrix-bound antithrombin III and by gel filtration. Thromb Res 1976;9:575–83.

[26] Clagett GP, Salzman EW, Wheeler HB, et al. Prevention of venous thromboembolism. Chest 1992;102(Suppl): 391S–407S.

[27] Hyers TM, Agnelli G, Hull RD, et al. Antithrombotic therapy for venous thromboembolic disease. Chest 1998;114(Suppl):561S–78S.

[28] Hyers TM, Agnelli G, Hull RD, et al. Antithrombotic therapy for venous thromboembolic disease. Chest 2001;119(Suppl):176S–93S.

[29] Levine M, Jent M, Hirsh J, et al. A comparison of low-molecular-weight heparin administered primarily at home with unfractionated heparin administered in the hospital for proximal deep-vein thrombosis. N Engl J Med 1996;334:677–81.

[30] Koopman MMW, Prandoni P, Piovella F, et al. Treatment of venous thrombosis with intravenous unfractionated heparin administered in the hospital as compared with subcutaneous low-molecular-weight heparin administered at home. N Engl J Med 1996; 334:682–7.

[31] Gould MK, Dembitzer AD, Sanders GD, et al. Low

molecular weight heparins compared with unfraction-ated heparin for treatment of acute deep venous thrombosis: A cost-effectiveness analysis. Ann Intern Med 1999;130:789–99.

[32] Wells PS, Kovacs MJ, Bormanis J, et al. Expanding eligibility for outpatient treatment of deep venous thrombosis and pulmonary embolism with low-molecular weight heparin: a comparison of patient self-injection with homecare injection. Arch Intern Med 1998; 158:1809–12.

[33] Meignan M, Rosso J, Gauthier H, et al. Systematic lung scans reveal a high frequency of silent pulmonary embolism in patients with proximal deep venous thrombosis. Arch Intern Med 2000;160:159–64.

[34] Schulman S, Granqvist S, Holmstrom M, et al. The duration of oral anticoagulant therapy after a second episode of venous thromboembolism. N Engl J Med 1997;336:393–8.

[35] Schulman S, Rhedin A-S, Lindmaker P, et al. A comparison of six weeks with six months of oral anticoagulant therapy after a first episode of idiopathic venous thromboembolism. N Engl J Med 1995;332: 1661–5.

[36] Kearon C, Gent M, Hirsh J, et al. Extended anticoagulation prevented recurrence after a first episode of idiopathic venous thromboembolism. N Engl J Med 1999; 340:901–7.

[37] The Urokinase Pulmonary Embolism Trial: a national cooperative study. Circulation 1973;47(Suppl):1–100.

[38] Ohman EM, Harrington RA, Cannon CP, et al. Intravenous thrombolysis in acute myocardial infarction. Chest 2001;119(Suppl):253S–77S.

[39] Konstantinides S, Geibel A, Heusel G, Heinrich F, Kasper W. Heparin plus alteplase compared with heparin alone in patients with submassive pulmonary embolism. N Engl J Med 2002;347:1143–50.

[40] Greenfield LJ, Michna BA. Twelve year clinical experience with the Greenfield vena cava filter. Surgery 1988;104:706–12.

[41] Geerts WH, Heit JA, Clagett GP, et al. Prevention of venous thromboembolism. Chest 2001;119(Suppl): 132S–75S.

[42] Kline A, Hughes LE, Campbell H, et al. Dextran 70 in prophylaxis of thromboembolic disease after surgery: a clinically oriented randomized, double-blind trial. BMJ 1975;2:109–12.

[43] Antiplatelet Trialists' Collaboration: Collaborative overview of randomised trials of antiplatelet therapy. III. Reduction in venous thrombosis and pulmonary embolism by antiplatelet prophylaxis among surgical and medical patients. BMJ 1994;308:235–46.

[44] Powers PJ, Gent M, Jay RM, et al. A randomized trial of less intense postoperative warfarin or aspirin therapy in the prevention of VTE after surgery for fractured hip. Arch Intern Med 1989;149:771–4.

[45] Graor RA, Stewart JH, Lotke PA, et al. RD heparin (ardeparin sodium) vs aspirin to prevent deep venous thrombosis after hip or knee replacement surgery. Chest 1992;102:118S.

[46] Lotke PA, Palevsky H, Keenan AM, et al. Aspirin and warfarin for thromboembolic disease after total joint arthroplasty. Clin Orthop 1996;324:251–8.

[47] Perez JV, Warwick DJ, Case CP, et al. Death after proximal femoral fracture: an autopsy study. Injury 1995;26:237–40.

[48] MacMahon S, Rodgers A, Collins R, et al. Antiplatelet therapy to prevent thrombosis after hip fracture: rationale for a randomised trial. J Bone Joint Surg 1994;76: 521–4.

[49] Pulmonary Embolism Prevention (PEP) Trial Collaborative Group (2000). Prevention of pulmonary embolism and deep vein thrombosis with low dose aspirin: Pulmonary Embolism Prevention (PEP) trial. Lancet 2000;355:1295–302.

[50] Comp PC, Spiro TE, Friedman RJ, et al. Prolonged enoxaparin therapy to prevent venous thromboembolism after primary hip or knee replacement. J Bone J Surg 2001;83A:336–45.

[51] Bergqvist D, Agnelli G, Cohen AT, et al. Duration of prophylaxis against venous thromboembolism with enoxaparin after surgery for cancer. N Engl J Med 2002;346:975–80.

[52] Warkentin TE, Levine MN, Hirsh J, et al. Heparin-induced thrombocytopenia (HIT) in patients treated with low molecular weight heparin or unfractionated heparin. N Engl J Med 1995;332:1330–5.

[53] Butson ARC. Intermittent pneumatic calf compression for prevention of deep venous thrombosis in general abdominal surgery. Am J Surg 1981;142:525–7.

[54] Hills NH, Pflug JJ, Jeyasingh K, et al. Prevention of deep vein thrombosis by intermittent pneumatic compression of the calf. BMJ 1972;1:131–5.

[55] Moser G, Krahenbuhl B, Barroussel R, et al. Mechanical versus pharmacologic prevention of deep venous thrombosis. Surg Gynecol Obstet 1981;152: 448–50.

[56] Wells PS, Lensing AWA, Hirsh J. Graduated compression stockings in the prevention of postoperative VTE: a meta-analysis. Arch Intern Med 1994;154:67–72.

[57] Turner GM, Cole SE, Brooks JH. The efficacy of graduated compression stockings in the prevention of deep vein thrombosis after major gynaecological surgery. Br J Obstet Gynaecol 1984;91:588–91.

[58] Allan A, Williams JT, Bolton JP, et al. The use of graduated compression stockings in the prevention of postoperative deep vein thrombosis. Br J Surg 1983;70:172–4.

[59] Verstraete M, Prentice CRM, Samama M, et al. A European view on the North American Fifth Consensus on Antithrombotic Therapy. Chest 2000;117: 1755–70.

[60] Nicolaides AN. Prevention of venous thromboembolism: European consensus statement. International Angiology 1992;11:151–9.

[61] Nicolaides AN, Berqvist D, Hull RD. Prevention of venous thromboembolism: International consensus statement. International Angiology 1997;16:1–38.

[62] Goldhaber SZ, Dunn K, MacDougall RC. New onset

of venous thromboembolism among hospitalized patients at Brigham and Women's Hospital is caused more often by prophylaxis failure than by withholding treatment. Chest 2000;118:1680–4.

[63] Stratton MA, Anderson FA, Bussey HI, et al. Prevention of venous thromboembolism: adherence to the 1995 American College of Chest Physicians consensus guidelines for surgical patients. Arch Intern Med 2000;160:4–40.

[64] Bratzler DW, Raskob GE, Murray CK, et al. Underuse of venous thromboembolism prophylaxis for general surgery patients: physicians practices in the community hospital setting. Arch Intern Med 1998;158:1909–12.

[65] Arnold DM, Kahn SR, Shrier I. Missed opportunities

for prevention of venous thromboembolism: an evaluation of the use of thromboprophylaxis guidelines. Chest 2001;120:1964–71.

[66] Wen DY, Hall WA. Complications of subcutaneous low-dose heparin therapy in neurosurgical patients. Surg Neurol 1998;50:521–5.

[67] Macdonald RL, Amidei C, Lin G, et al. Safety of perioperative subcutaneous heparin for prophylaxis of VTE in patients undergoing craniotomy. Neurosurgery 1999;45:245–52.

[68] McCarthy ST, Turner J. Low-dose subcutaneous heparin in the prevention of deep-vein thrombosis and pulmonary emboli following acute stroke. Age Ageing 1986;15:84–8.

CLINICS
IN CHEST
MEDICINE

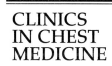

Clin Chest Med 24 (2003) 153–170

Clinical and laboratory evaluation of thrombophilia

Stephanie L. Perry, MD[a,b], Thomas L. Ortel, MD, PhD[b,c,*]

[a]*Division of Medical Oncology, Duke University Medical Center, Trent Drive, Durham, NC 27710, USA*
[b]*Division of Hematology, Duke University Medical Center, Trent Drive, Durham, NC 27710, USA*
[c]*Clinical Coagulation and Platelet Antibody Laboratories, Duke University Medical Center, Research Drive, Durham, NC 27710, USA*

Thrombophilia is defined as a predisposition toward thrombotic events, specifically, venous thrombotic events [1]. In addition to inherited and acquired disorders of hemostasis, environmental factors can place patients at increased risk for a first-time and recurrent venous thrombosis. This review begins with an overview of the more frequent causes of thrombophilia and then discusses how to proceed with a hypercoagulable work-up of patients with venous thrombosis. Considerations include which patients to screen for inherited disorders, what tests to include in the screening, when to perform the tests, and the impact of the results on the clinical management of the patient.

Overview of causes of thrombophilia

Inherited thrombophilia

The disorders listed in Table 1 account for the majority of patients with venous thrombosis and inherited thrombophilia. The identification of one or

This work was supported by a Midcareer Investigator Award in Patient-Oriented Research (K24 AI01603) from the NIH (TLO), a cooperative agreement (UR6/CCU420565-01) with the Hematologic Diseases Branch, Centers for Disease Control and Prevention (TLO), and by a Blood Banking and Related Areas Training Grant (T32-HL07057-25) from the NIH (SLP).

* Corresponding author. Division of Hematology, Duke University Medical Center, Box 3422, Stead Building, Room 0563, Durham, NC 27710.

E-mail address: ortel001@mc.duke.edu (T.L. Ortel).

more of these disorders may have an impact on therapeutic recommendations.

Activated protein C resistance/factor V Leiden

Activated protein C (APC) resistance is one of the most common inherited disorders of thrombophilia, accounting for almost 20% of cases of venous thrombosis (Table 1) [2]. The prevalence of factor V Leiden, the primary cause of APC resistance, is highest in European populations at approximately 2% to 7%, and much lower in Africans, Asians, and non-Caucasian Americans [3,4]. In the Leiden Thrombophilia Study (case-matched, controlled study), the estimated relative risk (RR) for venous thrombosis was 6 to 8 for heterozygotes [2] and 80 for homozygotes for factor V Leiden [5].

In 95% of cases, APC resistance is caused by a point mutation in the factor V gene, resulting in the substitution of a G for an A at position 506 [6,7]. This missense mutation changes one of three APC cleavage sites in the heavy chain of factor Va, leading to decreased proteolytic inactivation of factor Va and, consequently, increased thrombin generation [8,9]. Approximately 5% of all patients with APC resistance do not have factor V Leiden. These patients also have an increased risk for venous thrombosis, with a fourfold difference in risk between the highest and lowest quartiles of APC resistance [10].

Clinical data obtained from the Physicians' Health Study found that, during a mean follow-up period of 8.6 years, the RR for venous thromboembolism in healthy male subjects (aged 40–84 years) with factor V Leiden was 2.7 (confidence interval [CI], 1.3–5.6), which increased to 3.5 (CI, 1.5–8.4) if the event was spontaneous [11]. The risk for venous thrombosis was

The abnormal fibrinogens identified in these patients have demonstrated functional defects in fibrinogen conversion to fibrin and fibrin assembly [36]. Two mechanisms that have been proposed to explain the increased thrombotic risk owing to these malfunctioning fibrinogens include (1) defective thrombin binding to abnormal fibrin, leading to increased thrombin levels; and (2) defective stimulation of tissue plasminogen activator (tPA)–mediated fibrinolysis by the abnormal fibrin [37].

Slightly more than half (53%) of patients with dysfibrinogenemia are asymptomatic, 26% present with hemorrhage only, and 21% present with thrombosis with or without hemorrhage [35]. For patients with thrombosis, convincing evidence linking the abnormal fibrinogen with the clinical phenotype exists for only a limited number of individuals [37].

Hyperhomocysteinemia

The prevalence of mild-to-moderate elevations in plasma homocysteine levels among patients with venous thromboembolism is approximately 10% (see Table 1) [38]. Mild elevations in homocysteine are present in approximately 5% of normal adults [39].

Mild-to-moderate hyperhomocysteinemia is most frequently caused by gene defects in two enzymes involved in homocysteine metabolism. Homocysteine is the reduced form of methionine and undergoes intracellular metabolism through remethylation to methionine or transsulfuration to cystathione. The two enzymes involved are methylenetetrahydrofolate reductase (MTHFR) and cystathionine β-synthase (CBS), respectively. Slight elevations in homocysteine occur with heterozygous CBS deficiency, whereas higher homocysteine levels have been attributed to homozygosity for a thermolabile variant of the MTHFR gene (owing to a C to T substitution at position 677). The thermolabile mutation in MTHFR has a frequency of 5% to 12% in the Caucasian population and 1.4% in African Americans [40]. In contrast, heterozygous CBS deficiency is much less common, with a frequency of about 1 in 200 [41].

Elevated homocysteine levels have been shown to increase thrombin formation by several mechanisms, including enhancing factor XII and factor V activity, inhibiting thrombomodulin expression and protein C activation, increasing tissue factor expression, and decreasing the expression of heparan sulfate by the endothelium [42].

In a series of 67 patients with hyperhomocysteinemia and venous thrombotic events, 64% had DVT with or without pulmonary embolus, 24% had superficial venous thrombosis, and 12% had cerebral or mesenteric vein thrombosis [34]. In the Leiden Thrombophilia Study, the risk of an initial DVT was 2.5-fold higher for patients with elevated homocysteine levels above the 95th percentile [38]. Based on a meta-analysis of nine case–control studies, the pooled odds ratio for venous thromboembolism for patients with an elevated homocysteine level (above the 95th percentile) was 2.95 [43]. In a case–control study involving Taiwanese Chinese patients, the adjusted odds ratio was slightly higher (6.5) [44].

Elevated factor VIII

The prevalence of persistently elevated factor VIII levels is 25% among patients with venous thrombosis versus 11% in healthy control subjects (see Table 1) [45]. Several investigators have reported on a relationship between ABO blood type and factor VIII levels [46], and factor VIII is an acute phase reactant. The increase in factor VIII levels in patients with venous thromboembolism is persistent and independent of the acute phase response [47].

Factor VIII is a procofactor that accelerates the activation of factor X by factor IXa. The pathogenesis of elevated factor VIII levels and venous thrombosis is unclear. One possible mechanism is that elevated factor VIII levels increase the rate of thrombin formation. Another possible mechanism whereby elevated factor VIII levels could lead to an increased risk of thrombosis is by causing an acquired resistance to APC [48].

Elevated factor VIII concentrations (>150 IU/dL) were found to be an independent risk factor for venous thrombosis in the Leiden Thrombophilia Study, with an adjusted RR of 4.8 [45]. In a case–control study, familial clustering of elevated factor VIII levels was found among patients who had sustained a venous thrombotic event. The median age of the patient at the first thrombotic event was 41 years and ranged from 17 to 67 years. Of the 17 patients evaluated, clinical events included DVT in 16 patients, pulmonary embolus in 2 patients, DVT and pulmonary embolus in 2 patients, and inferior vena cava thrombosis in 1 patient. The event was spontaneous in 8 of the 17 patients (47%) [49].

Other causes of inherited thrombophilia

The thrombophilic disorders listed in Table 2 are also inherited, but their impact on therapeutic recommendations is less clear, and, in some cases, they are so uncommon that routine testing is impractical. These disorders are grouped into polymorphic changes, rare mutations and disorders, and quantitative abnormalities resulting in an increased thrombotic risk.

Table 2
Other causes of inherited thrombophilia

Disorder	Reference
Polymorphic changes	
Factor V HR2 haplotype	53,54
Rare mutations and disorders	
Homozygous homocystinuria	56
Thrombomodulin mutations	57
Reduced or defective plasminogen	59
Tissue plasminogen activator abnormalities	60
Heparin cofactor II deficiency	61
Quantitative coagulation factor and plasma	
protein abnormalities	
Elevated factor IX level	63
Elevated factor XI level	64
Factor XII deficiency	65
Elevated plasminogen activator inhibitor-1	66
Thrombin-activatable fibrinolysis	67
inhibitor deficiency	
Elevated lipoprotein (a) level	68,69

Polymorphic changes

Factor V HR2 genotype.   The HR2 allele of factor V encodes for several linked polymorphisms in the factor V gene that are associated with a slight decrease in the factor V level and decreased cofactor activity in the inactivation of factor VIIIa by APC [50,51]. The frequency of the haplotype in normal subjects (from Italy, India, and Somalia) is approximately 8% to 10% [52]. It has been reported to contribute to APC resistance in functional assays [52].

In a retrospective multicenter cohort study, there was no increased risk of venous thromboembolism for patients with the HR2 haplotype alone or in combination with deficiencies of ATIII, protein C, or protein S, or with the prothrombin gene mutation [53]. In contrast, patients heterozygous for factor V Leiden and HR2 had an increased RR for venous thromboembolism of 10.9 (CI, 2.9–40.6) compared with 4.2 (CI, 1.6–11.3) for patients with factor V Leiden alone [53]. Similarly, the Longitudinal Investigation of Thromboembolism Etiology (LITE) study found that the factor V HR2 haplotype alone did not increase the risk of venous thromboembolism, but patients with double heterozygosity for HR2 and factor V Leiden had an increased risk for idiopathic venous thromboembolism (odds ratio, 16.3; 95% CI, 1.7–159) [54].

Rare mutations and disorders

Homocystinuria.   A profound elevation in homocysteine levels owing to homozygous CBS deficiency is a rare cause of severe hyperhomocysteinemia or homocystinuria, with an estimated overall frequency of 1 in 344,000 worldwide [55]. A less common cause of homocystinuria is related to homozygous MTHFR deficiency. Clinical manifestations in these patients include early-onset venous and arterial thromboembolic events, ocular and skeletal abnormalities, and mental retardation. In untreated CBS deficiency, 50% of patients had thromboembolic events by age 30 years [56].

Thrombomodulin mutations.   Thrombomodulin is an endothelial cell membrane protein receptor for thrombin. Thrombin loses its procoagulant activity and acquires an increased ability to activate protein C when bound to thrombomodulin [22]. Point mutations in the thrombomodulin gene have been identified in several patients with venous thrombosis [57]. In the Paris Thrombosis Study (case–control study), there was no association between thrombosis and three of these mutations, although one was associated with varicose veins [58].

Plasminogen deficiency.   Plasminogen, a component of the fibrinolytic system, is converted to plasmin by tPA, urokinase, or both to digest fibrin clots. Several hundred cases of plasminogen deficiency have been described, in most cases associated with either a thromboembolic event or ligneous conjunctivitis. In a retrospective study, the prevalence of thrombotic events among patients from 20 kindreds with plasminogen deficiency was 23.6% [59]. Among healthy subjects, the prevalence of plasminogen deficiency is estimated at 1 in 250 [27], suggesting that many of these individuals are asymptomatic.

Tissue plasminogen activator abnormalities.   Tissue plasminogen activator activates plasminogen to plasmin. In one family with venous thrombosis, it was suggested that an imbalance between tPA and its inhibitor, plasminogen activator inhibitor-1 (PAI-1), resulted in a fibrinolytic disorder and increased thrombotic risk [60]. Several polymorphisms have been identified within the tPA gene locus, but none have been associated with an increased thrombotic risk [22].

Heparin cofactor II deficiency.   Heparin cofactor II specifically inhibits thrombin in the presence of heparin or dermatan sulfate. In one family, two members with reduced levels of heparin cofactor II had cerebrovascular events, and one had DVT in pregnancy [61]. Another study screened a cohort of 305 patients who had sustained a venous thromboembolism before 45 years of age and identified two unrelated patients with decreased levels of heparin cofactor II (0.65%) [62]. One patient had an upper extremity DVT and superficial venous thrombosis by age 28 years, and another sustained an acute cerebrovascular event at age 28 years and a DVT at age 42 years. Both patients had additional disorders; one was heterozygous for factor V Leiden and one for type I protein C deficiency [62].

Quantitative coagulation factor and plasma protein abnormalities

Elevated factor IX. Activated factor IX converts factor X to factor Xa in the presence of factor VIIIa, calcium ions, and a membrane surface. In the Leiden Thrombophilia Study, patients were screened for elevated factor IX levels using the 90th percentile as the cutoff [63]. After excluding for known inherited thrombophilias, the overall odds ratio for venous thrombosis and elevated factor IX levels was 2.5 (95% CI, 1.6–4.3). A dose–response relation was observed; for factor IX levels greater than 150 IU/dL, the adjusted odds ratio was 4.8 (95% CI, 2.3–10.1) [63].

Elevated factor XI. Activated factor XI converts factor IX to factor IXa. In the Leiden Thrombophilia Study, the adjusted odds ratio for DVT in patients with factor XI levels above the 90th percentile when compared with patients with factor XI levels less than or equal to the 90th percentile was 2.2 (95% CI, 1.5–3.2) [64]. A dose–response relationship was observed between the factor XI level and the risk for venous thrombosis, but the risk was not affected by other inheritable thrombophilias or the use of oral contraceptives [64].

Factor XII deficiency. Factor XII activates factor XI and is also involved in activation of the fibrinolytic pathway. Several reports have described patients with factor XII deficiency and venous thromboembolic events [65], but a causal relationship has not been established.

Elevated plasminogen activator inhibitor-1. Plasminogen activator inhibitor-1 regulates the activity of tPA, and elevated PAI-1 levels are the most common cause of impaired fibrinolytic function. One polymorphism of the PAI-1 gene characterized by a single G deletion/insertion variation (4G or 5G) increases the concentration and activity of the inhibitor. In a case–control study of patients with first episode DVT and no other thrombotic risk identified, the prevalence of elevated PAI-1 was higher in patients who were carriers of the 4G allele. The

prevalence was 57.9% in 4G/4G patients and 55.3% in 4G/5G patients compared with 28.6% in 5G/5G patients [66]. Among patients with DVT, the prevalence of reduced fibrinolytic activity owing to elevated PAI-1 was 45.7% [66].

Elevated thrombin-activatable fibrinolysis inhibitor. Thrombin-activatable fibrinolysis inhibitor (TAFI) is a protein that, when activated by thrombin, suppresses fibrinolysis. In the Leiden Thrombophilia Study, TAFI levels above the 90th percentile increased the risk for venous thrombosis by 1.7 (95% CI, 1.1–2.5) when compared with levels below the 90th percentile. The prevalence of elevated TAFI levels was 9% among healthy controls versus 14% in patients with first episode DVT [67].

Elevated lipoprotein(a) levels. Lipoprotein (a) interferes with fibrinolysis by competing with plasminogen for binding to fibrin. In a multicenter study, the risk of venous thrombosis was 3.2 (95% CI, 1.9–5.3) for patients with lipoprotein (a) levels greater than 30 mg/dL when compared with levels below this cutoff. A dose–response effect was noted. Patients who were also positive for factor V Leiden and had elevated lipoprotein (a) levels had an odds ratio for venous thrombosis of 9.8 (95% CI, 2.4–40.7). The prevalence of elevated levels in healthy controls was 7% [68]. In a case–control study of children, the risk of venous thromboembolism for children with lipoprotein (a) levels greater than 30 mg/dL was 7.2 (95% CI, 3.7–14.5) [69].

Acquired thrombophilia

In addition to inherited prothrombotic states, a variety of acquired conditions can modulate an individual's risk for thrombosis. These acquired thrombophilic risk factors include medical conditions such as malignancy and inflammatory bowel disease, therapeutic agents, and environmental factors such as travel and trauma (Table 3).

Malignancy

Malignancies, especially adenocarcinomas, brain tumors, and myeloproliferative disorders, are associated with thrombotic complications [70]. In a case-controlled population study, the prevalence of malignancy was 11% for patients with DVT compared with 7.5% for age-matched individuals without thrombosis after approximately 5 years of follow-up [71]. In a prospective study, 3% of patients with spontaneous venous thrombosis were diagnosed with malignancy at presentation compared with none of the patients

Table 3
Acquired causes of venous thromboembolism

Causes	Reference
Malignancy	70
Paroxysmal nocturnal hemoglobinuria	73
Nephrotic syndrome	74,75
Inflamatory bowel disease	76
Antiphospholipid antibodies	82
Beçhet's syndrome	87
Systemic lupus erythematous	89
Pregnancy/postpartum	93
Travel	100
Trauma	99
Surgery	98
Therapy related	
Hormonal agents	
Oral contraceptives	102
Hormone replacement	109
Tamoxifen/raloxifene	110,111
Chemotherapy/thalidomide	70,112
Heparin-induced thrombocytopenia	113
Obesity	117,118
Hypertension	117
Smoking	117,118

with secondary causes of thrombosis. After 2 years, the risk for a malignancy was 2.3 (95% CI, 1.0–5.2) for patients with spontaneous versus secondary venous thrombosis [72]. Clinically, patients with malignancies may present with less common thrombotic manifestations, including migratory thrombophlebitis, nonbacterial thrombotic endocarditis, or portal or hepatic vein thrombosis.

The pathogenesis of developing thrombotic events may be caused by tumor cell activation of tissue factor directly through interactions with factor VIIa or indirectly by stimulating mononuclear cells. Other prothrombotic mechanisms include endothelial cell activation by tumor cells, quantitative and qualitative platelet defects, including thrombocytosis [70], and venous stasis from immobility, venous obstruction, or increased blood viscosity.

Paroxysmal nocturnal hemoglobinuria

Paroxysmal nocturnal hemoglobinuria is an acquired clonal disorder of hematopoietic stem cells. In a cohort study of 220 patients with the condition, the incidence of venous thrombosis was 28%, and thrombosis was the most significant risk factor for poor survival [73]. Patients presented with Budd-Chiari syndrome (44%), central nervous system thrombosis (29%), DVT (29%), and other sites of thrombosis (8%). The median age at presentation was 33 years [73].

Nephrotic syndrome

Patients with nephrotic syndrome have an increased tendency to experience venous thromboembolism, with an estimated incidence ranging from 10% to 40%. Thrombotic complications involve the superficial veins, veins of the lower extremity and pelvis, inferior vena cava, and, most commonly, the renal vein [74]. The point prevalence of renal vein thrombosis was 48% in one series of patients with nephrotic syndrome [75].

The pathogenesis of thromboembolic complications in nephrotic syndrome is thought to involve two mechanisms. First, glomerular hyperpermeability results in renal degradation and urinary loss of proteins such as ATIII, free protein S, plasminogen, α_2-antiplasmin, and albumin. Second, the hemostatic system is activated within the kidney. Monocytes and macrophages in the glomeruli, stimulated by T lymphocytes, can express tissue factor; and glomerular capillaries, damaged by immune complex deposition, can activate the coagulation system [74].

Inflammatory bowel disease

Inflammatory bowel disease, including Crohn's disease and ulcerative colitis, is associated with an increased risk of venous thromboembolism. In a case-controlled cohort, the incidence RR of venous thromboembolic events based on approximately 20,000 patient-years of follow-up was 4.7 (95% CI, 3.5–6.6) for DVT and 2.9 (95% CI, 1.8–4.7) for pulmonary embolus in Crohn's disease, and 2.8 (95% CI, 2.1–3.7) for DVT and 3.6 (95% CI, 2.5–5.2) for pulmonary embolus in ulcerative colitis [76]. No clear mechanism has been proposed for this increase in venous thromboembolism. One study found that 63.6% of patients with Crohn's disease had free protein S levels below the normal range [77]. Another study found that mean factor VII levels, lipoprotein (a), and fibrinogen were significantly higher in patients with Crohn's disease when compared with normal controls. Among patients with ulcerative colitis, only the mean factor VII level was significantly higher than in normal controls [78].

Antiphospholipid antibodies

Antiphospholipid antibodies, including anticardiolipin antibodies and lupus anticoagulants, are a heterogeneous group of immunoglobulins directed against protein–phospholipid complexes, predominantly prothrombin and β_2-glycoprotein I. In the normal population, the frequency of elevated anticardiolipin antibody levels is approximately 2% to 4%, and lupus anticoagulants are generally less frequent [79]. Lupus anticoagulants are detected in

8.5% to 14% of patients with venous thromboembolism [80,81].

Patients with antiphospholipid antibody syndrome present with thrombosis, pregnancy loss, or thrombocytopenia. In a prospective cohort of patients observed for 4 years, the prevalence of thrombotic complications was 2.5% per patient-year. Half were venous events, including DVT (53%), pulmonary embolus (23%), superficial venous thrombosis (18%), and hepatic vein thrombosis (6%) [82]. Antiphospholipid antibodies also have been reported among patients with cerebral venous thrombosis [83].

The pathogenesis of venous thrombosis among patients with antiphospholipid antibodies is unclear. Thrombotic complications occur more frequently with elevated antibody levels to β_2-glycoprotein I [84] and prothrombin [85]. Proposed thrombotic mechanisms include the inhibition of natural anticoagulant pathways (APC, ATIII), the inhibition of fibrinolysis, and endothelial cell activation [86].

Other rheumatologic disorders

Behçet's disease is a systemic vasculitis characterized by recurrent orogenital ulcers, uveitis, and skin lesions. In a case series of 113 patients with Behçet's disease, 44 (38.9%) had DVT, most commonly affecting the lower extremities. Deficiencies of protein C, protein S, or ATIII, APC resistance, anticardiolipin antibodies, or anti–β_2-glycoprotein I antibodies did not correlate with thrombosis in Behçet's disease [87]. The pathogenesis of venous thrombosis among patients with Behçet's disease is most likely caused by endothelial cell damage from the vasculitis, resulting in a prothrombotic state [88].

Systemic lupus erythematosus is also associated with thrombotic complications [89]. In most patients with this disease, the increased frequency of thromboembolic complications is associated with the presence of antiphospholipid antibodies. The prevalence rate for anticardiolipin antibodies in patients with systemic lupus erythematosus ranges from 50% to 60% [90]. Other risk factors that contribute to the increased thrombotic risk in these patients include elevated homocysteine levels [91] and factor V Leiden [92].

Pregnancy

Pregnant women have a risk for venous thromboembolism that is five times higher than the risk for nonpregnant women [93]. The incidence of venous thromboembolism in pregnancy and the postpartum period has been estimated at 71 to 85 events per 100,000 deliveries [94,95]. The incidence of pulmonary embolus is approximately 15 events per 100,000 deliveries, 7 antenatal and 8 postnatal [94]. The incidence of intracranial venous thrombosis is approximately 11.4 events per 100,000 deliveries [96]. The risk for DVT increases during the course of pregnancy, with almost half of all events occurring during the third trimester [97]. During pregnancy, the left leg is affected in 84% of patients with DVT. The pathogenesis of venous thrombosis during pregnancy and postpartum includes venous stasis caused by the gravid uterus and increased venous distension, damage to the pelvic vessels at delivery, increases in coagulation factors, decreases in protein S, and inhibition of fibrinolysis [94].

Surgery

The total incidence of DVT in surgical patients who receive no thromboprophylaxis varies according to the type of surgery performed. The incidence is approximately 25% in general surgery patients, 16% in gynecologic surgery patients, 54% in patients undergoing total hip replacement, 64% in patients undergoing total knee replacement, and 22% in neurosurgery patients [98]. Even with optimal thromboprophylaxis (low molecular weight heparin), the incidence of DVT ranges from approximately 6% in general surgery patients to 30% in patients undergoing knee replacement [98]. The incidence of symptomatic venous thromboembolism is generally lower, with clinically recognized pulmonary embolus occurring in 1.6% of general surgery patients, 0.9% of which is fatal [98].

Trauma

The incidence of DVT among patients with major trauma exceeds 50%, with fatal pulmonary embolus occurring in 0.4% to 2.0%. In patients who survive past the first day of a traumatic event, pulmonary embolus is the third most common cause of death [98]. A prospective study of venous thromboembolism after major trauma identified five independent risk factors for DVT: older age, blood transfusions, surgery, femur or tibia fracture, and spinal cord injury [99].

Travel

In a prospective case–control study, travel was reported to be a risk factor for a venous thromboembolic event. Patients who had traveled within the preceding 4 weeks and for longer than 4 hours had an odds ratio of having a venous thrombotic event of 3.98 (95% CI, 1.9–8.4) [100]. A retrospective review of cases of severe pulmonary embolus occurring within 1 hour after arrival to the Charles de Gaulle airport revealed that, for persons traveling more than 5000 km, the incidence of venous thromboembolism was 1.5 cases per 1 million persons compared with 0.01 case per 1 million persons traveling less than 5000 km [101]. A dose–response effect was observed, with the incidence of pulmonary embolism increasing with the distance traveled. Proposed mechanisms include venous stasis from immobility, hemoconcentration from dehydration, and impaired fibrinolysis and activation of coagulation from decreased oxygen tension and ambient pressure [101].

Therapy-related

Oral contraceptives are the most common transient risk factor for venous thromboembolism in young women. The annual incidence for DVT has been reported to be 2 to 3 cases per 10,000 women on oral contraceptives compared with 0.8 case per 10,000 women not on oral contraceptives [102]. The risk of fatal pulmonary embolus has been estimated to be 10.5 events per 1 million woman-years, with a relative risk of death from pulmonary embolus of 9.6 (95% CI, 3.1–29.1) [103]. The estrogen content and the type of progestin are important in increasing the risk of venous thrombosis. A 5-year case–control study found that the risk of venous thromboembolism increased with higher estrogen content. In addition, the risk for a thromboembolic event was higher during the first year of therapy when compared with subsequent years [104]. When second-generation (levonorgestrel or norgestimate) and third-generation (desogestrel or gestodene) progestins were compared with nonuse, the odds ratios for venous thromboembolism were 2.9 and 4.0, respectively [104]. Mechanisms of venous thrombosis related to the use of oral contraceptives include increases in procoagulant factors, decreases in ATIII and protein S, and diminished activity of APC [105,106].

Ovarian hyperstimulation syndrome (OHSS) is a rare complication of fertility medication and occurs during 2% to 6% of treatment cycles. OHSS is characterized by ovarian enlargement, liver and renal dysfunction, hypoalbuminemia, hydrothorax, ascites, hemoconcentration, and venous thrombosis. Venous thrombosis has been reported in the lower extremities, axillary vein, subclavian vein, cerebral veins, and the jugular system. Hemoconcentration and the development of a hyperviscous state may lead to the increased thrombotic risk [107].

Hormone replacement therapy also increases the risk of venous thromboembolism. The Heart and Estrogen/Progestin Replacement Study (HERS) was a randomized, blinded, placebo-controlled trial with 4.1 years of follow-up. Women (mean age at baseline, 67 ± 7 years) randomized to receive 0.625 mg of

conjugated equine estrogens and 2.5 mg of medroxyprogesterone acetate daily sustained 4.6 DVTs and 2.0 PEs per 1000 person-years versus 1.6 DVTs and 0.7 PEs for women on placebo [108,109]. In HERS II, these patients were observed for an additional 2.7 years in an open-labeled fashion. Women receiving hormone therapy sustained 4.2 DVTs and 2.1 pulmonary emboli per 1000 person-years versus 3.4 DVTs and 0.7 pulmonary emboli in women receiving placebo. For the 6.8 years of follow-up, the unadjusted intention-to-treat relative hazard of venous thromboembolism for women receiving hormone replacement therapy was 2.08 (95% CI, 1.28–3.40) [109].

Tamoxifen inhibits the action of estrogen on breast tissue and is used in the treatment of breast cancer. For women less than 50 years of age in the Breast Cancer Prevention Trial, the overall relative risk of pulmonary embolus for women receiving tamoxifen was 3.01 (95% CI, 1.15–9.27). For all ages, the overall relative risk for DVT was 1.6 (95% CI, 0.91–2.86) [110]. Raloxifene, a selective estrogen receptor modulator, is used in the prophylaxis and treatment of patients with osteoporosis. In one study, the relative risk of sustaining a venous thromboembolic event was 3.1 (95% CI, 1.5–6.2) for women receiving raloxifene [111].

In several studies, patients with cancer were at a higher risk for venous thrombosis while receiving chemotherapy (4% to 15%) when compared with the risk after chemotherapy (0% to 2%) [70]. Drugs that immediately damage the vascular endothelium include bleomycin, carmustine, BCNU, and vincristine. Chemotherapy agents can also interact with natural anticoagulants. For example, L-asparaginase decreases ATIII levels, which may contribute to the thrombotic risk with this drug [70]. In addition, when given with combination chemotherapy, thalidomide increases the risk for DVT. DVT occurred in 28% of patients with multiple myeloma who received combination chemotherapy with thalidomide compared with 4% of patients who received combination chemotherapy alone ($P = 0.002$) [112]. The mechanism remains unclear.

Heparin-induced thrombocytopenia occurs in approximately 2% to 3% of patients receiving unfractionated heparin for 5 or more days [113]. Approximately one third of patients with heparin-induced thrombocytopenia will present with a thromboembolic complication, most commonly pulmonary embolus [114]. In addition, the risk for a thromboembolic complication remains high even after the heparin has been discontinued [115]. In one study, the odds ratio for a proximal DVT was 27.0 (95% CI, 5.4–141) and for a pulmonary embolus, 93.4 (95% CI, 5.7–1374) [116]. In patients with heparin-induced thrombocytopenia, thrombotic events can precede the development of thrombocytopenia [116].

Other risk factors

In the Nurses' Health Study cohort, obesity, hypertension, and cigarette smoking were found to be risk factors for pulmonary embolus [117]. When compared with the leanest individuals (body mass index [BMI] < 21.9 kg/m^2), women with a BMI greater than or equal to 29.0 kg/m^2 had a RR for pulmonary embolus of 3.2 (95% CI, 1.7–6.0). The RR for pulmonary embolus was 3.3 (95% CI, 1.7–6.5) for women who smoked 35 cigarettes or more daily when compared with women who never smoked. After adjusting for BMI, hypertension was also associated with an increased risk for pulmonary embolus at 1.9 (95% CI, 1.2–2.8) [117]. In a prospective cohort study of men, cigarette smoking and waist circumference were found to be risk factors for venous thromboembolism [118]. The adjusted RR for venous thromboembolism for men in the highest decile of waist circumference (≥100 cm) when compared with men with a waist circumference less than 100 cm was 3.92 (95% CI, 2.1–7.29). For men who smoked more than 15 cigarettes a day, the adjusted RR for a venous thromboembolism was 2.82 (95% CI, 1.3–6.13) when compared with the risk for nonsmokers [118].

Combined risks for thrombophilia

Combined inherited thrombophilic disorders

In a retrospective cohort of patients with first episode DVT, the risk for a recurrent venous thrombotic event for patients with a combined factor V Leiden mutation and prothrombin gene mutation was higher than the risk for factor V Leiden alone or for neither mutation. For patients with the combined defect who sustained a spontaneous first event, the risk was higher at 5.4 (95% CI, 2.0–14.1) [119].

Factor V Leiden also has been reported to affect the clinical phenotype in families with protein C deficiency [120], protein S deficiency [121], and ATIII deficiency [122]. In all families, the coinheritance of more than one risk factor resulted in an increased thrombotic risk for the individuals affected. Factor V Leiden has been reported to modulate the thrombotic risk in patients with homocystinuria [123], homozygosity for the thermolabile MTHFR polymorphism [124], elevated lipoprotein (a) levels [68], and the factor V HR2 genotype [53].

Combined inherited and acquired thrombophilic disorders

The presence of one or more inherited hypercoagulable states is associated with an increased thrombotic risk during pregnancy. In a case–control study, the RR for women during pregnancy and the postpartum period with factor V Leiden mutation was 9.3 (95% CI, 5.1–16.9); the RR for women with the prothrombin gene mutation was 15.2 (95% CI, 4.2–52.6). In pregnant women with the factor V Leiden and the prothrombin gene mutation, the estimated odds ratio was 107 [125]. In a retrospective cohort study, the frequency of venous thromboembolism during pregnancy was 4.1% in women with a deficiency of ATIII, protein C, or protein S versus 0.5% in women with no deficiency [126].

The risk of venous thrombosis in women with either factor V Leiden or the prothrombin gene mutation is increased by the use of oral contraceptives [127,128]. Similarly, the use of hormone replacement therapy in women with factor V Leiden is associated with an increased thrombotic risk [129]. Factor V Leiden has been reported to increase the risk for thrombosis in patients with antiphospholipid antibodies [130]. In contrast, factor V Leiden does not seem to increase the risk for venous thromboembolism in patients undergoing joint replacement surgery [131] or with cancer [132]. Nonetheless, patients with cancer and venous thromboembolism have an increased frequency of acquired APC resistance [133].

Considerations in the evaluation of thrombophilia

The annual incidence of venous thrombosis is approximately 1 event per 1000 persons per year, with an annual incidence in children of 1event per 100,000 and in the elderly of 1 event per 100 [134,135]. This disparity reflects the increased risk of venous thrombosis from acquired conditions and environmental factors (see Table 3) and the interaction of these conditions and factors with underlying inherited thrombophilic disorders. Before 1993, the known inherited thrombophilic disorders included dysfibrinogenemia and deficiencies of ATIII, protein C, and protein S, and only 5% to 20% of patients with idiopathic venous thrombosis were diagnosed with an inherited thrombophilic disorder [136]. Since the discovery of APC resistance in 1993 and the prothrombin gene mutation in 1996, it is estimated that more than half of the patients with clinical characteristics of thrombophilia are diagnosed with at least one inherited thrombophilic disorder [137]. Considerations in the evaluation of patients include the impact of the cause of venous thrombosis on the duration and intensity of anticoagulant therapy for the individual patient and the identification of potential inherited risk factors for family members. Recommendations for the duration of anticoagulant therapy are based on weighing the morbidity and mortality of a recurrent venous thrombotic event against the risk of a hemorrhagic complication. The following sections summarize the authors' approach to evaluating a patient with a venous thromboembolic event for an underlying hypercoagulable state.

Clinical parameters to assist in the decision to evaluate a patient for thrombophilia

History

The assessment of a patient with venous thromboembolism begins with the history. Important information includes the patient's age at the time of the event, his or her ethnicity, and the clinical presentation (location of thrombus, severity of the event, circumstances surrounding the event). One should determine whether there have been prior thrombotic events, and whether they have occurred in the setting of acquired risk factors such as surgery or other variables (see Table 3). Patients should be questioned about routine cancer screening appropriate for age and personal habits such as smoking. In women, questions regarding the use of oral contraceptives, pregnancies, prior miscarriages, and hormonal replacement therapy need to be addressed. A detailed family history is essential. If a family member has sustained a thromboembolic event, the age of that family member and the circumstances surrounding the event need to be determined. A familial history of multiple spontaneous abortions or stillbirths can provide clues to familial antiphospholipid antibody syndrome (with or without systemic lupus erythematosus).

Physical examination

Thorough cardiovascular, pulmonary, and abdominal examinations should be performed as part of a complete physical. The extremities should be examined for chronic venous stasis changes, skin ulcers, and livedo reticularis. Older patients with an apparent idiopathic venous thromboembolism should be evaluated carefully for malignancy.

Laboratory assessment

Testing for inherited or acquired thrombophilia

Patients should be suspected of having, and should be tested for, an inherited thrombophilia if they experience venous thrombosis at 50 years of age or younger,

if they have a history of recurrent or unprovoked events, if they sustain a thrombotic event in an unusual site (eg, cerebral or mesenteric), or if they have a positive family history for venous thromboembolism, particularly at a younger age [138,139]. Screening asymptomatic family members for an inherited thrombophilic disorder is controversial [140,141]. Asymptomatic family members often inquire about screening when they might be exposed to known acquired risk factors, such as surgery or pregnancy, or when deciding about the use of oral contraceptives or other hormonal agents. In these situations, screening family members of symptomatic carriers of ATIII, protein C, or protein S deficiency or factor V Leiden is reasonable [142,143]. Screening asymptomatic individuals with no personal or family history of venous thromboembolism is generally not recommended, even when the individual may be potentially exposed to one or more acquired risk factors.

Recommended tests for evaluation of an inherited thrombophilic disorder

All patients should undergo a routine laboratory evaluation (eg, serum chemistries, complete blood count with review of the blood film, baseline prothrombin time and activated partial thromboplastin time) before starting any therapy to establish baseline values. These tests may also provide certain clues concerning possible acquired disorders (eg, myeloproliferative disorders, lupus anticoagulants). When clinically indicated, laboratory evaluation for an inherited risk factor should include testing for those disorders that are most strongly associated with an increased thrombotic risk (see Table 1). One should test for antiphospholipid antibodies, given that the presence of these antibodies may affect the duration of therapy. Additional testing for the selected hypercoagulable states listed in Table 2 should generally be reserved for patients in whom an inherited thrombophilic state is strongly suspected and in whom screening for the more common thrombophilic disorders has been unrevealing.

When to perform laboratory tests

Although there are no consensus recommendations concerning when a hypercoagulable work-up should be performed, several practical issues should be kept in mind when ordering these tests. First, the results of some of the tests can be affected during an acute thromboembolic event, including transient drops in ATIII, protein C, and protein S levels [144,145], transient elevations in factor VIII, and transient disappearance of antiphospholipid antibodies. Second, several of the assays are affected by the therapy used to treat the thromboembolic event, including a transient drop in ATIII levels following a bolus of heparin [144] and decreased levels of protein C and protein S while on warfarin therapy. Third, even if the work-up is limited to the tests listed in Table 1 and an assay for anti-phospholipid antibodies, the cost of an evaluation for thrombophilia can easily exceed $1000. Because the identification of a hypercoagulable state has the most impact on the duration of therapy, the authors generally perform these tests in the outpatient setting when the patient is clinically stable. Essentially all of the tests, with the exceptions of assays for protein C and protein S (and factor IX), can be performed while the patient is on warfarin therapy. When clinically indicated, the authors have discontinued warfarin and treated patients with low molecular weight heparin until testing for protein C and protein S could be performed.

Analysis of the clinical and laboratory data

Applying data in the patient with thrombosis

The impacts of different hypercoagulable states on the duration of anticoagulation therapy are summarized in Table 4. If a venous thromboembolic event is spontaneous or associated with the more common thrombophilic disorders, there is a trend to treat patients with anticoagulants for an increasing duration of time (Table 4). It is less clear how to incorporate the causes of inherited thrombophilia listed in Table 2, although the presence of one or more of these risk factors in addition to one of the more common risk factors listed in Table 1 may lean one toward a more prolonged course of therapy. For patients with an active malignancy, the current treatment guidelines are to continue anticoagulant therapy indefinitely, or until the tumor has been effectively treated (Table 4).

For some hypercoagulable states, additional therapy may be indicated. Patients with hyperhomocysteinemia or the thermolabile MTHFR polymorphism may benefit from folic acid supplementation [17]. Markedly elevated lipoprotein (a) levels can be treated with niacin, but there are no data suggesting that lowering elevated lipoprotein (a) levels will decrease the risk for recurrent thrombosis. These therapies would be performed in addition to anticoagulation therapy in a patient with a thrombotic event and may need to be continued after the course of anticoagulation therapy has been completed.

Benefits and risks of screening asymptomatic individuals

There are several potential benefits from screening asymptomatic individuals. Individuals who test positive for an abnormality may be able to take measures that will lessen their risk for a thrombotic event, such as avoiding prolonged immobilization or choosing not to use hormonal agents. These individuals could receive education on the signs and symptoms of thrombosis. With this awareness, they might seek medical attention sooner. During times of increased risk (surgery, pregnancy), individuals could be monitored more closely and potentially receive more

Table 4
Impact of clinical and laboratory evaluation on anticoagulation therapy for venous thrombosis

Duration of therapy	Clinical/laboratory evaluation	References
3–6 Months	Reversible or time-limited major risk factor (major surgery, trauma, or medical illness)	17,139,150
6 Months	Weak risk factor (estrogen use, long distance travel, minor trauma) and no inherited or acquired thrombophilia	138,139,150
6 Months (may consider extended therapy)	Unprovoked thrombotic event and no inherited/acquired thrombophilia or patient heterozygous for factor V Leiden or prothrombin 20210 gene mutation	17,138,139,150
12 Months to indefinite	Recurrent unprovoked events with no inherited/acquired thrombophilia Unprovoked thrombotic events with antithrombin III, protein C, or protein S deficiency, or homozygous factor V Leiden, double heterozygosity, combined thrombophilias, antiphospholipid antibody syndrome, active malignancy, life-threatening event (near fatal pulmonary embolus, cerebral or visceral venous thrombus), or ongoing risk factor	17,138,139,150

aggressive thromboprophylaxis. For individuals who test negative, their anxiety of having an event may be decreased.

There also are potential risks from screening asymptomatic individuals. Asymptomatic individuals who test positive for an inherited disorder could potentially experience discrimination and loss of privacy. Individuals could potentially be turned down for insurance coverage or not be considered for employment because they are at potentially increased risk for venous thromboembolism. Currently, there are no standard treatment guidelines for the treatment of asymptomatic individuals, even in high-risk situations; therefore, this information may merely provoke unnecessary anxiety.

Summary

Thrombophilia is the predisposition to venous thromboembolism and is caused by inherited and acquired factors, alone or in combination. With the discovery of APC resistance and the prothrombin gene mutation, more than half of all patients with clinical characteristics of thrombophilia are now diagnosed with an inherited disorder. The hypercoagulable work-up of patients with venous thromboembolism is important, because the causes can influence the duration and management of anticoagulation therapy, as well as affect other decisions regarding life and health issues.

References

[1] The British Committee for Standards in Haematology. Guidelines on the investigation and management of thrombophilia. J Clin Pathol 1990;43:703–10.

[2] Koster T, Rosendaal FR, De Ronde H, Briët E, Vandenbroucke JP, Bertina RM. Venous thrombosis due to poor anticoagulant response to activated protein C: Leiden Thrombophilia Study. Lancet 1993;342: 1503–6.

[3] Rees DC, Cox M, Clegg JB. World distribution of factor V Leiden. Lancet 1995;346:1133–4.

[4] Ridker PM, Miletich JP, Hennekens CH, Buring JE. Ethnic distribution of factor V Leiden in 4047 men and women: implications for venous thromboembolism screening. JAMA 1997;277:1305–7.

[5] Rosendaal FR, Koster T, Vandenbroucke JP, Reitsma PH. High risk of thrombosis in patients homozygous for factor V Leiden (activated protein C resistance). Blood 1995;85:1504–8.

[6] Zoller B, Dahlback B. Linkage between inherited resistance to activated protein C and factor V gene mutation in venous thrombosis. Lancet 1994;343: 1536–8.

[7] Bertina RM, Koeleman BPC, Koster T, Rosendaal FR, Dirven RJ, De Ronde H, et al. Mutation in blood coagulation factor V associated with resistance to activated protein C. Nature 1994;369:64–7.

[8] Heeb MJ, Kojima Y, Greengard JS, Griffin JH. Activated protein C resistance: molecular mechanisms based on studies using purified Gln506-factor V. Blood 1995;85:3405–11.

[9] Kalafatis M, Haley PE, Lu D, Bertina RM, Long GL, Mann KG. Proteolytic events that regulate factor V activity in whole plasma from normal and activated protein C (APC)–resistant individuals during clotting: an insight into the APC-resistance assay. Blood 1996;87:4695–707.

[10] de Visser MC, Rosendaal FR, Bertina RM. A reduced sensitivity for activated protein C in the absence of factor V Leiden increases the risk of venous thrombosis. Blood 1999;93:1271–6.

[11] Ridker PM, Hennekens CH, Lindpaintner K, Stampfer MJ, Eisenberg PR, Miletich JP. Mutation in the gene coding for coagulation factor V and the risk of myocardial infarction, stroke, and venous thrombosis in apparently healthy men. N Engl J Med 1995;332: 912–7.

[12] Simioni P, Prandoni P, Lensing AW, Scudeller A, Sardella C, Prins MH, et al. The risk of recurrent venous thromboembolism in patients with an Arg506→Gln mutation in the gene for factor V (factor V Leiden). N Engl J Med 1997;336:399–403.

[13] Martinelli I, Cattaneo M, Panzeri D, Mannucci PM. Low prevalence of factor V:Q506 in 41 patients with isolated pulmonary embolism. Thromb Haemost 1997;77:440–3.

[14] Levoir D, Emmerich J, Alhenc-Gelas M, Dumontier I, Petite JP, Fiessinger JN, et al. Portal vein thrombosis and factor V Arg 506 to Gln mutation. Thromb Haemost 1995;73:550–1.

[15] de Moerloose P, Wutschert R, Heinzmann M, Perneger T, Reber G, Bounameaux H. Superficial vein thrombosis of lower limbs: influence of factor V Leiden, factor II G20210A and overweight. Thromb Haemost 1998;80:239–41.

[16] Martinelli I, Landi G, Merati G, Cella R, Tosetto A, Mannucci PM. Factor V gene mutation is a risk factor for cerebral venous thrombosis. Thromb Haemost 1996;75:393–4.

[17] Seligsohn U, Lubetsky A. Genetic susceptibility to venous thrombosis. N Engl J Med 2001;344:1222–31.

[18] Rosendaal FR, Doggen CJM, Zivelin A, Arruda VR, Aiach M, Siscovick DS, et al. Geographic distribution of the 20210G to A prothrombin variant. Thromb Haemost 1998;79:706–8.

[19] Poort SR, Rosendaal FR, Reitsma PH, Bertina RM. A common genetic variation in the 3′-untranslated region of the prothrombin gene is associated with elevated plasma prothrombin levels and an increase in venous thrombosis. Blood 1996;88:3698–703.

[20] Butenas S, Van't Veer C, Mann KG. "Normal" thrombin generation. Blood 1999;94:2169–78.

[21] Smirnov MD, Safa O, Esmon NL, Esmon CT. Inhibition of activated protein C anticoagulant activity by prothrombin. Blood 1999;94:3839–46.

[22] Lane DA, Grant PJ. Role of hemostatic gene polymorphisms in venous and arterial thrombotic disease. Blood 2000;95:1517–32.

[23] Kyrle PA, Mannhalter C, Beguin S, Stumpflen A, Hirschl M, Weltermann A, et al. Clinical studies and thrombin generation in patients homozygous or heterozygous for the G20210A mutation in the prothrombin gene. Arterioscler Thromb Vasc Biol 1998; 18:1287–91.

[24] Simioni P, Prandoni P, Lensing AW, Manfrin D, Tormene D, Gavasso S, et al. Risk for subsequent venous thromboembolic complications in carriers of the prothrombin or the factor V gene mutation with a first episode of deep vein thrombosis. Blood 2000;96: 3329–33.

[25] Shen MC, Lin JS, Tsay W. High prevalence of antithrombin III, protein C and protein S deficiency, but no factor V Leiden mutation in venous thrombophilic Chinese patients in Taiwan. Thromb Res 1997;87: 377–85.

[26] Tait RC, Walker ID, Perry DJ, Islam SI, Daly ME, McCall F, et al. Prevalence of antithrombin deficiency in the healthy population. Br J Haematol 1994;87: 106–12.

[27] Lane DA, Mannucci PM, Bauer KA, Bertina RM, Bochkov NP, Boulyjenkov V, et al. Inherited thrombophilia. Part 1. Thromb Haemost 1996;76:651–62.

[28] Finazzi G, Caccia R, Barbui T. Different prevalence of thromboembolism in the subtypes of congenital antithrombin III deficiency: review of 404 cases. Thromb Haemost 1987;58:1094.

[29] Pabinger I, Schneider B. Thrombotic risk in hereditary antithrombin III, protein C, or protein S deficiency: a cooperative, retrospective study. Gesellschaft fur Thrombose- und Hamostaseforschung (GTH) Study Group on Natural Inhibitors. Arterioscler Thromb Vasc Biol 1996;16:742–8.

[30] Boyer C, Wolf M, Vedrenne J, Meyer D, Larrieu MJ. Homozygous variant of antithrombin III: AT III Fontainebleau. Thromb Haemost 1986;56:18–22.

[31] Miletich J, Sherman L, Broze Jr G. Absence of thrombosis in subjects with heterozygous protein C deficiency. N Engl J Med 1987;317:991–6.

[32] Reitsma PH, Bernardi F, Doig RG, Gandrille S, Greengard JS, Ireland H, et al. Protein C deficiency: a database of mutations, 1995 update. Thromb Haemost 1995;73:876–89.

[33] Seligsohn U, Berger A, Abend M, Rubin L, Attias D, Zivelin A, et al. Homozygous protein C deficiency manifested by massive venous thrombosis in the newborn. N Engl J Med 1984;310:559–62.

[34] De Stefano V, Finazzi G, Mannucci PM. Inherited thrombophilia: pathogenesis, clinical syndromes, and management. Blood 1996;87:3531–44.

[35] McDonagh J. Dysfibrinogenemia and other disorders of fibrinogen structure or function. In: Colman RW, Hirsh J, Marder VJ, Clowes AW, George JN, editors. Hemostasis and thrombosis. basic principles and clinical practice. 4th edition. Philadelphia: Lippincott Williams & Wilkins; 2001. p. 855–92.

[36] Mosesson MW. Dysfibrinogenemia and thrombosis. Semin Thromb Hemost 1999;25:311–9.

[37] Haverkate F, Samama M. Familial dysfibrinogenemia and thrombophilia. Thromb Haemost 1995;73: 151–61.

[38] den Heijer M, Koster T, Blom HJ, Bos GMJ, Briet E, Reitsma PH, et al. Hyperhomocysteinemia as a risk ractor for deep vein thrombosis. N Engl J Med 1996; 334:759–62.

[39] Kang SS, Wong PW, Malinow MR. Hyperhomocysteinemia as a risk factor for occlusive vascular disease. Annu Rev Nutr 1992;12:279–98.

[40] Arruda VR, von Zuben PM, Chiaparini LC, Annichino-Bizzacchi JM, Costa FF. The mutation Ala677 → Val in the methylene tetrahydrofolate reductase gene: a risk factor for arterial disease and venous thrombosis. Thromb Haemost 1997;77:818–21.

[41] Marz W, Nauck M, Wieland H. The molecular mechanisms of inherited thrombophilia. Z Kardiol 2000; 89:575–86.

[42] Welch GN, Loscalzo J. Homocysteine and atherothrombosis. N Engl J Med 1998;338:1042–50.

[43] Ray JG. Meta-analysis of hyperhomocysteinemia as a risk factor for venous thromboembolic disease. Arch Intern Med 1998;158:2101–6.

[44] Hsu TS, Hsu LA, Chang CJ, Sun CF, Ko YL, Kuo CT, et al. Importance of hyperhomocysteinemia as a risk factor for venous thromboembolism in a Taiwanese population: a case-control study. Thromb Res 2001;102:387–95.

[45] Koster T, Blann AD, Briet E, Vandenbroucke JP, Rosendaal FR. Role of clotting factor VIII in effect of von Willebrand factor on occurrence of deep vein thrombosis. Lancet 1995;345:152–5.

[46] Kamphuisen PW, Eikenboom JCJ, Bertina RM. Elevated factor VIII levels and the risk of thrombosis. Arterioscler Thromb Vasc Biol 2001;21:731–8.

[47] O'Donnell J, Mumford AD, Manning RA, Laffan M. Elevation of FVIII:C in venous thromboembolism is persistent and independent of the acute phase response. Thromb Haemost 2000;83:10–3.

[48] Kamphuisen PW, Eikenboom JC, Bertina RM. Elevated factor VIII levels and the risk of thrombosis. Arterioscler Thromb Vasc Biol 2001;21:731–8.

[49] Schambeck CM, Hinney K, Haubitz I, Mansouri TB, Wahler D, Keller F. Familial clustering of high factor VIII levels in patients with venous thromboembolism. Arterioscler Thromb Vasc Biol 2001;21:289–92.

[50] Lunghi B, Iacoviello L, Gemmati D, Dilasio MG, Castoldi E, Pinotti M, et al. Detection of new polymorphic markers in the factor V gene: association with factor V levels in plasma. Thromb Haemost 1996;75:45–8.

[51] Hoekema L, Castoldi E, Tans G, Girelli D, Gemmati D, Bernardi F, et al. Functional properties of factor V and factor Va encoded by the R2-gene. Thromb Haemost 2001;85:75–81.

[52] Bernardi F, Faioni EM, Castoldi E, Lunghi B, Castaman G, Sacchi E, et al. A factor V genetic component differing from factor V R506Q contributes to the activated protein C resistance phenotype. Blood 1997; 90:1552–7.

[53] Faioni EM, Franchi F, Bucciarelli P, Margaglione M, De SV, Castaman G, et al. Coinheritance of the HR2 haplotype in the factor V gene confers an increased risk of venous thromboembolism to carriers of factor V R506Q (factor V Leiden). Blood 1999;94:3062–6.

[54] Folsom AR, Cushman M, Tsai MY, Aleksic N, Heckbert SR, Boland LL, et al. A prospective study of venous thromboembolism in relation to factor V Leiden and related factors. Blood 2002;99:2720–5.

[55] Gaustadnes M, Ingerslev J, Rutiger N. Prevalence of congenital homocystinuria in Denmark. N Engl J Med 1999;340:1513.

[56] Mudd SH, Skovby F, Levy HL, Pettigrew KD, Wilcken B, Pyeritz RE, et al. The natural history of homocystinuria due to cystathionine beta-synthase deficiency. Am J Hum Genet 1985;37:1–31.

[57] Ohlin AK, Marlar RA. Thrombomodulin gene defects in families with thromboembolic disease–a report on four families. Thromb Haemost 1999;81:338–44.

[58] Le Flem L, Mennen L, Aubry ML, Aiach M, Scarabin J, Emmerich J, et al. Thrombomodulin promoter mutations, venous thrombosis, and varicose veins. Arterioscler Thromb Vasc Biol 2001;21:445–51.

[59] Sartori MT, Patrassi GM, Theodoridis P, Perin A, Pietrogrande F, Girolami A. Heterozygous type I plasminogen deficiency is associated with an increased risk for thrombosis: a statistical analysis in 20 kindreds. Blood Coagul Fibrinolysis 1994;5:889–93.

[60] Pizzo SV, Fuchs HE, Doman KA, Petruska DB, Berger Jr H. Release of tissue plasminogen activator and its fast-acting inhibitor in defective fibrinolysis. Arch Intern Med 1986;146:188–91.

[61] Tran TH, Marbet GA, Duckert F. Association of hereditary heparin cofactor II deficiency with thrombosis. Lancet 1985;2(8452):413–4.

[62] Bernardi F, Legnani C, Micheletti F, Lunghi B, Ferraresi P, Palareti G, et al. A heparin cofactor II mutation (HCII Rimini) combined with factor V Leiden or type I protein C deficiency in two unrelated thrombophilic subjects. Thromb Haemost 1996;76:505–9.

[63] van Hylckama V, van der Linden I, Bertina RM, Rosendaal FR. High levels of factor IX increase the risk of venous thrombosis. Blood 2000;95:3678–82.

[64] Meijers JC, Tekelenburg WL, Bouma BN, Bertina RM, Rosendaal FR. High levels of coagulation factor XI as a risk factor for venous thrombosis. N Engl J Med 2000;342:696–701.

[65] Halbmayer W-M, Mannhalter C, Feichtinger C, Rubi M, Fischer M. The prevalence of factor XII deficiency in 103 orally anticoagulated outpatients suffering from recurrent venous and/or arterial thromboembolism. Thromb Haemost 1992;68:285–90.

[66] Sartori MT, Wiman B, Vettore S, Dazzi F, Girolami A, Patrassi GM. 4G/5G polymorphism of PAI-1 gene promoter and fibrinolytic capacity in patients with deep vein thrombosis. Thromb Haemost 1998;80: 956–60.

[67] van Tilburg NH, Rosendaal FR, Bertina RM. Thrombin activatable fibrinolysis inhibitor and the risk for deep vein thrombosis. Blood 2000;95:2855–9.

[68] von Depka M, Nowak-Gottl U, Eisert R, Dieterich C, Barthels M, Scharrer I, et al. Increased lipoprotein (a) levels as an independent risk factor for venous thromboembolism. Blood 2000;96:3364–8.

[69] Nowak-Gottl U, Junker R, Hartmeier M, Koch HG, Munchow N, Assmann G, et al. Increased lipoprotein(a) is an important risk factor for venous thromboembolism in childhood. Circulation 1999;100: 743–8.

[70] Piccioli A, Prandoni P, Ewenstein BM, Goldhaber SZ. Cancer and venous thromboembolism. Am Heart J 1996;132:850–5.

[71] Nordstrom M, Lindblad B, Anderson H, Bergqvist D, Kjellstrom T. Deep venous thrombosis and occult malignancy: an epidemiological study. BMJ 1994; 308:891–4.

[72] Prandoni P, Lensing AWA, Büller HR, Cogo A, Prins MH, Cattelan AM, et al. Deep vein thrombosis and the incidence of subsequent symptomatic cancer. N Engl J Med 1992;327:1128–33.

[73] Socie G, Mary JY, de Gramont A, Rio B, Leporrier M, Rose C, et al. Paroxysmal nocturnal haemoglobinuria: long-term follow-up and prognostic factors. French Society of Haematology. Lancet 1996;348: 573–7.

[74] Sagripanti A, Barsotti G. Hypercoagulability, intraglomerular coagulation, and thromboembolism in nephrotic syndrome. Nephron 1995;70:271–81.

[75] Wagoner RD, Stanson AW, Holley KE, Winter CS. Renal vein thrombosis in idiopathic membranous glomerulopathy and nephrotic syndrome: incidence and significance. Kidney Int 1983;23:368–74.

[76] Bernstein CN, Blanchard JF, Houston DS, Wajda A. The incidence of deep venous thrombosis and pulmonary embolism among patients with inflammatory bowel disease: a population-based cohort study. Thromb Haemost 2001;85:430–4.

[77] Aadland E, Odegaard OR, Roseth A, Try K. Free protein S deficiency in patients with chronic inflammatory bowel disease. Scand J Gastroenterol 1992; 27:957–60.

[78] Hudson M, Chitolie A, Hutton RA, Smith MS, Pounder RE, Wakefield AJ. Thrombotic vascular risk factors in inflammatory bowel disease. Gut 1996; 38:733–7.

[79] Petri M. Diagnosis of antiphospholipid antibodies. Rheum Dis Clin North Am 1994;20:443–69.

[80] Ginsberg JS, Wells PS, Brill-Edwards P, Donovan D, Moffatt K, Johnston M, et al. Antiphospholipid anti-

bodies and venous thromboembolism. Blood 1995; 86:3685–91.

[81] Simioni P, Prandoni P, Zanon E, Saracino MA, Scudeller A, Villalta S, et al. Deep venous thrombosis and lupus anticoagulant: a case-control study. Thromb Haemost 1996;76:187–9.

[82] Finazzi G, Brancaccio V, Moia M, Ciavarella N, Mazzucconi MG, Schinco P, et al. Natural history and risk factors for thrombosis in 360 patients with antiphospholipid antibodies: a four year prospective study from the Italian registry. Am J Med 1996;100:530–6.

[83] Carhuapoma JR, Mitsias P, Levine SR. Cerebral venous thrombosis and anticardiolipin antibodies. Stroke 1997;28:2363–9.

[84] Tsutsumi A, Matsuura E, Ichikawa K, Fujisaku A, Mukai M, Kobayashi S, et al. Antibodies to β_2-glycoprotein I and clinical manifestations in patients with systemic lupus erythematosus. Arthritis Rheum 1996; 39:1466–74.

[85] Forastiero RR, Martinuzzo ME, Cerrato GS, Kordich LO, Carreras LO. Relationship of anti-β_2-glycoprotein I and antiprothrombin antibodies to thrombosis and pregnancy loss in patients with antiphospholipid antibodies. Thromb Haemost 1997;78:1008–14.

[86] Roubey RAS. Immunology of the antiphospholipid antibody syndrome. Arthritis Rheum 1996;39: 1444–54.

[87] Houman MH, Ben GI, Khiari BSI, Lamloum M, Ben Ahmed M, Miled M. Deep vein thrombosis in Behçet's disease. Clin Exp Rheumatol 2001;19:S48–50.

[88] Leiba M, Sidi Y, Gur H, Leiba A, Ehrenfeld M. Behçet's disease and thrombophilia. Ann Rheum Dis 2001;60:1081–5.

[89] Petri M. Thrombosis and systemic lupus erythematosus: the Hopkins lupus cohort prospective study. Scand J Rheumatol 1996;25:191–3.

[90] Shapiro SS. The lupus anticoagulant/antiphospholipid syndrome. Annu Rev Med 1996;47:533–53.

[91] Petri M, Roubenoff R, Dallal GE, Nadeau MR, Selhub J, Rosenberg IH. Plasma homocysteine as a risk factor for atherothrombotic events in systemic lupus erythematosus. Lancet 1996;348:1120–4.

[92] Fijnheer R, Horbach DA, Donders RC, Vile H, von Oort E, Nieuwenhuis HK, et al. Factor V Leiden, antiphospholipid antibodies and thrombosis in systemic lupus erythematosus. Thromb Haemost 1996; 76:514–7.

[93] Toglia MR, Weg JG. Venous thromboembolism during pregnancy. N Engl J Med 1996;335:108–14.

[94] McColl MD, Ramsay JE, Tait RC, Walker ID, McCall F, Conkie JA, et al. Risk factors for pregnancy associated venous thromboembolism. Thromb Haemost 1997;78:1183–8.

[95] Simpson EL, Lawrenson RA, Nightingale AL, Farmer RD. Venous thromboembolism in pregnancy and the puerperium: incidence and additional risk factors from a London perinatal database. Br J Obstet Gynaecol 2001;108:56–60.

[96] Lanska DJ, Kryscio RJ. Stroke and intracranial venous thrombosis during pregnancy and puerperium. Neurology 1998;51:1622–8.

[97] Ray JG, Chan WS. Deep vein thrombosis during pregnancy and the puerperium: a meta-analysis of the period of risk and the leg of presentation. Obstet Gynecol Surv 1999;54:265–71.

[98] Geerts WH, Heit JA, Clagett GP, Pineo GF, Colwell CW, Anderson FAJ, et al. Prevention of venous thromboembolism. Chest 2001;119:132S–75S.

[99] Geerts WH, Code KI, Jay RM, Chen E, Szalai JP. A prospective study of venous thromboembolism after major trauma. N Engl J Med 1994;331:1601–6.

[100] Ferrari E, Chevallier T, Chapelier A, Baudouy M. Travel as a risk factor for venous thromboembolic disease: a case-control study. Chest 1999;115:440–4.

[101] Lapostolle F, Surget V, Borron SW, Desmaizieres M, Sordelet D, Lapandry C, et al. Severe pulmonary embolism associated with air travel. N Engl J Med 2001;345:779–83.

[102] Rosendaal FR, Helmerhorst FM, Vandenbroucke JP. Oral contraceptives, hormone replacement therapy and thrombosis. Thromb Haemost 2001;86:112–23.

[103] Parkin L, Skegg DC, Wilson M, Herbison GP, Paul C. Oral contraceptives and fatal pulmonary embolism. Lancet 2000;355:2133–4.

[104] Lidegaard O, Edstrom B, Kreiner S. Oral contraceptives and venous thromboembolism: a five-year national case-control study. Contraception 2002;65: 187–96.

[105] Vandenbroucke JP, Rosing J, Bloemenkamp KW, Middeldorp S, Helmerhorst FM, Bouma BN, et al. Oral contraceptives and the risk of venous thrombosis. N Engl J Med 2001;344:1527–35.

[106] Rosing J, Middeldorp S, Curvers J, Christella M, Thomassen LG, Nicolaes GA, et al. Low-dose oral contraceptives and acquired resistance to activated protein C: a randomised cross-over study. Lancet 1999;354:2036–40.

[107] Lamon D, Chang CK, Hruska L, Kerlakian G, Smith JM. Superior vena cava thrombosis after in vitro fertilization: case report and review of the literature. Ann Vasc Surg 2000;14:283–5.

[108] Hulley S, Grady D, Bush T, Furberg C, Herrington D, Riggs B, et al. Randomized trial of estrogen plus progestin for secondary prevention of coronary heart disease in postmenopausal women: Heart and Estrogen/progestin Replacement Study (HERS) Research Group. JAMA 1998;280:605–13.

[109] Hulley S, Furberg C, Barrett-Connor E, Cauley J, Grady D, Haskell W, et al. Noncardiovascular disease outcomes during 6.8 years of hormone therapy: Heart and Estrogen/progestin Replacement Study follow-up (HERS II). JAMA 2002;288:58–66.

[110] Fisher B, Costantino JP, Wickerham DL, Redmond CK, Kavanah M, Cronin WM, et al. Tamoxifen for prevention of breast cancer: report of the National Surgical Adjuvant Breast and Bowel Project P-1 Study. J Natl Cancer Inst 1998;90:1371–88.

[111] Cummings SR, Eckert S, Krueger KA, Grady D,

Powles TJ, Cauley JA, et al. The effect of raloxifene on risk of breast cancer in postmenopausal women: results from the MORE randomized trial. Multiple Outcomes of Raloxifene Evaluation. JAMA 1999; 281:2189–97.

[112] Zangari M, Anaissie E, Barlogie B, Badros A, Desikan R, Gopal AV, et al. Increased risk of deep vein thrombosis in patients with multiple myeloma receiving thalidomide and chemotherapy. Blood 2001;98: 1614–5.

[113] Warkentin TE, Chong BH, Greinacher A. Heparin-induced thrombocytopenia: towards consensus. Thromb Haemost 1998;79:1–7.

[114] Warkentin TE. Clinical presentation of heparin-induced thrombocytopenia. Semin Hematol 1998;35: 9–16.

[115] Warkentin TE, Kelton JG. A 14-year study of heparin-induced thrombocytopenia. Am J Med 1996;101: 502–7.

[116] Warkentin TE, Levine MN, Hirsh J, Horsewood P, Roberts RS, Gent M, et al. Heparin-induced thrombocytopenia in patients treated with low-molecular-weight heparin or unfractionated heparin. N Engl J Med 1995;332:1330–5.

[117] Goldhaber SZ, Grodstein F, Stampfer MJ, Manson JE, Colditz GA, Speizer FE, et al. A prospective study of risk factors for pulmonary embolism in women. JAMA 1997;277:642–5.

[118] Hansson PO, Eriksson H, Welin L, Svardsudd K, Wilhelmsen L. Smoking and abdominal obesity: risk factors for venous thromboembolism among middle-aged men. "The study of men born in 1913". Arch Intern Med 1999;159:1886–90.

[119] De Stefano V, Martinelli I, Mannucci PM, Paciaroni P, Chiusolo P, Casorelli I, et al. The risk of recurrent deep vein thrombosis among heterozygous carriers of both factor V Leiden and the G20210A prothrombin mutation. N Engl J Med 1999;341:801–6.

[120] Koeleman BPC, Reitsma PH, Allaart CF, Bertina RM. Activated protein C resistance as an additional risk factor for thrombosis in protein C–deficient families. Blood 1994;84:1031–5.

[121] Zoller B, Berntsdotter A, de Frutos PG, Dahlback B. Resistance to activated protein C as an additional genetic risk factor in hereditary deficiency of protein S. Blood 1995;85:3518–23.

[122] van Boven HH, Reitsma PH, Rosendaal FR, Bayston V, Chowdhury V, Bauer KA, et al. Factor V Leiden (FV R506Q) in families with inherited antithrombin deficiency. Thromb Haemost 1996;75:417–21.

[123] Mandel H, Brenner B, Berant M, Rosenberg N, Lanir N, Jakobs C, et al. Coexistence of hereditary homocystinuria and factor V Leiden: effect on thrombosis. N Engl J Med 1996;334:763–8.

[124] Salomon O, Steinberg DM, Zivelin A, Gitel S, Dardik R, Rosenberg N, et al. Single and combined prothrombotic factors in patients with idiopathic venous thromboembolism: prevalence and risk assessment. Arterioscler Thromb Vasc Biol 1999;19:511–8.

[125] Gerhardt A, Scharf RE, Beckmann MW, Struve S, Bender HG, Pillny M, et al. Prothrombin and factor V mutations in women with a history of thrombosis during pregnancy and the puerperium. N Engl J Med 2000;342:374–80.

[126] Friederich PW, Sanson BJ, Simioni P, Zanardi S, Huisman MV, Kindt I, et al. Frequency of pregnancy-related venous thromboembolism in anticoagulant factor–deficient women: implications for prophylaxis. Ann Intern Med 1996;125:955–60.

[127] Vandenbroucke JP, Koster T, Briet E, Reitsma PH, Bertina RM, Rosendaal FR. Increased risk of venous thrombosis in oral contraceptive users who are carriers of factor V Leiden mutation. Lancet 1994;344: 1453–7.

[128] Martinelli I, Taioli E, Bucciarelli P, Akhavan S, Mannucci PM. Interaction between the G20210A mutation of the prothrombin gene and oral contraceptive use in deep vein thrombosis. Arterioscler Thromb Vasc Biol 1999;19:700–3.

[129] Herrington DM, Vittinghoff E, Howard TD, Major DA, Owen J, Reboussin DM, et al. Factor V Leiden, hormone replacement therapy, and risk of venous thromboembolic events in women with coronary disease. Arterioscler Thromb Vasc Biol 2002;22:1012–7.

[130] Hansen KE, Kong DF, Moore KD, Ortel TL. Risk factors associated with thrombosis in subjects with antiphospholipid antibodies. J Rheumatol 2001;28: 2018–24.

[131] Ryan DH, Crowther MA, Ginsberg JS, Francis CW. Relation of factor V Leiden genotype to risk for acute deep venous thrombosis after joint replacement surgery. Ann Intern Med 1998;128:270–6.

[132] Otterson GA, Monahan BP, Harold N, Steinberg SM, Frame JN, Kaye FJ. Clinical significance of the FV:Q506 mutation in unselected oncology patients. Am J Med 1996;101:406–12.

[133] Haim N, Lanir N, Hoffman R, Haim A, Tsalik M, Brenner B. Acquired activated protein C resistance is common in cancer patients and is associated with venous thromboembolism. Am J Med 2001;110:91–6.

[134] Rosendaal FR. Thrombosis in the young: epidemiology and risk factors. A focus on venous thrombosis. Thromb Haemost 1997;78:1–6.

[135] Rosendaal FR. Risk factors for venous thrombosis: prevalence, risk, and interaction. Semin Hematol 1997;34:171–87.

[136] Koeleman BP, Reitsma PH, Bertina RM. Familial thrombophilia: a complex genetic disorder. Semin Hematol 1997;34:256–64.

[137] Middeldorp S, Büller HR, Prins MH, Hirsh J. Approach to the thrombophilic patient. In: Colman RW, Hirsh J, Marder VJ, Clowes AW, George JN, editors. Hemostasis and thrombosis. basic principles and clinical practice. 4th edition. Philadelphia: Lippincott Williams & Wilkins; 2001. p. 1085–100.

[138] Bauer KA. The thrombophilias: well-defined risk factors with uncertain therapeutic implications. Ann Intern Med 2001;135:367–73.

[139] Hirsh J, Lee AY. How we diagnose and treat deep vein thrombosis. Blood 2002;99:3102–10.

[140] Mannucci PM. Genetic hypercoagulability: prevention suggests testing family members. Blood 2001; 98:21–2.

[141] Green D. Genetic hypercoagulability: screening should be an informed choice. Blood 2001;98:20.

[142] Simioni P, Tormene D, Prandoni P, Zerbinati P, Gavasso S, Cefalo P, et al. Incidence of venous thromboembolism in asymptomatic family members who are carriers of factor V Leiden: a prospective cohort study. Blood 2002;99:1938–42.

[143] Simioni P, Sanson BJ, Prandoni P, Tormene D, Friederich PW, Girolami B, et al. Incidence of venous thromboembolism in families with inherited thrombophilia. Thromb Haemost 1999;81:198–202.

[144] Lane DA, Olds RR, Thein S-L. Antithrombin and its deficiency states. Blood Coagul Fibrinolysis 1992;3: 315–41.

[145] Bauer KA. Hypercoagulable states. In: Hoffman R, Benz EJ, Shattil SJ, Furie B, Cohen HJ, Silberstein LE, et al, editors. Hematology: basic principles and practice. 3rd edition. New York: Churchill Livingstone; 2000. p. 2009–39.

[146] van Boven HH, Vandenbroucke JP, Briet E, Rosendaal FR. Gene–gene and gene–environment interactions determine risk of thrombosis in families with inherited antithrombin deficiency. Blood 1999;94: 2590–4.

[147] Koster T, Rosendaal FR, Briet E, van der Meer FJ, Colly LP, Trienekens PH, et al. Protein C deficiency in a controlled series of unselected outpatients: an infrequent but clear risk factor for venous thrombosis (Leiden Thrombophilia Study). Blood 1995;85: 2756–61.

[148] Makris M, Leach M, Beauchamp NJ, Daly ME, Cooper PC, Hampton KK, et al. Genetic analysis, phenotypic diagnosis, and risk of venous thrombosis in families with inherited deficiencies of Protein S. Blood 2000;95:1935–41.

[149] Makris M, Rosendaal FR, Preston FE. Familial thrombophilia: genetic risk factors and management. J Intern Med 1997;740(Suppl):9–15.

[150] Hyers TM, Agnelli G, Hull RD, Morris TA, Samama M, Tapson V, et al. Antithrombotic therapy for venous thromboembolic disease. Chest 2001;119:176S–93S.

CLINICS
IN CHEST
MEDICINE

Index

A

ACCP. *See American College of Chest Physicians (ACCP) consensus statement on antithrombotic therapy.*

Acute venous thromboembolism
thrombolytic therapy for
local and systemic, **73–90**. *See also Deep venous thrombosis; Pulmonary embolism.*

Age
as factor in venous thromboembolism, 1–2

American College of Chest Physicians (ACCP) consensus statement on antithrombotic therapy, **137–149**. *See also Venous thromboembolism, treatment of, ACCP consensus statement related to.*
evolution of, 140–142, 142–144
future directions related to, 146
impact of, 144–146
perceptions of, 144–146
rules of evidence in, 137–140

Angiography
pulmonary
in pulmonary embolism diagnosis, 13–14
in venous thromboembolism in ICU patients, 114
spiral CT
in pulmonary embolism diagnosis, 14–16

Antibody(ies)
antiphospholipid
thrombophilia caused by, 157–158

Anticoagulant(s)
cessation of
recurrent venous thromboembolism after
risk factors for, 63–66
for venous thromboembolism
ACCP consensus statement related to, **137–149**
bleeding associated with
risk factors for, 66

duration of
comparisons of, 67–68

Antiphospholipid antibodies
thrombophilia due to, 157–158

Antithrombin
heparin and, 41–44

Antithrombin III deficiency
thrombophilia caused by, 152–153

Aspirin
in venous thromboembolism prevention
ACCP consensus statement related to, 143

B

Bleeding
during anticoagulation therapy
risk factors for, 66

C

Calf vein thrombosis
treatment of
ACCP consensus statement related to, 142

Cancer
recurrent venous thromboembolism associated with, 64

Cardiac arrest
thrombolytic therapy for, 83

Catheter(s)
central venous
as factor in venous thromboembolism, 5

Central venous catheters
as factor in venous thromboembolism, 5

Chemotherapy agents
thrombophilia caused by, 159

Chest radiography
in acute pulmonary embolism diagnosis, 29–30

doi:10.1016/S0272-5231(03)00009-1